T0343330

2011 YEAR BOOK OF ONCOLOGY®

The 2011 Year Book Series

Year Book of Anesthesiology and Pain Management™: Drs Chestnut, Abram, Black, Gravlee, Lien, Mathru, and Roizen

Year Book of Cardiology®: Drs Gersh, Cheitlin, Elliott, Gold, Graham, and Thourani

Year Book of Critical Care Medicine®: Drs Dellinger, Parrillo, Balk, Dorman, Dries, and Zanotti-Cavazzoni

Year Book of Dermatology and Dermatologic Surgery™: Dr Del Rosso

Year Book of Diagnostic Radiology®: Drs Osborn, Abbara, Elster, Manaster, Oestreich, Offiah, Rosado de Christenson, Stephens, and Walker

Year Book of Emergency Medicine®: Drs Hamilton, Bruno, Handly, Mullin, Quintana, and Ramoska

Year Book of Endocrinology®: Drs Schott, Apovian, Clarke, Eugster, Ludlam, Meikle, Schinner, Schteingart, and Toth

Year Book of Gastroenterology™: Drs Talley, DeVault, Harnois, Murray, Pearson, Philcox, Picco, and Smith

Year Book of Hand and Upper Limb Surgery®: Drs Yao and Steinmann

Year Book of Medicine®: Drs Barker, Garrick, Gersh, Khardori, LeRoith, Panush, Talley, and Thigpen

Year Book of Neonatal and Perinatal Medicine®: Drs Fanaroff, Benitz, Donn, Neu, Papile, Polin, and Van Marter

Year Book of Neurology and Neurosurgery®: Drs Klimo and Rabinstein

Year Book of Obstetrics, Gynecology, and Women's Health®: Drs Dungan and Shulman

Year Book of Oncology®: Drs Arceci, Bauer, Chiorean, Gordon, Lawton, Murphy, Thigpen, and Tsao

Year Book of Ophthalmology®: Drs Rapuano, Cohen, Flanders, Fudemberg, Hammersmith, Milman, Myers, Nagra, Nelson, Penne, Pyfer, Sergott, Shields, Talekar, and Vander

Year Book of Orthopedics®: Drs Morrey, Beauchamp, Huddleston, Swiontkowski, and Trigg

Year Book of Otolaryngology-Head and Neck Surgery®: Drs Sindwani, Balough, Franco, Gapany, and Mitchell

Year Book of Pathology and Laboratory Medicine®: Drs Raab, Parwani, Bejarano, and Bissell

Year Book of Pediatrics®: Dr Stockman

Year Book of Plastic and Aesthetic Surgery™: Drs Miller, Gosain, Gurtner, Gutowski, Ruberg, Salisbury, and Smith

Year Book of Psychiatry and Applied Mental Health®: Drs Talbott, Ballenger, Buckley, Frances, Krupnick, and Mack

Year Book of Pulmonary Disease®: Drs Barker, Jones, Maurer, Raza, Tanoue, and Willsie

Year Book of Sports Medicine®: Drs Shephard, Cantu, Feldman, Jankowski, Khan, Lebrun, Nieman, Pierrynowski, and Rowland

Year Book of Surgery®: Drs Copeland, Behrns, Daly, Eberlein, Fahey, Huber, Klodell, Mozingo, and Pruett

Year Book of Urology®: Drs Andriole and Coplen

Year Book of Vascular Surgery®: Drs Moneta, Gillespie, Starnes, and Watkins

2011

The Year Book of ONCOLOGY®

Editor-in-Chief

Robert J. Arceci, MD, PhD

King Fahd Professor of Pediatric Oncology, Johns Hopkins University, Johns Hopkins Hospital, Baltimore, Maryland

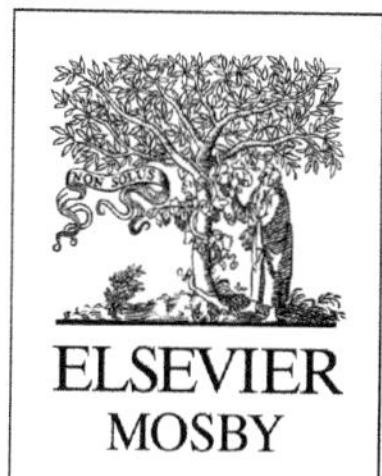

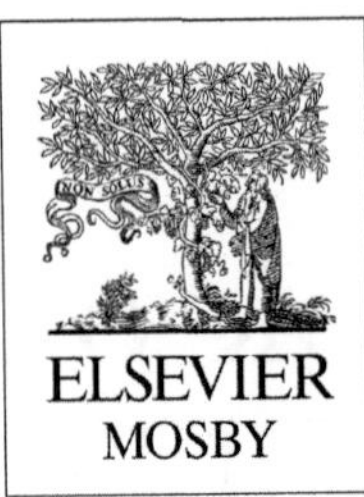

Vice President, Continuity: Kimberly Murphy
Editor: Yonah Korngold
Production Supervisor, Electronic Year Books: Donna M. Skelton
Electronic Article Manager: Emily Ogle
Illustrations and Permissions Coordinator: Dawn Vohsen

2011 EDITION

Composition by TNQ Books and Journals Pvt Ltd, India

Printed and bound by CPI Group (UK) Ltd, Croydon, CR0 4YY

Transferred to Digital Print 2011

Editorial Office:
Elsevier
Suite 1800
1600 John F. Kennedy Blvd.
Philadelphia, PA 19103-2899

International Standard Serial Number: 1040-1741
International Standard Book Number: 978-0-323-08420-8

Associate Editors

Thomas L. Bauer II, MD
Chief, Thoracic Surgery, Helen F. Graham Cancer Center, Christiana Care, Clinical Assistant Professor of Surgery, Jefferson Medical College, Adjunct Assistant Professor of Biological Sciences, University of Delaware, Senior Scholar, Jefferson School of Population Health, Newark, Delaware

E. Gabriela Chiorean, MD
Assistant Professor of Medicine, Medical Director, Gastrointestinal Oncology Program, Indiana University Melvin and Bren Simon Cancer Center, Indianapolis, Indiana

Michael S. Gordon, MD
Associate Professor of Clinical Medicine, University of Arizona College of Medicine, President, Premiere Oncology of Arizona, Scottsdale, Arizona

Colleen A. Lawton, MD
Professor of Radiation Oncology, Director of Residency Program, Department of Radiation Oncology, Medical College of Wisconsin, Milwaukee, Wisconsin

Barbara A. Murphy, MD
Professor of Medicine, Director, Cancer Supportive Care Program, Director, Head and Neck Research Program, Vanderbilt-Ingram Cancer Center, Nashville, Tennessee

James Tate Thigpen, MD
Professor of Medicine and Director, Division of Oncology, University of Mississippi Medical Center, Jackson, Mississippi

Anne S. Tsao, MD
Associate Professor, Director, Mesothelioma Program, Director, Thoracic Chemo-Radiation Program, University of Texas M.D. Anderson Cancer Center, Department of Thoracic/Head & Neck Medical Oncology, Houston, Texas

Contributors

Elizabeth S. Bloom, MD
Associate Professor of Radiation Oncology, Division of Radiation Oncology, The University of Texas M.D. Anderson Cancer Center, The University of Texas MD Anderson Cancer Center Radiation Treatment Center at Bellaire, Houston, Texas

Thomas A. Buchholz, MD
Professor and Chair, Department of Radiation Oncology, The University of Texas M.D. Anderson Cancer Center, Houston, Texas

Shine Chang, PhD
Professor of Epidemiology, Director, Cancer Prevention Research Training Program, The University of Texas M.D. Anderson Cancer Center, Houston, Texas

Steven J. Chmura, MD, PhD
Assistant Professor, Department of Radiation and Cellular Oncology, University of Chicago Medical Center, Chicago, Illinois

Amy C. Degnim, MD
Associate Professor of Surgery, Mayo Clinic, Rochester, Minnesota

Nancy E. De La Fuente, BS
Graduate Research Assistant, Department of Epidemiology, Cancer Prevention Research Training Program, The University of Texas M.D. Anderson Cancer Center, Houston, Texas

Senem Demirci, MD
Department of Radiation Oncology, Ege University Faculty of Medicine, Izmir, Turkey

Desiree D'Angelo Donovan, DO
Department of Surgery, Christiana Care Health System, Newark, Delaware

Paige L. Dorn, MD
Resident, Department of Radiation and Cellular Oncology, University of Chicago Medical Center, Chicago, Illinois

Francisco J. Esteva, MD, PhD
Professor, Department of Breast Medical Oncology, Director, Breast Cancer Translational Research Laboratory, The University of Texas M.D. Anderson Cancer Center, Houston, Texas

Stephen A. Feig, MD
Chief, Breast Imaging, UCI Medical Center, Orange, California; Professor of Radiology, University of California Irvine, Irvine, California

Karen A. Gelmon, MD, FRCPC
Professor of Medicine, University of British Columbia, Medical Oncologist, British Columbia Cancer Agency, Vancouver Cancer Centre, Vancouver, British Columbia, Canada

Yun Gong, MD
Associate Professor, Department of Surgery, University of Minnesota, Minneapolis, Minnesota

Ana Maria Gonzalez-Angulo, MD, MSc
Associate Professor, Departments of Breast Medical Oncology and Systems Biology, The University of Texas M.D. Anderson Cancer Center, Houston, Texas

Bruce G. Haffty, MD
Professor and Chairman, Department of Radiation Oncology, UMDNJ-Robert Wood Johnson Medical School; Associate Director, The Cancer Institute of New Jersey, New Brunswick, New Jersey

Steven E. Harms, MD
Radiologist, The Breast Center of Northwest Arkansas, Fayetteville, Arkansas; Clinical Professor, Department of Radiology, University of Arkansas for Medical Sciences, Little Rock, Arkasas

Kathleen C. Horst, MD
Assistant Professor, Department of Radiation Oncology, Stanford University, Stanford, California

Daniel C. Hughes, PhD
Assistant Professor, Institute for Health Promotion, The University of Texas Health Science Center San Antonio, San Antonio, Texas

Kelly K. Hunt, MD
Resident, Department of Radiation Oncology, University of Michigan, Ann Arbor, Michigan

Jennifer K. Litton, MD
Assistant Professor, Breast Medical Oncology, The University of Texas M.D. Anderson Cancer Center, Houston, Texas

Lawrence B. Marks, MD
Professor and Chairman, Department of Radiation Oncology, University of North Carolina, Chapel Hill, North Carolina

Cynthia M. Mojica, PhD, MPH
Assistant Professor, Institute for Health Promotion, The University of Texas Health Science Center San Antonio, San Antonio, Texas

Meena S. Moran, MD
Associate Professor, Yale University School of Medicine, New Haven, Connecticut

Susan G. Orel Roth, MD
Professor of Radiology, Department of Radiology, University of Pennsylvania, Philadelphia, Pennsylvania

Joseph E. Panoff, MD
Department of Radiation Oncology, University of Miami Miller School of Medicine, Miami, Florida

Kanwal P. S. Raghav, MD
Fellow, Division of Cancer Medicine, The University of Texas M.D. Anderson Cancer Center, Houston, Texas

William M. Sikov, MD
Clinical Associate Professor of Medicine, Department of Internal Medicine, Warren Alpert Medical School of Brown University, Providence, Rhode Island

Richard L. Theriault, DO, MBA
Professor, Department of Breast Medical Oncology, The University of Texas M.D. Anderson Cancer Center, Houston, Texas

Jamie L. Wagner, DO
Assistant Professor, Department of Surgical Oncology, The University of Texas M.D. Anderson Cancer Center, Houston, Texas

Gary J. Whitman, MD
Professor of Radiology, Department of Diagnostic Radiology, The University of Texas M.D. Anderson Cancer Center, Houston, Texas

David J. Winchester, MD
Clinical Professor of Surgery, University of Chicago Pritzker School of Medicine, Chief, Division of General Surgery and Chair of Surgical Oncology, NorthShore University HealthSystem, Evanston, Illinois

Jean L. Wright, MD
Assistant Professor of Clinical Radiation Oncology, Department of Radiation Oncology, University of Miami Miller School of Medicine, Miami, Florida

Table of Contents

Journals Represented

Journals represented in this YEAR BOOK are listed below.

AJR American Journal of Roentgenology
Annals of Surgery
Annals of Surgical Oncology
Annals of Thoracic Surgery
Archives of Physical Medicine and Rehabilitation
Blood
British Journal of Cancer
British Journal of Radiology
British Journal of Surgery
Cancer
Clinical Cancer Research
Cancer Research
Clinical Oncology Clinical Plastic Surgery
Diabetes Care
European Journal of Cancer
Gastrointestinal Endoscopy
Gynecology Oncology
International Journal of Radiation Oncology Biology Physics
Journal of Clinical Oncology
Journal of the American College of Cardiology
Journal of the American College of Surgeons
Journal of the American Medical Association
Journal of the National Cancer Institute
Journal of Urology
Lancet
Lancet Oncology
Leukemia
Nature
Nature Genetics
New England Journal of Medicine
Oncologist
Oncology
Radiotherapy & Oncology
Science
Thorax

STANDARD ABBREVIATIONS

The following terms are abbreviated in this edition: acquired immunodeficiency syndrome (AIDS), cardiopulmonary resuscitation (CPR), central nervous system (CNS), cerebrospinal fluid (CSF), computed tomography (CT), deoxyribonucleic acid (DNA), electrocardiography (ECG), health maintenance organization (HMO), human immunodeficiency virus (HIV), intensive care unit (ICU), intramuscular (IM), intravenous (IV), magnetic resonance (MR) imaging (MRI), ribonucleic acid (RNA), ultrasound (US), and ultraviolet (UV).

Note

The Year Book of Oncology is a literature survey service providing abstracts of articles published in the professional literature. Every effort is made to assure the accuracy of the information presented in these pages. Neither the editors nor the publisher of the Year Book of Oncology can be responsible for errors in the original materials. The editors' comments are their own opinions. Mention of specific products within this publication does not constitute endorsement.

To facilitate the use of the Year Book of Oncology as a reference tool, all illustrations and tables included in this publication are now identified as they appear in the original article. This change is meant to help the reader recognize that any illustration or table appearing in the Year Book of Oncology may be only one of many in the original article. For this reason, figure and table numbers will often appear to be out of sequence within the Year Book of Oncology.

1 Supportive Care

Randomized, Double-Blind Study of Denosumab Versus Zoledronic Acid in the Treatment of Bone Metastases in Patients With Advanced Cancer (Excluding Breast and Prostate Cancer) or Multiple Myeloma

Henry DH, Costa L, Goldwasser F, et al (Joan Karnell Cancer Ctr, Philadelphia, PA; Hosp de Santa Maria and Instituto de Medicina Molecular, Lisboa, Portugal; Teaching Hosp Cochin, Paris, France; et al)

J Clin Oncol 29:1125-1132, 2011

Purpose.—This study compared denosumab, a fully human monoclonal anti-receptor activator of nuclear factor kappa-B ligand antibody, with zoledronic acid (ZA) for delaying or preventing skeletal-related events (SRE) in patients with advanced cancer and bone metastases (excluding breast and prostate) or myeloma.

Patients and Methods.—Eligible patients were randomly assigned in a double-blind, double-dummy design to receive monthly subcutaneous denosumab 120 mg (n = 886) or intravenous ZA 4 mg (dose adjusted for renal impairment; n = 890). Daily supplemental calcium and vitamin D were strongly recommended. The primary end point was time to first on-study SRE (pathologic fracture, radiation or surgery to bone, or spinal cord compression).

Results.—Denosumab was noninferior to ZA in delaying time to first on-study SRE (hazard ratio, 0.84; 95% CI, 0.71 to 0.98; $P = .0007$). Although directionally favorable, denosumab was not statistically superior to ZA in delaying time to first on-study SRE ($P = .03$ unadjusted; $P = .06$ adjusted for multiplicity) or time to first-and-subsequent (multiple) SRE (rate ratio, 0.90; 95% CI, 0.77 to 1.04; $P = .14$). Overall survival and disease progression were similar between groups. Hypocalcemia occurred more frequently with denosumab. Osteonecrosis of the jaw occurred at similarly low rates in both groups. Acute-phase reactions after the first dose occurred more frequently with ZA, as did renal adverse events and elevations in serum creatinine based on National Cancer Institute Common Toxicity Criteria for Adverse Events grading.

Conclusion.—Denosumab was noninferior (trending to superiority) to ZA in preventing or delaying first on-study SRE in patients with advanced cancer metastatic to bone or myeloma. Denosumab represents a potential novel treatment option with the convenience of subcutaneous administration and no requirement for renal monitoring or dose adjustment.

▶ Denosumab is a fully humanized monoclonal antibody directed against receptor activator of nuclear factor κβ ligand to disrupt the cycle of bone resorption associated with bone metastases. This is one of 3 reports of phase III trials comparing denosumab with zoledronic acid. This particular one is in patients with either myeloma or solid tumors other than breast or prostate cancer and at reduced risk of skeletal-related events including pathologic fracture, surgery for cancer-related bone events, radiation to bone, or spinal cord compression. This study showed noninferiority of denosumab compared with zoledronic acid and a strong trend for superiority. In a further analysis, superiority of denosumab was shown in patients with solid tumors after removal of the patients with myeloma. The trials in breast and prostate cancer each showed superiority for denosumab. All 3 studies called for a pooled analysis, which also showed superiority for denosumab. These 3 trials led to the approval of denosumab by the Food and Drug Administration for use in all patients with solid tumor with bone metastases. Because the drug is superior to zoledronic acid in reducing the risk of skeletal-related events, it should be the treatment of choice. In the case of multiple myeloma, an ongoing phase III trial with an accrual target of 1500 patients with multiple myeloma should eventually determine whether the drug should be used in patients with this disease.

J. T. Thigpen, MD

2 Breast Cancer

General Issues

Weight Lifting for Women at Risk for Breast Cancer–Related Lymphedema: A Randomized Trial

Schmitz KH, Ahmed RL, Troxel AB, et al (Univ of Pennsylvania School of Medicine and Abramson Cancer Ctr, Philadelphia; Univ of Minnesota Med School, Minneapolis; et al)

JAMA 304:2699-2705, 2010

Context.—Clinical guidelines for breast cancer survivors without lymphedema advise against upper body exercise, preventing them from obtaining established health benefits of weight lifting.

Objective.—To evaluate lymphedema onset after a 1-year weight lifting intervention vs no exercise (control) among survivors at risk for breast cancer–related lymphedema (BCRL).

Design, Setting, and Participants.—A randomized controlled equivalence trial (Physical Activity and Lymphedema trial) in the Philadelphia metropolitan area of 154 breast cancer survivors 1 to 5 years postunilateral breast cancer, with at least 2 lymph nodes removed and without clinical signs of BCRL at study entry. Participants were recruited between October 1, 2005, and February 2007, with data collection ending in August 2008.

Intervention.—Weight lifting intervention included a gym membership and 13 weeks of supervised instruction, with the remaining 9 months unsupervised, vs no exercise.

Main Outcome Measures.—Incident BCRL determined by increased arm swelling during 12 months (≥5% increase in interlimb difference). Clinician-defined BCRL onset was also evaluated. Equivalence margin was defined as doubling of lymphedema incidence.

Results.—A total of 134 participants completed follow-up measures at 1 year. The proportion of women who experienced incident BCRL onset was 11% (8 of 72) in the weight lifting intervention group and 17% (13 of 75) in the control group (cumulative incidence difference [CID], −6.0%; 95% confidence interval [CI], −17.2% to 5.2%; *P* for equivalence = .04). Among women with 5 or more lymph nodes removed, the proportion who experienced incident BCRL onset was 7% (3 of 45) in the weight lifting intervention group and 22% (11 of 49) in the control group (CID, −15.0%; 95% CI, −18.6% to −11.4%; *P* for equivalence = .003). Clinician-defined BCRL onset occurred in 1 woman in the weight lifting intervention group and 3 women in the control group (1.5% vs 4.4%, *P* for equivalence = .12).

Conclusion.—In breast cancer survivors at risk for lymphedema, a program of slowly progressive weight lifting compared with no exercise did not result in increased incidence of lymphedema.

Trial Registration.—clinicaltrials.gov Identifier: NCT00194363.

▶ Schmitz and colleagues have shed new light on the benefits of resistance training, particularly progressive weight training, for breast cancer survivors at risk for lymphedema. For far too long, breast cancer survivors have been encouraged to engage in less activity and limit the use of the affected arm out of fear of developing the condition and uncertainty about personal risk and safety. However, such advice often results in physical deconditioning of the arm[1] and prevents breast cancer survivors from reaping the benefits of increased activity. In this study, Schmitz and colleagues provide compelling evidence that properly designed, supervised progressive weight training is not only safe but also may be protective against developing lymphedema. It is important to note that lymphedema is now and will continue to be a frequent and serious unwanted complication for breast cancer survivors, even those who undergo sparing procedures, such as sentinel node biopsy. Therefore, the importance of research aimed at finding effective modalities that reduce the likelihood of lymphedema while enhancing survivors' physical and mental well-being cannot be overstated.

This study is the latest in a continuum of research conducted by Schmitz and colleagues on the efficacy of weight training for lymphedema. In the initial pilot study, the team found no evidence that a 6-month progressive weight lifting program among breast cancer survivors (n = 45) precipitated lymphedema incidence or worsened symptoms of those *with* lymphedema.[2] Previously published results for the current study[3] showed favorable results: increased strength, reduced symptoms, and decreased incidence of exacerbation of lymphedema in 145 breast cancer survivors *with* stable arm lymphedema enrolled in a 1-year progressive weight lifting randomized controlled trial. Continuing with this study, the team assessed the 1-year progressive weight lifting randomized controlled trial results of 154 breast cancer survivors *without* clinical signs of breast cancer–related lymphedema. Survivors in the intervention group participated in 13 weeks of supervised exercise sessions and twice-weekly unsupervised sessions thereafter for up to 1 year. Fitness trainers were available to help participants adhere to the exercise plan, safely increase or decrease weight, and monitor arm swelling. Control group participants received part of the intervention (gym membership and 13 weeks of supervised exercise sessions) after the 1-year study period. The team found no evidence that breast cancer survivors who engaged in weight lifting were at increased risk of lymphedema.

It is important to note some of the strengths of this study. First, intensive and comprehensive training the trainers on the progressive weight lifting protocol, followed by a period of checking for protocol fidelity, greatly enhanced the safety and internal validity of the study. Second, the program was not only progressive (ie, weight was increased after participants successfully managed a given weight) but was also regressive, that is, participants regressed to a lower weight if they missed a set number of sessions. Third, progression from supervised sessions in small groups for the first 13 weeks to independent sessions for the remainder of the study period most likely enhanced the participants' perceived efficacy to perform the weight training and contributed to the high completion rate over a 1-year period.

The strengths should be viewed with the consideration of some limitations. Lymphedema can suddenly occur years after treatment,[4] often with no clear precipitating factor.[5] Therefore, longer-term studies involving weight training with very long follow-up are needed in the future. In addition, as the authors pointed out, corresponding gains in strength were not directly explainable by changes in lean mass. It may be that most of the gains in strength were the results of neuromuscular recruitment mechanisms rather than incremental gains in lean mass. Again, more research is needed. Last, future research might be conducted in low-income and/or ethnic minority breast cancer survivors, as women in this sample were well-educated, self-motivated, and primarily non-Hispanic white (with a small number of African Americans).

The primary objective of this pivotal study was to test the safety of a properly designed 1-year progressive weight lifting program for breast cancer survivors who underwent axillary lymph node dissection. This study, consistent with earlier work, provides strong evidence that breast cancer survivors can confidently participate in weight training and thus gain the benefits of such a program (strength, body mass changes, etc). Still, as the authors have correctly pointed out, additional research is needed before we can convincingly say that resistance training prevents lymphedema. The authors should be lauded for their continued exemplary research and are urged to continue providing scientific evidence of the efficacy of properly designed exercise for women at risk for lymphedema.

D. C. Hughes, PhD
C. M. Mojica, PhD, MPH

References

1. Schmitz KH. Balancing lymphedema risk: exercise versus deconditioning for breast cancer survivors. *Exerc Sport Sci Rev.* 2010;38:17-24.
2. Ahmed RL, Thomas W, Yee D, Schmitz KH. Randomized controlled trial of weight training and lymphedema in breast cancer survivors. *J Clin Oncol.* 2006; 24:2765-2772.
3. Schmitz KH, Ahmed RL, Troxel A, et al. Weight lifting in women with breast-cancer-related lymphedema. *N Engl J Med.* 2009;361:664-673.
4. Petrek JA, Heelan MC. Incidence of breast carcinoma-related lymphedema. *Cancer.* 1998;83:2776-2881.
5. Rockson SG. Precipitating factors in lymphedema: myths and realities. *Cancer.* 1998;83:2814-2816.

Effect of Active Resistive Exercise on Breast Cancer–Related Lymphedema: A Randomized Controlled Trial

Kim DS, Sim Y-J, Jeong HJ, et al (Kosin Univ College of Medicine, Busan, Republic of Korea)

Arch Phys Med Rehabil 91:1844-1848, 2010

Objective.—To investigate the differences between the effects of complex decongestive physiotherapy with and without active resistive exercise for the treatment of patients with breast cancer–related lymphedema (BCRL).

Design.—Randomized control-group study.

Setting.—An outpatient rehabilitation clinic.

Participants.—Patients (N=40) with diagnosed BCRL.

Interventions.—Patients were randomly assigned to either the active resistive exercise group or the nonactive resistive exercise group. In the active resistive exercise group, after complex decongestive physiotherapy, active resistive exercise was performed for 15min/d, 5 days a week for 8 weeks. The nonactive resistive exercise group performed only complex decongestive physiotherapy.

Main Outcome Measures.—The circumferences of the upper limbs (proximal, distal, and total) for the volume changes, and the Short Form-36 version 2 questionnaire for the quality of life (QOL) at pretreatment and 8 weeks posttreatment for each patient.

Results.—The volume of the proximal part of the arm was significantly more reduced in the active resistive exercise group than that of the nonactive resistive exercise group ($P<.05$). In the active resistive exercise group, there was significantly more improvement in physical health and general health, as compared with that of the nonactive resistive exercise group ($P<.05$).

Conclusions.—For the treatment of patients with BCRL, active resistive exercise with complex decongestive physiotherapy did not cause additional swelling, and it significantly reduced proximal arm volume and helped improve QOL.

▶ Treatment of BCRL remains a difficult conversation between physicians and patients because there are many unknowns related to the effectiveness of available interventions. Patients often modify their work and lifestyle habits in hopes of preventing the development of lymphedema and for fear of worsening the symptoms of BCRL. Furthermore, current treatment options for BCRL are limited and have variable outcomes.

In this study reported by Kim and colleagues, the authors address the role of active resistance exercise in women undergoing treatment for BCRL. A total of 40 breast cancer survivors diagnosed with BCRL by a selected physician all received complex decongestive therapy and were randomized to participate in active resistance exercise or receive no further intervention. The patients randomized to participate in active resistance exercise performed the exercises for 15 minutes a day, 5 days a week, for a total of 8 weeks. Change in the affected arm was assessed via a calculation of volume using arm circumference measurements. The authors report that proximal arm volume was significantly reduced in the group that completed the exercises compared with the nonactive resistance exercise group. However, no significant reduction between groups was seen in distal and total arm volumes. After 8 weeks of treatment, QOL was improved in both groups, although the exercise group had significant improvements in physical and general health categories compared with the nonactive resistance group.

The small sample size and the method the investigators used to calculate arm volumes are significant limitations of this study. It is difficult to infer from these data that active resistance exercise can improve BCRL outcomes; it does not, however, appear to worsen it. There was variability between the 2 groups with respect to the onset of lymphedema, in that those who did not participate in active resistance exercise tended to have BCRL for a longer period of time before the intervention, and it is not clear how many prior interventions were employed in each group. It appears that both groups benefited from treatment in terms of QOL, and this may be the most important message that we can relay to our patients with BCRL.

Patients undergoing treatment for breast cancer are at varying risk for developing lymphedema and should be educated on how their individual risk may differ from that of other patients with breast cancer. Prevention strategies for those at highest risk are certainly needed, and further assessment of how currently available treatment methods impact short- and long-term outcomes in individuals living with BCRL deserves more attention. Using active resistance exercise may be one approach, incorporated into a multifaceted anatomic and physiologic treatment strategy, to improve QOL and potentially reduce arm volumes in individuals with BCRL. More data are desperately needed to formulate the best prevention and treatment regimens to relieve patients with breast cancer from the morbidity of lymphedema.

J. L. Wagner, DO
K. K. Hunt, MD

Safety of pregnancy following breast cancer diagnosis: A meta-analysis of 14 studies

Azim HA Jr, Santoro L, Pavlidis N, et al (Jules Bordet Inst, Brussels, Belgium; European Inst of Oncology, Milan, Italy; Univ of Ioannina, Greece; et al)
Eur J Cancer 47:74-83, 2011

Background.—Due to the rising trend of delaying pregnancy to later in life, more women are diagnosed with breast cancer before completing their families. Therefore, enquiry into the feasibility and safety of pregnancy following breast cancer diagnosis is on the rise. Available evidence suggests that women with a history of breast cancer are frequently advised against future conception for fear that pregnancy could adversely affect their breast cancer outcome. Hence, we conducted a meta-analysis to understand the effect of pregnancy on overall survival of women with a history of breast cancer.

Methods.—Two of the authors independently performed a literature search up to September 2009 with no language restrictions. Eligible studies were published retrospective control-matched, population-based and hospital-based studies that have addressed the impact of pregnancy on the overall survival of women with history of breast cancer. Pooling of data was done using the random effect model. Unpublished statistics from three studies were obtained to perform further subgroup and sensitivity analyses. This included examining the effect of pregnancy according to age at diagnosis, healthy mother effect, type of study, nodal status and other parameters.

Results.—Fourteen studies were included in this meta-analysis (1244 cases and 18,145 controls). Women who got pregnant following breast cancer diagnosis had a 41% reduced risk of death compared to women who did not get pregnant [PRR: 0.59 (90% confidence interval (CI): 0.50–0.70)]. This difference was seen irrespective of the type of the study and particularly in women with history of node-negative disease. In a subgroup analysis, we compared the outcome of women with history of breast cancer who became pregnant to breast cancer patients who did not get pregnant and were known to be free of relapse. In this analysis, we did not find significant differences in survival between either group [PRR: 0.85; 95% CI: 0.53–1.35].

Conclusions.—This study confirms that pregnancy in women with history of breast cancer is safe and does not compromise their overall survival. Hence, breast cancer survivors should not be denied the opportunity of future conception.

► How do we advise young women with breast cancer about fertility, future pregnancies, and breast cancer recurrence risks? When the patient is in the office, stressed about her diagnosis and potential treatments, what evidence can we use to respond?

This study by Azim and colleagues provides meaningful clinical guidance for patients and physicians. Pregnancy after breast cancer does not increase the risk of dying from breast cancer. Fertility and the potential for future pregnancies need to be discussed as part of the patient's treatment plan. Endocrine therapy, if appropriate, needs to be reviewed. The hazards of recurrence based on disease characteristics and the potential timing of recurrence need to be reviewed so the patient can make an informed decision regarding any future pregnancy.

This study reports on a carefully constructed, detailed meta-analysis assessing the impact of pregnancy following successful treatment for primary breast carcinoma in young women, and it will certainly help the clinician and reassure patients. The authors provide a well-defined search strategy, data collection, and analysis of previously published studies of pregnancy following treatment for primary breast cancer. All the studies included cases and controls. The authors used the Preferred Reporting Items for Systematic Reviews and Meta-analyses method to identify studies for this analysis. Of 6132 studies,

14 met the authors' criteria for inclusion in the meta-analysis. The end point assessed was overall survival in the pregnant population versus the control population of women with breast cancer who did not become pregnant. The 1244 women who became pregnant were compared with 18 145 control patients. The results show a substantial reduction in the risk of dying from breast cancer in the women who became pregnant after successful breast cancer treatment.

The authors specifically controlled for the healthy mother effect by analyzing case-matched control studies in which the cases and controls were known to be free of relapse. A substantial reduction in the relative risk of death was reported for women with node-negative disease: the pooled relative risk was 0.63 in the node-negative group and 0.96 in the node-positive group. No deleterious effect of a subsequent pregnancy was seen for any group. Although the authors point out limitations of their study (eg, it is based on published retrospective data and does not include biological parameters, such as estrogen receptor [ER] or human epidermal growth factor receptor 2 status, that are important in breast cancer prognosis), the conclusions are substantiated. Counseling against pregnancy is not appropriate for women who have had successful treatment for primary breast cancer and remain fertile.

Fertility assessment and discussions regarding future pregnancy should be part of the individual counseling and treatment planning for young women with primary breast cancer. Recommendations for pregnancy termination are not appropriate for women who have had primary breast cancer and a subsequent pregnancy. The authors note that detailed information regarding pregnancy outcome and breastfeeding for this population has not been well described, so specific recommendations must be particularized for the individual patient.

Young women with a diagnosis of primary breast cancer are being successfully treated, and many have good outcomes. Frequently, clinicians are faced with the need to discuss fertility and pregnancy subsequent to successful treatment for breast cancer. Recommendations prohibiting subsequent pregnancy are not warranted. Termination of pregnancy to improve breast cancer–specific survival has no role in younger women who become pregnant after successful treatment for primary breast cancer. Guidance regarding the use of endocrine therapy, that is, tamoxifen, for those with ER-positive tumors should include a discussion of the potential risks or harms of discontinuing treatment in order to become pregnant.

R. L. Theriault, DO, MBA
J. K. Litton, MD

Long-Term Metformin Use Is Associated With Decreased Risk of Breast Cancer

Bodmer M, Meier C, Krähenbühl S, et al (Univ Hosp Basel, Switzerland; et al)
Diabetes Care 33:1304-1308, 2010

Objective.—To evaluate whether use of oral hypoglycemic agents is associated with an altered breast cancer risk in women.

Research Design and Methods.—Using the U.K.-based General Practice Research Database, we conducted a nested case-control analysis among 22,621 female users of oral antidiabetes drugs with type 2 diabetes. We evaluated whether they had an altered risk of breast cancer in relation to use of various types of oral hypoglycemic agents. Case and control patients with a recorded diagnosis of type 2 diabetes were matched on age, calendar time, and general practice, and the multivariate conditional logistic regression analyses were further adjusted for use of oral antidiabetes drugs, insulin, estrogens, smoking BMI, diabetes duration, and HbA1c (A1C).

Results.—We identified 305 case patients with a recorded incident diagnosis of breast cancer. The mean ± SD age was 67.5 ± 10.5 years at the time of the cancer diagnosis. Long-term use of ≥40 prescriptions (>5 years) of metformin, based on 17 exposed case patients and 120 exposed control patients, was associated with an adjusted odds ratio of 0.44 (95% CI 0.24–0.82) for developing breast cancer compared with no use of metformin. Neither short-term metformin use nor use of sulfonylureas or other antidiabetes drugs was associated with a materially altered risk for breast cancer.

Conclusions.—A decreased risk of breast cancer was observed in female patients with type 2 diabetes using metformin on a long-term basis.

▶ Metformin is a fascinating drug. Although it was initially approved for the treatment of type 2 diabetes, preclinical studies and retrospective clinical series have suggested that metformin may have antitumor activity in breast cancer and other solid tumors. Patients with breast cancer and type 2 diabetes treated with metformin had higher rates of complete pathologic response to neoadjuvant chemotherapy than women who had not taken metformin.[1] Proposed mechanisms of its antitumor action include improved insulin resistance and upregulation of adenosine monophosphate–activated protein kinase activity, which interferes with cancer cell metabolism. The epidemiologic data regarding metformin as a chemoprevention agent are limited.

As reported in this article, Bodmer and colleagues conducted one of the largest case-control studies to address the role of antidiabetic treatments in the risk of breast cancer. Four controls were identified for each breast cancer case, and they were matched by all the known risk factors and concomitant medications. Overall, there was no difference in the risk of breast cancer based on metformin use versus no use. However, when metformin use was stratified by exposure duration, a significant trend emerged. Women who filled 40 or more metformin prescriptions had a 56% reduction in the risk of breast cancer (odds ratio, 0.44; 95% confidence interval, 0.24-0.82; $P = .01$).

This is an interesting, hypothesis-generating observational study that supports clinical trials of metformin as a novel chemoprevention agent. Ongoing studies are also testing a potential therapeutic role of metformin in combination with other therapies in patients with advanced breast cancer.

F. J. Esteva, MD, PhD

Reference

1. Jiralerspong S, Palla SL, Giordano SH, et al. Metformin and pathologic complete responses to neoadjuvant chemotherapy in diabetic patients with breast cancer. *J Clin Oncol.* 2009;27:3297-3302.

Epidemiology

Associations of Breast Cancer Risk Factors With Tumor Subtypes: A Pooled Analysis From the Breast Cancer Association Consortium Studies

Yang XR, Chang-Claude J, Goode EL, et al (Natl Cancer Inst, Rockville, MD; German Cancer Res Ctr, Heidelberg, Germany; Mayo Clinic, Rochester, MN; et al)

J Natl Cancer Inst 103:250-263, 2011

Background.—Previous studies have suggested that breast cancer risk factors are associated with estrogen receptor (ER) and progesterone receptor (PR) expression status of the tumors.

Methods.—We pooled tumor marker and epidemiological risk factor data from 35 568 invasive breast cancer case patients from 34 studies participating in the Breast Cancer Association Consortium. Logistic regression models were used in case—case analyses to estimate associations between epidemiological risk factors and tumor subtypes, and case—control analyses to estimate associations between epidemiological risk factors and the risk of developing specific tumor subtypes in 12 population-based studies. All statistical tests were two-sided.

Results.—In case—case analyses, of the epidemiological risk factors examined, early age at menarche (≤12 years) was less frequent in case patients with PR^- than PR^+ tumors ($P = .001$). Nulliparity ($P = 3 \times 10^{-6}$) and increasing age at first birth ($P = 2 \times 10^{-9}$) were less frequent in ER^- than in ER^+ tumors. Obesity (body mass index [BMI] ≥ 30 kg/m^2) in younger women (≤50 years) was more frequent in ER^-/PR^- than in ER^+/PR^+ tumors ($P = 1 \times 10^{-7}$), whereas obesity in older women (>50 years) was less frequent in PR^- than in PR^+ tumors ($P = 6 \times 10^{-4}$). The triple-negative ($ER^-/PR^-/HER2^-$) or core basal phenotype (CBP; triple-negative and cytokeratins [CK]5/6$^+$ and/or epidermal growth factor receptor [EGFR]$^+$) accounted for much of the heterogeneity in parity-related variables and BMI in younger women. Case-control analyses showed that nulliparity, increasing age at first birth, and obesity in younger women showed the expected associations with the risk of ER^+ or PR^+ tumors but not triple-negative (nulliparity vs parity, odds ratio [OR] = 0.94, 95% confidence interval [CI] = 0.75 to 1.19, $P = .61$; 5-year increase in age at first full-term birth, OR = 0.95, 95% CI = 0.86 to 1.05, $P = .34$; obesity in younger women, OR = 1.36, 95% CI = 0.95 to 1.94, $P = .09$) or CBP tumors.

Conclusions.—This study shows that reproductive factors and BMI are most clearly associated with hormone receptor-positive tumors and suggest that triple-negative or CBP tumors may have distinct etiology.

▶ Over the past 2 decades, the progress achieved in breast cancer research has been remarkable. In particular, the concept that breast cancer is a monolithic disease crumbles faster and faster all the time, with new technologies and large consortium projects revealing important differences between breast cancer subtypes and their risk factors. For years, we knew that not all breast cancers were similar in microscopic appearance, growth trajectory, and response to therapy. Now, thanks to pooled studies like this one by Yang and colleagues, we have insights that open doors to therapeutic and prevention strategies tailored to such subtypes—a major advance in the battle against cancer—because we are now able to recognize differences between breast cancers at a molecular and biochemical level.

As critical as these findings are for drawing attention to differences in the risk factors for breast cancer subtypes of varying aggressiveness, gaps in our knowledge persist. For example, whether the patterns reported are evident for nonwhite women remains to be determined, as the analysis included mostly white women (92%). Also, the impact of hormone replacement therapy (HRT) use on the risk for specific breast cancer subtypes was not addressed and is a major limitation given the putative link between HRT and ER^+ breast cancer development.

Finally, these results draw attention to our lack of detailed understanding of the underlying mechanisms of ER and PR in both normal and neoplastic tissue. Future research efforts oriented toward expanding our fundamental knowledge of the roles of and relationship between ER and PR would enhance breast cancer research considerably.

N. E. De La Fuente, BS
S. Chang, PhD

Prognostic Factors

Identification of a low-risk subgroup of HER-2-positive breast cancer by the 70-gene prognosis signature

Knauer M, Cardoso F, Wesseling J, et al (The Netherlands Cancer Inst/Antoni van Leeuwenhoek Hosp, Plesmanlaan, Amsterdam; Institut Jules Bordet, Brussels, Belgium)
Br J Cancer 103:1788-1793, 2010

Background.—Overexpression of HER-2 is observed in 15–25% of breast cancers, and is associated with increased risk of recurrence. Current guidelines recommend trastuzumab and chemotherapy for most HER-2-positive patients. However, the majority of patients does not recur and might thus be overtreated with adjuvant systemic therapy. We investigated whether the 70-gene MammaPrint signature identifies HER-2-positive patients with favourable outcome.

Methods.—In all, 168 T1–3, N0–1, HER-2-positive patients were identified from a pooled database, classified by the 70-gene signature as good or poor prognosis, and correlated with long-term outcome. A total of 89 of these patients did not receive adjuvant chemotherapy.

Results.—In the group of 89 chemotherapy-naive patients, after a median follow-up of 7.4 years, 35 (39%) distant recurrences and 29 (33%) breast cancer-specific deaths occurred. The 70-gene signature classified 20 (22%) patients as good prognosis, with 10-year distant disease-free survival (DDFS) of 84%, compared with 69 (78%) poor prognosis patients with 10-year DDFS of 55%. The estimated hazard ratios (HRs) were 4.5 (95% confidence interval (CI) 1.1–18.7, $P = 0.04$) and 3.8 (95% CI 0.9–15.8, $P = 0.07$) for DDFS and breast cancer-specific survival (BCSS), respectively. In multivariate analysis adjusted for known prognostic factors and hormonal therapy, HRs were 5.8 (95% CI 1.3–26.7, $P = 0.03$) and 4.7 (95% CI 1.0–21.7, $P = 0.05$) for DDFS and BCSS, respectively.

Interpretation.—The 70-gene prognosis signature is an independent prognostic indicator that identifies a subgroup of HER-2-positive early breast cancer with a favourable long-term outcome.

▶ The *HER-2* oncogene is amplified in about 25% of breast cancers and is a significant predictor of both overall survival and time to relapse.[1] Over-expression of *HER-2* is associated with significant benefit from adjuvant chemotherapy.[2] The Herceptin Adjuvant trial also demonstrated a hazard ratio of 0.49 (95% confidence interval [CI], 0.38-0.63; $P < .0001$) for time to distant recurrence with trastuzumab compared with observation.[3] Combined analysis of 2 American trials (the National Surgical Adjuvant Breast and Bowel Project trial B-31 and the North Central Cancer Treatment Group trial N9831) showed an absolute difference of 4.8% (95% CI, 0.6%-9.0%) in overall survival and 18.2% (95% CI, 12.7%-23.7%) in disease-free survival at 4 years with the addition of trastu-zumab to chemotherapy for *HER-2*-positive tumors.[4] These trials have established trastuzumab-based adjuvant chemotherapy as the cornerstone of therapy in *HER-2*-positive breast cancers. As a result, the National Comprehensive Cancer Network[5] and the International Consensus Panel on the Primary Therapy of Early Breast Cancer[6] recommend trastuzumab-based adjuvant chemotherapy for all women with either *HER-2*-positive, node-positive disease or *HER-2*-positive, node-negative disease with tumor sizes less than 1 cm (T1c or above) and the consideration of trastuzumab for T1b tumors (6-10 mm), especially those that are hormone receptor negative.

In this retrospective analysis, Knauer and colleagues concluded that the 70-gene MammaPrint prognosis signature is an independent prognostic factor and can identify a subgroup of *HER-2*-positive early breast cancer with a favorable long-term outcome. The suggested clinical implication is that less-intensive therapy in such good-prognosis patients should be evaluated, as there is the potential to spare them from aggressive chemotherapy. These are exciting data that should be reviewed cautiously and subjected to appropriate validation.

Although the therapeutic implications suggested here are intriguing, it is important to consider the great benefit of modern adjuvant anti-HER-2 therapies: their significant synergism with chemotherapy; this benefit was evident even in patients who we believed had low-risk tumors.[4] In general, *HER-2*-positive tumors have aggressive biological characteristics and poor prognosis, and even when treating hormone receptor–positive tumors, one would feel hesitant to deny chemotherapy because *HER-2* expression is associated with resistance to endocrine therapy and poor outcomes.[7] On the other hand, there are the toxic effects of chemotherapy and trastuzumab, but in general, these are modest and may be considered by some patients as an acceptable risk when compared with the risk of cancer recurrence.

The 70-gene expression profile (MammaPrint/Amsterdam signature) was validated in earlier analyses but was not evaluated in the *HER-2*-positive population as an independent group.[8,9] This and the limited number of patients are major limitations of Knauer and colleagues' study.

The Microarray In Node-negative Disease May Avoid Chemotherapy trial[10] is the right approach to validating this signature prospectively and has an interesting, novel design that accounts for the main clinical and pathologic characteristics of breast cancer. The data presented in this article are intriguing and should at least be reproduced; the study definitively opens the door to better patient selection for aggressive therapies in *HER-2*-positive breast cancer.

K. P. S. Raghav, MD
A. M. Gonzalez-Angulo, MD, MSc

References

1. Slamon DJ, Clark GM, Wong SG, Levin WJ, Ullrich A, McGuire WL. Human breast cancer: correlation of relapse and survival with ampli-fication of the HER-2/neu oncogene. *Science*. 1987;235:177-182.
2. Muss HB, Thor AD, Berry DA, et al. c-erbB-2 expression and response to adjuvant therapy in women with node-positive early breast cancer. *N Engl J Med*. 1994;330:1260-1266.
3. Piccart-Gebhart MJ, Procter M, Leyland-Jones B, et al. Herceptin Adjuvant (HERA) Trial Study Team. Trastuzumab after adjuvant chemo-therapy in HER-2-positive breast cancer. *N Engl J Med*. 2005;353:1659-1672.
4. Romond EH, Perez EA, Bryant J, et al. Trastuzumab plus adjuvant chemotherapy for operable HER-2-positive breast cancer. *N Engl J Med*. 2005;353:1673-1684.
5. National Comprehensive Cancer Network (NCCN) guidelines, http://www.nccn.org. Accessed January 25, 2011.
6. Goldhirsch A, Ingle JN, Gelber RD, Coates AS, Thürlimann B, Senn HJ, et al. Panel members. Thresholds for therapies: highlights of the St Gallen International Expert Consensus on the primary therapy of early breast cancer 2009. *Ann Oncol*. 2009;20:1319-1329.
7. Carlomagno C, Perrone F, Gallo C, et al. c-erb B2 overexpression decreases the benefit of adjuvant tamoxifen in early-stage breast cancer without axillary lymph node metastases. *J Clin Oncol*. 1996;14:2702-2708.
8. van de Vijver MJ, He YD, van't Veer LJ, et al. A gene-expression signature as a predictor of survival in breast cancer. *N Engl J Med*. 2002;347:1999-2009.
9. Buyse M, Loi S, van't Veer L, et al. TRANSBIG Consortium. Validation and clinical utility of a 70-gene prognostic signature for women with node-negative breast cancer. *J Natl Cancer Inst*. 2006;98:1183-1192.
10. MINDACT trial (NCT00433589), http://clinicaltrials.gov. Accessed January 25, 2011.

Early Stage and Adjuvant Therapy

17ß-Hydroxysteroid dehydrogenase type 1 as predictor of tamoxifen response in premenopausal breast cancer

Källström A-C, Salme R, Rydén L, et al (Helsingborg Hosp, Sweden; Linköping Univ, Sweden; Lund Univ, Sweden)

Eur J Cancer 46:892-900, 2010

17ß-Hydroxysteroid dehydrogenases (17HSDs) are involved in the local regulation of sex steroids. 17HSD1 converts oestrone (E1) to the more potent oestradiol (E2) and 17HSD2 catalyses the reverse reaction. The aim of this study was to investigate the expression of these enzymes in premenopausal breast cancers and to analyse if they have any prognostic or tamoxifen predictive value. Premenopausal patients with invasive breast cancer, stage II (UICC), were randomised to either 2 years of adjuvant tamoxifen ($n = 276$) or no tamoxifen ($n = 288$). The median follow-up was 13.9 years (range 10.5–17.5). The expression of 17HSD1 and 17HSD2 was analysed with immunohistochemistry using tissue microarrays. The enzyme expression level (−/+/++/+++) was successfully determined in 396 and 373 tumours, respectively. Women with hormone-receptor positive tumours, with low levels (−/+/++) of 17HSD1, had a 43% reduced risk of recurrence, when treated with tamoxifen (Hazard Ratio (HR) = 0.57; 95% confidence interval (CI), 0.37–0.86; $p = 0.0086$). On the other hand high expression (+++) of 17HSD1 was associated with no significant difference between the two treatment arms (HR = 0.91; 95% CI, 0.43–1.95; $p = 0.82$). The interaction between 17HSD1 and tamoxifen was significant during the first 5 years of follow-up ($p = 0.023$). In the cohort of systemically untreated patients no prognostic importance was observed for 17HSD1. We found no predictive or prognostic value for 17HSD2. This is the first report of 17HSD1 in a cohort of premenopausal women with breast cancer randomised to tamoxifen. Our data suggest that 17HSD1 might be a predictive factor in this group of patients.

► An association between likelihood of benefit from tamoxifen and levels of 17β-hydroxysteroid dehydrogenases (17HSDs) has been previously reported. This study is different in that it focuses on premenopausal rather than postmenopausal women. The subjects were 564 participants in a trial of adjuvant tamoxifen versus no tamoxifen in premenopausal women with hormone-receptor positive tumors. Tamoxifen was given for 2 years. Two different doses of tamoxifen were used: 20 mg po daily and 40 mg po daily; but the effects of the different doses were not examined. At the time of this retrospective translational research study, the median follow-up of the patients was 13.9 years. Women with low expression of 17HSD1, which converts oestrone to oestradiol, benefited from tamoxifen (hazard ratio [HR] = 0.57, $P = .0086$), whereas women with high levels of 17HSD1 did not benefit (HR = 0.91, $P = .82$). The investigators found no prognostic value for 17HSD1, only the above-noted predictive value for the efficacy of tamoxifen. Additionally, the greatest effect of tamoxifen in the 17HSD1 low expressors was in those patients who also had high expression of progesterone receptor. 17HSD2 had no prognostic or predictive value in the study. This study, therefore, suggests that 17HSD1 may be a useful factor in predicting which patients would benefit from treatment with tamoxifen.

There are a couple of caveats that must be taken into consideration in determining the usefulness of the observations in this trial. First, the study was retrospective; hence, the data should be considered more as hypothesis generating than as establishing a standard of care. Second, the investigators themselves suggest that the mechanism for the observed effect may be that those patients with low 17HSD1 have low levels of oestradiol, which in turn makes the tamoxifen, which is thought to act through competition with estradiom for the estrogen receptor, more effective with less estradio with which to compete. If this is correct, higher doses of tamoxifen might overcome the effect of high levels of 17HSD1. This study included 2 different dose levels of tamoxifen, one twice as much as the other. One is left with the question as to whether the observed effects would be substantially different if all patients had received the higher dose of 40 mg. What ultimate clinical role 17HSD1 will play in determining whether a patient needs tamoxifen or not must await validation of these observations in a prospective trial.

J. T. Thigpen, MD

Alteration of Topoisomerase II–Alpha Gene in Human Breast Cancer: Association with Responsiveness to Anthracycline-Based Chemotherapy

Press MF, Sauter G, Buyse M, et al (Univ of Southern California, Los Angeles, CA; Univ of California Los Angeles; City of Hope Natl Med Ctr, Duarte, CA; et al)

J Clin Oncol 29:859-867, 2011

Purpose.—Approximately 35% of *HER2*-amplified breast cancers have coamplification of the topoisomerase II-alpha (*TOP2A*) gene encoding an enzyme that is a major target of anthracyclines. This study was designed to evaluate whether *TOP2A* gene alterations may predict incremental responsiveness to anthracyclines in some breast cancers.

Methods.—A total of 4,943 breast cancers were analyzed for alterations in *TOP2A* and *HER2*. Primary tumor tissues from patients with metastatic breast cancer treated in a trial of chemotherapy plus/minus trastuzumab were studied for amplification/deletion of *TOP2A* and *HER2* as a test set followed by evaluation of malignancies from two separate, large trials for changes in these same genes as a validation set. Association between these alterations and clinical outcomes was determined.

Results.—Test set cases containing *HER2* amplification treated with doxorubicin and cyclophosphamide (AC) plus trastuzumab, demonstrated longer progression-free survival compared to those treated with AC alone ($P = .0002$). However, patients treated with AC alone whose tumors contain *HER2/TOP2A* coamplification experienced a similar improvement in survival ($P = .004$). Conversely, for patients treated with paclitaxel, *HER2/TOP2A* coamplification was not associated with improved outcomes. These observations were confirmed in a larger validation set, where *HER2/TOP2A* coamplification was again associated with longer survival when only anthracycline-containing chemotherapy was used for treatment compared with outcome in *HER2*-positive cancers lacking *TOP2A* coamplification.

Conclusion.—In a study involving nearly 5,000 breast malignancies, both test set and validation set demonstrate that *TOP2A* coamplification, not *HER2* amplification, is the clinically useful predictive marker of an incremental response to anthracycline-based chemotherapy. Absence of *HER2/TOP2A* coamplification may indicate a more restricted efficacy advantage for breast cancers than previously thought.

▶ *HER2* amplification has, since 1998, marked a group of patients as having breast cancer that requires treatment that is different from the treatment for those that do not overexpress *HER2*. In particular, *HER2* amplification has been associated with better patient outcomes in those treated with an anthracycline and with trastuzumab. More recently, interest has focused on *TOP2A* gene alterations in association with *HER2* overexpression as a marker for anthracycline sensitivity. Studies have variously reported that only those patients with coamplification of both *HER2* and *TOP2A* benefit from an anthracycline more so than with regimens not containing an anthracycline. This study reports an attempt to clarify the issue by evaluating the coamplification as a marker of anthracycline sensitivity. When one puts these results together with results from previous literature on this topic, the following conclusions would seem reasonable. (1) There is little evidence for an advantage of using anthracyclines in patients who do not exhibit coamplification of *HER2* and *TOP2A*. (2) In patients with *HER2* amplification without *TOP2A* coamplification, the use of trastuzumab with chemotherapy yields improved progression-free survival and overall survival, but it is not necessary to use anthracycline-based chemotherapy to achieve this. (3) In patients with coamplification of both *HER2* and *TOP2A*, inclusion of an anthracycline confers improved progression-free survival and overall survival even in the absence of trastuzumab. (4) In patients who do not overexpress *HER2*, there is no advantage to an anthracycline-based regimen.

J. T. Thigpen, MD

Dose-Dense Chemotherapy in Nonmetastatic Breast Cancer: A Systematic Review and Meta-analysis of Randomized Controlled Trials

Bonilla L, Ben-Aharon I, Vidal L, et al (Rabin Med Ctr, Petah Tikva, Israel)

J Natl Cancer Inst 102:1845-1854, 2010

Background.—Dose-dense chemotherapy has become a mainstay regimen in the adjuvant setting for women with high-risk breast cancer. We performed a systematic review and meta-analysis of the existing data from randomized controlled trials regarding the efficacy and toxicity of the dose-dense chemotherapy approach in nonmetastatic breast cancer.

Methods.—Randomized controlled trials that compared a dose-dense chemotherapy protocol with a standard chemotherapy schedule in the neoadjuvant or adjuvant setting in adult women older than 18 years with breast cancer were identified by searching The Cochrane Cancer Network register of trials, The Cochrane Library, and LILACS and MEDLINE databases (from January 1966 to January 2010). Hazard ratios (HRs) of death and recurrence and relative risks of adverse events were estimated and pooled. All statistical tests were two-sided.

Results.—Ten trials met the inclusion criteria and were classified into two categories based on trial methodology. Three trials enrolling 3337 patients compared dose-dense chemotherapy with a conventional chemotherapy schedule (similar agents). Patients who received dose-dense chemotherapy had better overall survival (HR of death = 0.84, 95% confidence interval [CI] = 0.72 to 0.98, P = .03) and better disease-free survival (HR of recurrence or death = 0.83, 95% CI = 0.73 to 0.94, P = .005) than those on the conventional schedule. No benefit was observed in patients with hormone receptor–positive tumors. Seven trials enrolling 8652 patients compared dose-dense chemotherapy with regimens that use standard intervals but with different agents and/or dosages in the treatment arms. Similar results were obtained for these trials with respect to overall survival (HR of death = 0.85, 95% CI = 0.75 to 0.96, P = .01) and disease-free survival (HR of recurrence or death = 0.81, 95% CI = 0.73 to 0.88, $P < .001$). The rate of nonhematological adverse events was higher in the dose-dense chemotherapy arms than in the conventional chemotherapy arms.

Conclusion.—Dose-dense chemotherapy results in better overall and disease-free survival, particularly in women with hormone receptor-negative breast cancer. However, additional data from randomized controlled trials are needed before dose-dense chemotherapy can be considered as the standard of care.

▶ For the past 3 decades, oncologists have generally held that dose and schedule were important in determining the efficacy of chemotherapy. Results of a CALGB trial in breast cancer demonstrated that dose-dense therapy (single agents or combinations given in sequence at shorter interval than conventional therapy supported by growth factors) compared with conventional therapy produces superior disease-free and overall survival. Over the past 15 years, 10 phase III trials comparing dose dense therapy to conventional therapy have been published. This article presents a meta-analysis of these 10 trials to determine the level of any advantage associated with dose-dense therapy. The data show that dose-dense therapy is associated with a better disease-free survival (hazard ratio [HR] = 0.83, P = .005) and overall survival (HR = 0.84, P = .03) than conventional therapy. This establishes dose-dense therapy as a valid approach. Before such an approach becomes the standard of care, however, 3 caveats must be addressed. First, 7 of the 10 trials did not use the same agents in the dose-dense and conventional arms. This introduces additional variables that must be accounted for before a definitive conclusion can be reached about the dose-dense approach. Second, the small number of trials included in this meta-analysis leaves open the possibility that conclusions are subject to publication bias (negative trials not published because they were negative). Finally, it is clear that not all patients benefit from a dose-dense approach. For example, essentially half the patient population, those with HR + disease, do not gain an advantage from this approach. Further studies are needed to characterize fully the patient population that is likely to benefit before this becomes the standard of care.

J. T. Thigpen, MD

HER2, *TOP2A*, and TIMP-1 and Responsiveness to Adjuvant Anthracycline-Containing Chemotherapy in High-Risk Breast Cancer Patients

Ejlertsen B, Jensen M-B, Nielsen KV, et al (Danish Breast Cancer Cooperative Group Statistical Ctr, Copenhagen, Denmark; Copenhagen Univ Hosp, Denmark; Dako A/S, Glostrup, Denmark; et al)

J Clin Oncol 28:984-990, 2010

Purpose.—To evaluate whether the combination of HER2 with TIMP-1 (HT) or *TOP2A* with TIMP-1 (2T) more accurately identifies patients who benefit from cyclophosphamide, epirubicin, and fluorouracil (CEF) compared with cyclophosphamide, methotrexate, and fluorouracil (CMF) than these markers do when analyzed individually.

Patients and Methods.—The Danish Breast Cancer Cooperative Group (DBCG) 89D trial randomly assigned 980 high-risk Danish breast cancer patients to CMF or CEF. Archival tumor tissue was analyzed TIMP-1, and HER2-negative and TIMP-1 immunoreactive tumors were classified as HT nonresponsive and otherwise HT responsive. Similarly, the 2T panel was constructed by combining *TOP2A* and TIMP-1; tumors with normal *TOP2A* status and TIMP-1 immunoreactivity were classified as 2T-nonresponsive and otherwise 2T-responsive.

Results.—In total, 623 tumors were available for analysis, of which 154 lacked TIMP-1 immunoreactivity, 188 were HER2 positive, and 139 had a *TOP2A* aberration. HT status was a statistically significant predictor of benefit from CEF compared with CMF ($P_{interaction} = .036$ for invasive disease–free survival [IDFS] and .047 for overall survival [OS]). The 269 (43%) patients with a 2T-responsive profile had a significant reduction in IDFS events (adjusted hazard ratio, 0.48; 95% CI, 0.34 to 0.69; $P < .001$) and OS events (adjusted hazard ratio, 0.54; 95% CI, 0.38 to 0.77; $P < .001$). 2T status was a highly significant predictor of benefit from CEF compared with CMF ($P_{interaction} < .0001$ for IDFS and .004 for OS).

Conclusion.—The 2T profile is a more accurate predictor of incremental benefit from anthracycline-containing chemotherapy than HER2, TIMP-1, or *TOP2A* individually, and compared with these, 2T classifies a larger proportion of patients as sensitive to anthracyclines.

► Continuing the theme of looking for biological markers that will identify those patients most likely to benefit from anthracyclines, this study looks at *TOP2A* and

TIMP-1 in addition to HER2. The study uses a 980-patient phase III trial comparing cyclophosphamide, epirubicin, and fluorouracil (CEF) with cyclophosphamide, methotrexate, and fluorouracil (CMF) as a basis for the trial. The bottom line is that abnormalities of either or both of *TOP2A* and TIMP-1 represent better predictors of anthracycline sensitivity than the commonly HER2 status. The importance of this observation is that we can now avoid giving an anthracycline with all of the attendant risks of cardiotoxicity to a number of patients who otherwise would have received the anthracycline in the belief that anthracycline-based combinations are better than alternatives such as CMF. This is supported by another article reviewed herein that suggested that coamplification of HER2 and *TOP2A* represented a better marker of anthracycline sensitivity than HER2 status alone. Both this article and the one reviewed earlier[1] point out indirectly that assessment of the meaning of specific biologic abnormalities is far more complex than simply assessing the status of a single marker and thus led to the conclusion that we have to accrue a great deal more information before we can accurately predict optimal treatment from the biologic profile. This does not mean that we shouldn't use the information we have at hand now to benefit (hopefully) patients now, but it does mean that we have to reassess constantly our treatment paradigms in light of expanding biologic data.

J. T. Thigpen, MD

Reference

1. Press MF, Sauter G, Buyse M, et al. Alteration of topoisomerase II-alpha gene in human breast cancer: association with responsiveness to anthracycline-based chemotherapy. *J Clin Oncol.* 2011;29:859-867.

Longer Therapy, Iatrogenic Amenorrhea, and Survival in Early Breast Cancer

Swain SM, Jeong J-H, Geyer CE Jr, et al (Natl Surgical Adjuvant Breast and Bowel Project (NSABP), Washington, DC; Univ of Pittsburgh, PA; et al)
N Engl J Med 362:2053-2065, 2010

Background.—Chemotherapy regimens that combine anthracyclines and taxanes result in improved disease-free and overall survival among women with operable lymph-node–positive breast cancer. The effectiveness of concurrent versus sequential regimens is not known.

Methods.—We randomly assigned 5351 patients with operable, node-positive, early-stage breast cancer to receive four cycles of doxorubicin and cyclophosphamide followed by four cycles of docetaxel (sequential ACT); four cycles of doxorubicin and docetaxel (doxorubicin–docetaxel); or four cycles of doxorubicin, cyclophosphamide, and docetaxel (concurrent ACT). The primary aims were to examine whether concurrent ACT was more effective than sequential ACT and whether the doxorubicin–docetaxel regimen would be as effective as the concurrent-ACT regimen.

The secondary aims were to assess toxic effects and to correlate amenorrhea with outcomes in premenopausal women.

Results.—At a median follow-up of 73 months, overall survival was improved in the sequential-ACT group (8-year overall survival, 83%) as compared with the doxorubicin–docetaxel group (overall survival, 79%; hazard ratio for death, 0.83; P=0.03) and the concurrent-ACT group (overall survival, 79%; hazard ratio, 0.86; P=0.09). Disease-free survival was improved in the sequential-ACT group (8-year disease-free survival, 74%) as compared with the doxorubicin–docetaxel group (disease-free survival, 69%; hazard ratio for recurrence, a second malignant condition, or death, 0.80; P=0.001) and the concurrent-ACT group (disease-free survival, 69%; hazard ratio, 0.83; P=0.01). The doxorubicin–docetaxel regimen showed noninferiority to the concurrent-ACT regimen for overall survival (hazard ratio, 0.96; 95% confidence interval, 0.82 to 1.14). Overall survival was improved in patients with amenorrhea for 6 months or more across all treatment groups, independently of estrogen-receptor status.

Conclusions.—Sequential ACT improved disease-free survival as compared with doxorubicin–docetaxel or concurrent ACT, and it improved overall survival as compared with doxorubicin–docetaxel. Amenorrhea was associated with improved survival regardless of the treatment and estrogen-receptor status. (ClinicalTrials.gov number, NCT00003782.)

▶ A survival advantage with the use of chemotherapy that includes taxanes and anthracyclines in patients with lymph node–positive yet operable breast cancer has been well documented. The sequencing of the chemotherapy (concurrent vs sequential regimens) has shown improvement in disease-free and overall survival. Which of these methods of chemotherapy delivery is best was not known and was the basis for this phase III, randomized trial. Patients in this trial were randomly assigned to: (1) doxorubicin and cyclophosphamide (AC) for 4 cycles followed by 4 cycles of docetaxel (T); or (2) doxorubicin and docetaxel for 4 cycles; or (3) doxorubicin and cyclophosphamide plus docetaxel (ACT) for 4 cycles.

The results confirm that that sequential AC for 4 cycles followed by T for 4 cycles provides the best outcome in terms of disease-free and overall survival. The question one still must grapple with is why is this the case? Certainly in the concurrent ACT treatment there was dose reduction in the docetaxel compared with the AC for 4 cycles followed by T for 4 cycles arm of the study. Also, in the concurrent ACT arm, there was a dose reduction of the doxorubicin compared with that of the sequential group. The authors do a reasonable job of addressing these concerns. But the remaining question is related to amenorrhea. These authors have confirmed that increased time of amenorrhea in premenopausal females (> 6 months) is associated with improvements in survival end points. So another reason for the sequential chemotherapy being better than the concurrent may be related to time of amenorrhea. The relative importance of each of these aspects of the chemotherapeutic regimens needs further investigation. For now, these data confirm sequential ACT as the gold standard for operable lymph node–positive breast cancer.

C. A. Lawton, MD

Long-Term Benefits of 5 Years of Tamoxifen: 10-Year Follow-Up of a Large Randomized Trial in Women at Least 50 Years of Age With Early Breast Cancer

Hackshaw A, Roughton M, Forsyth S, et al (Cancer Res UK and Univ College London Cancer Trials Centre)
J Clin Oncol 29:1657-1663, 2011

Purpose.—The Cancer Research UK "Over 50s" trial compared 5 and 2 years of tamoxifen in women with early breast cancer. Results are reported after median follow-up of 10 years.

Patients and Methods.—Between 1987 and 1997, 3,449 patients age 50 to 81 years with operable breast cancer who had been taking 20 mg of tamoxifen for 2 years were randomly assigned to either stop or continue for an additional 3 years, if they were alive and recurrence free. Data on recurrences, new tumors, deaths, and cardiovascular events were obtained (April 2010).

Results.—There were 1,103 recurrences, 755 deaths as a result of breast cancer, 621 cardiovascular (CV) events, and 236 deaths as a result of CV events. Fifteen years after starting treatment, for every 100 women who received tamoxifen for 5 years, 5.8 fewer experienced recurrence, compared with those who received tamoxifen for 2 years. The risk of contralateral breast cancer was significantly reduced (hazard ratio, 0.70; 95% CI, 0.48 to 1.00). Among women age 50 to 59 years, there was a 35% reduction in CV events ($P = .005$) and 59% reduction in death as a result of a CV event ($P = .02$); in older women, the effect was much smaller and not statistically significant.

Conclusion.—Taking tamoxifen for the recommended 5 years reduces the risk of recurrence or contralateral breast cancer 15 years after starting treatment. It also lowers the risk of CV disease and death as a result of a CV event, particularly among those age 50 to 59 years. Women should therefore be encouraged to complete the full course. Although aromatase inhibitors improve disease-free survival, tamoxifen remains a cheap and highly effective alternative, particularly in developing countries.

▶ For women older than 50 who have ER-positive breast cancer, the use of hormonal therapy for 5 years as adjuvant treatment is reasonably well established. The original agent used in this setting in large clinical trials was tamoxifen, although recent evidence of a superior effect with aromatase inhibitors has led to the replacement of tamoxifen with an aromatase inhibitor. This study provides long-term follow-up of patients randomly assigned to either 2 or 5 years of tamoxifen on 1 of the earlier trials. Among a total of 3449 women in the randomization, the use of 5 rather than 2 years of tamoxifen led to a 5.8% reduction in recurrences. The beneficial effects associated with prolonged use of tamoxifen were greatest in the younger women on the trial (ages 50 to 59). In addition, this study shows a marked reduction in risk of cardiovascular events (35%) and of death related to cardiovascular events (59%). One reasonably assumes that at least the beneficial effects seen with regard to the reduction in recurrence of the breast cancer will hold for the use of 5 years of aromatase inhibitors, the current standard of care in the United States.

J. T. Thigpen, MD

Pathologic Complete Response in Breast Cancer Patients Receiving Anthracycline- and Taxane-Based Neoadjuvant Chemotherapy: Evaluating the Effect of Race/Ethnicity

Chavez-MacGregor M, Litton J, Chen H, et al (The Univ of Texas M D Anderson Cancer Ctr, Houston; et al)

Cancer 116:4168-4177, 2010

Background.—The current study was conducted to evaluate the influence of race/ethnicity and tumor subtype in pathologic complete response (pCR) following treatment with neoadjuvant chemotherapy.

Methods.—A total of 2074 patients diagnosed with breast cancer between 1994 and 2008 who were treated with neoadjuvant anthracycline-and taxanebased chemotherapy were included. pCR was defined as no residual invasive cancer in the breast and axilla. The Kaplan-Meier product-limit was used to calculate survival outcomes. Cox proportional hazards models were fitted to determine the relationship of patient and tumor variables with outcome.

Results.—The median patient age was 50 years; 14.6% of patients were black, were 15.2% Hispanic, 64.3% were white, and 5.9% were of other race. There were no differences in pCR rates among race/ethnicity (12.3% in black, 14.2% in Hispanics, 12.3% in whites, and 11.5% in others, $P = .788$). Lack of pCR, breast cancer subtype, grade 3 tumors, and lymphovascular invasion were associated with worse recurrence-free survival (RFS) and overall survival (OS) ($P \leq .0001$). Differences in RFS by race/ethnicity were noted in the patients with hormone receptor-positive disease ($P = .007$). On multivariate analysis, Hispanics had improved RFS (hazard ratio [HR], 0.69; 95% confidence interval [95% CI], 0.49-0.97) and OS (HR, 0.63; 95% CI, 0.41-0.97); blacks had a trend toward worse outcomes (RFS: HR, 1.28 [95% CI, 0.97-1.68] and OS: HR, 1.32 [95% CI, 0.97-1.81]) when compared with whites.

Conclusions.—In this cohort of patients, race/ethnicity was not found to be significantly associated with pCR rates. On a multivariate analysis, improved outcomes were observed in Hispanics and a trend toward worse outcomes in black patients, when compared with white patients. Further research was needed to explore the potential differences in biology and outcomes (Figs 1 and 2).

▶ Beyond its clinical utility, the value of neoadjuvant chemotherapy lies in the utility of response in the breast and regional nodes for predicting the likelihood of the eradication of occult metastatic disease, as reflected in RFS and OS. While some of the factors that impact response to neoadjuvant chemotherapy are well known, patients with high-grade, hormone receptor-negative

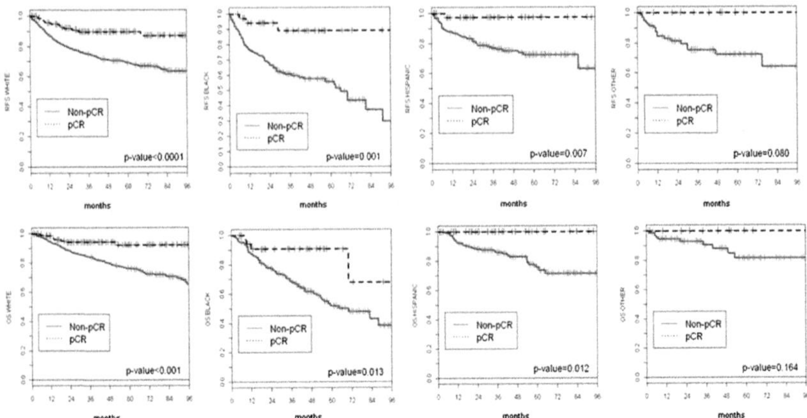

FIGURE 1.—Recurrence-free survival (RFS) and overall survival (OS) by pathologic complete response (pCR) are shown according to race/ethnicity. (Reprinted from Chavez-MacGregor M, Litton J, Chen H, et al. Pathologic complete response in breast cancer patients receiving anthracycline- and taxane-based neoadjuvant chemotherapy: evaluating the effect of race/ethnicity. *Cancer.* 2010;116:4168-4177. Copyright 2010 American Cancer Society. This material is reproduced with permission of Wiley-Liss, Inc., a subsidiary of John Wiley & Sons, Inc.)

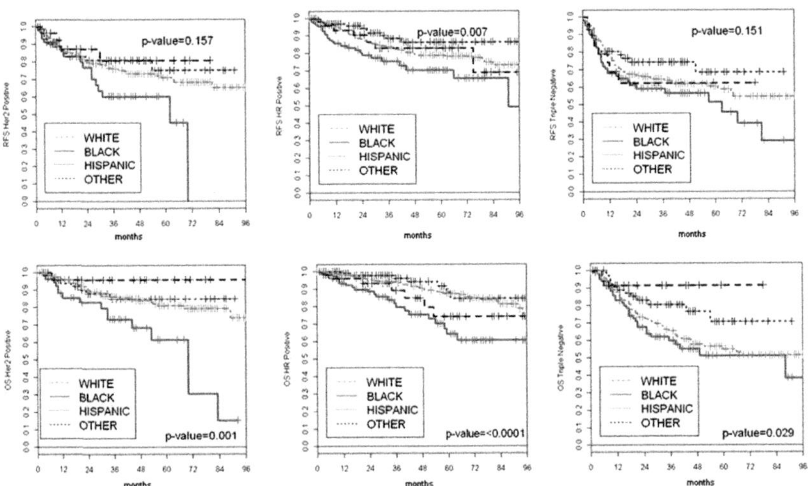

FIGURE 2.—Recurrence-free survival (RFS) and overall survival (OS) are shown by tumor subtype and race/ethnicity. HER-2 indicates human epidermal growth factor receptor 2; HR, hormone receptor. (Reprinted from Chavez-MacGregor M, Litton J, Chen H, et al. Pathologic complete response in breast cancer patients receiving anthracycline- and taxane-based neoadjuvant chemotherapy: evaluating the effect of race/ethnicity *Cancer.* 2010;116:4168-4177. Copyright 2010 American Cancer Society. This material is reproduced with permission of Wiley-Liss, Inc., a subsidiary of John Wiley & Sons, Inc.)

and/or human epidermal growth factor receptor 2 (HER2)-positive, and earlier-stage cancers are more likely to achieve a pCR than those with low-grade, hormone receptor—positive/HER2-negative, or locally advanced cancers; the identification of tumor- or patient-associated factors that influence response within receptor-defined subsets is a high priority for current and future neoadjuvant trials, with the hope that this will lead to novel and effective targeted therapies. When differences in response to neoadjuvant chemotherapy and prognosis between groups of patients are noted, it is important to determine if these reflect differences in biology or other confounding factors.

The impact of race and ethnicity on breast cancer response to treatment and prognosis is multifactorial: variations in tumor and host biology, socioeconomic factors, and cultural differences reflected in attitudes toward the medical profession and compliance all likely play a role. In the United States, this is complicated further by the heterogeneity of racial and ethnic groups and by the intermixing of these groups, thereby making it all the more important that we strive to detect biological factors common to a particular racial or ethnic group that could affect individuals who no longer identify themselves as part of that group.

This article by Chavez-MacGregor and colleagues is a retrospective review of 2074 patients treated at The University of Texas MD Anderson Cancer Center. The authors assessed the impact of patient-reported race and ethnicity, categorized as black, Hispanic, non-Hispanic white, and other, on rates of pCR, RFS, and OS following anthracycline- and taxanebased neoadjuvant chemotherapy. Patients with HER2-positive or triple-negative breast cancers had higher pCR rates (22.6% and 19.4%, respectively) than patients with hormone receptor–positive cancers (5%). Patients who achieved a pCR had excellent 5-year RFS and OS rates, which did not differ by racial/ethnic group. Likewise, pCR rates did not differ by racial/ethnic group, even though black patients were much more likely to have high-grade (72% vs 62% for all other patient groups) or triple-negative (33% vs 22%) cancers, which suggests that these factors may have been offset by a higher proportion of stage III disease (47% vs 37%).

Given the incidence of poor prognostic features in black patients, it is not surprising that their RFS and OS rates were inferior to those in other racial/ethnic groups, but it is remarkable that the largest disparity was seen in those with hormone receptor–positive disease. Given that all patients received similar neoadjuvant chemotherapy, this suggests either that hormone receptor–positive disease in black patients is more likely to harbor adverse biological features not overpowered by chemotherapy or that other factors are involved. In contrast, Hispanic patients had higher RFS and OS rates than non-Hispanic whites despite similar baseline prognostic features and pCR rates. The authors note that this is consistent with what has been referred to as the "Hispanic paradox," an epidemiological observation that Hispanics in the United States tend to have better health outcomes than would be predicted given their socioeconomic indicators.

This retrospective review is valuable because of its size; the extent of the demographic, prognostic, pathologic, and follow-up data available; and the relative homogeneity of the treatment administered. These results underscore the need to ensure accrual of adequate numbers of black and Hispanic patients to ongoing and future neoadjuvant studies to identify unfavorable and favorable biologic factors in these patient groups. In addition, since this analysis cannot exclude the possibility that differences in administration of postoperative radiation and/or adjuvant endocrine therapy may have contributed to the inferior outcomes in the black patients, even among patients treated at the same institution, we are reminded of the importance of ensuring that all patients have access to potentially lifesaving treatments and monitoring and promoting patient compliance.

Enthusiasm for large breast cancer adjuvant treatment studies has waned with the realization that only the fraction of patients who were destined to relapse with standard treatment are truly informative as to the value of a novel treatment approach. In contrast, with neoadjuvant therapy, response can be assessed in all participants and correlated with results from tissue and blood samples obtained prior to and during treatment. The goal is to separate patients who are likely to do well with standard treatment from those in whom novel therapies must be considered and, just as important, those in whom toxic therapy can be abbreviated or even omitted. While awareness that patients from different racial or ethnic groups have divergent prognoses is important, identifying the biological and other factors that underlie those differences should prove more useful in the long run.

W. M. Sikov, MD

Breast Conserving Therapy

Long-Term Results of Hypofractionated Radiation Therapy for Breast Cancer

Whelan TJ, Pignol J-P, Levine MN, et al (McMaster Univ and Juravinski Cancer Centre, Hamilton, Toronto, Canada; Odette Cancer Centre, Toronto, Canada; et al)

N Engl J Med 362:513-520, 2010

Background.—The optimal fractionation schedule for whole-breast irradiation after breast-conserving surgery is unknown.

Methods.—We conducted a study to determine whether a hypofractionated 3-week schedule of whole-breast irradiation is as effective as a 5-week schedule. Women with invasive breast cancer who had undergone breast-conserving surgery and in whom resection margins were clear and axillary lymph nodes were negative were randomly assigned to receive whole-breast irradiation either at a standard dose of 50.0 Gy in 25 fractions over a period of 35 days (the control group) or at a dose of 42.5 Gy in 16 fractions over a period of 22 days (the hypofractionated-radiation group).

Results.—The risk of local recurrence at 10 years was 6.7% among the 612 women assigned to standard irradiation as compared with 6.2% among the 622 women assigned to the hypofractionated regimen (absolute difference, 0.5 percentage points; 95% confidence interval [CI], −2.5 to 3.5). At 10 years, 71.3% of women in the control group as compared with 69.8% of the women in the hypofractionated-radiation group had a good or excellent cosmetic outcome (absolute difference, 1.5 percentage points; 95% CI, −6.9 to 9.8).

Conclusions.—Ten years after treatment, accelerated, hypofractionated whole-breast irradiation was not inferior to standard radiation treatment in women who had undergone breast-conserving surgery for invasive breast cancer with clear surgical margins and negative axillary nodes. (ClinicalTrials.gov number, NCT00156052.)

▶ Breast-conserving treatment for patients with invasive breast cancer has been a standard approach for decades. Its equivalence to mastectomy in terms of cancer control and overall survival is no longer questioned. Patients who choose breast-conserving treatment are as a standard subjected to 5 to 6 weeks of whole-breast irradiation plus a boost to the tumor site for an additional 5 to 6 days. The goal of this course of treatment is to eradicate the disease while maintaining breast cosmesis.

One way to improve on this treatment would be to deliver the radiation over a shorter period of time while still maintaining good cosmesis and cancer control. Much of the partial breast radiation therapy work has done just that, but the data are immature. These authors have designed a phase III trial for node-negative breast cancer patients who had clear margins after lumpectomy and randomized them to standard 5 weeks of whole-breast radiation therapy using 50 Gy in 25 fractions versus a hypofractionated 3-week course of 42.5 Gy in 16 fractions.

The 10-year results published in this article show that this hypofractionated option appears to be equal to the standard option in terms of breast control and cosmesis. In addition, there is a large convenience and cost savings to these hypofractionated schedules. These data do not apply to all breast cancer patients but should be seriously considered as an option for node-negative patients with surgically clear margins after lumpectomy.

C. A. Lawton, MD

Patient selection for accelerated partial-breast irradiation (APBI) after breast-conserving surgery: Recommendations of the Groupe Européen de Curiethérapie-European Society for Therapeutic Radiology and Oncology (GEC-ESTRO) breast cancer working group based on clinical evidence (2009)

Polgár C, On behalf of the GEC-ESTRO breast cancer working group (Natl Inst of Oncology, Budapest, Hungary; et al)

Radiother Oncol 94:264-273, 2010

Purpose.—To give recommendations on patient selection criteria for the use of accelerated partial-breast irradiation (APBI) based on available clinical evidence complemented by expert opinion.

Methods and Materials.—Overall, 340 articles were identified by a systematic search of the PubMed database using the keywords "partial-breast irradiation" and "APBI". This search was complemented by searches of reference lists of articles and handsearching of relevant conference abstracts and book chapters. Of these, 3 randomized and 19 prospective non-randomized studies with a minimum median follow-up time of 4 years were identified. The authors reviewed the published clinical evidence on APBI, complemented by relevant clinical and pathological studies of standard breast-conserving therapy and, through a series of personal communications, formulated the recommendations presented in this article.

Results.—The GEC-ESTRO Breast Cancer Working Group recommends three categories guiding patient selection for APBI: (1) a low-risk group for whom APBI outside the context of a clinical trial is an acceptable treatment option; including patients ageing at least 50 years with unicentric, unifocal, pT1–2 (≤30 mm) pN0, non-lobular invasive breast cancer without the presence of an extensive intraductal component (EIC) and lympho-vascular invasion (LVI) and with negative surgical margins of at least 2 mm, (2) a high-risk group, for whom APBI is considered contraindicated; including patients ageing ≤40 years; having positive margins, and/or multicentric or large (>30 mm) tumours, and/or EIC positive or LVI positive tumours, and/or 4 or more positive lymph nodes or unknown axillary status (pNx), and (3) an intermediate-risk group, for whom APBI is considered acceptable only in the context of prospective clinical trials.

Conclusions.—These recommendations will provide a clinical guidance regarding the use of APBI outside the context of a clinical trial before large-scale randomized clinical trial outcome data become available. Furthermore they should promote further clinical research focusing on controversial issues in the treatment of early-stage breast carcinoma.

▶ The standard of care for organ preservation in breast cancer consists of whole breast irradiation following lumpectomy plus a boost to the tumor bed. Any alternative treatment for breast conservation must be compared with this standard. Accelerated partial breast irradiation (APBI) has gained popularity as its results in well-selected patients appear comparable with standard whole breast radiation therapy. The key to the success of APBI (as with many new modes of treatment) is patient selection. The Groupe Européen de Curiethérapie-European Society for Therapeutic Radiology and Oncology Breast Cancer Working Group is to be commended for developing these patient selection guidelines for APBI. These guidelines will help patients and their physicians select APBI if it is appropriate for them and hopefully help deselect APBI if inappropriate. We await the results of large randomized trials to validate this type of treatment for breast conservation and to validate these guidelines.

C. A. Lawton, MD

Axillary Management

Axillary Dissection vs No Axillary Dissection in Women With Invasive Breast Cancer and Sentinel Node Metastasis: A Randomized Clinical Trial

Giuliano AE, Hunt KK, Ballman KV, et al (John Wayne Cancer Inst at Saint John's Health Ctr, Santa Monica, CA; M D Anderson Cancer Ctr, Houston, TX; Mayo Clinic Rochester, MN; et al)

JAMA 305:569-575, 2011

Context.—Sentinel lymph node dissection (SLND) accurately identifies nodal metastasis of early breast cancer, but it is not clear whether further nodal dissection affects survival.

Objective.—To determine the effects of complete axillary lymph node dissection (ALND) on survival of patients with sentinel lymph node (SLN) metastasis of breast cancer.

Design, Setting, and Patients.—The American College of Surgeons Oncology Group Z0011 trial, a phase 3 noninferiority trial conducted at 115 sites and enrolling patients from May 1999 to December 2004. Patients were women with clinical T1-T2 invasive breast cancer, no palpable adenopathy, and 1 to 2 SLNs containing metastases identified by frozen section, touch preparation, or hematoxylin-eosin staining on permanent section. Targeted enrollment was 1900 women with final analysis after 500 deaths, but the trial closed early because mortality rate was lower than expected.

Interventions.—All patients underwent lumpectomy and tangential whole-breast irradiation. Those with SLN metastases identified by SLND were randomized to undergo ALND or no further axillary treatment. Those randomized to ALND underwent dissection of 10 or more nodes. Systemic therapy was at the discretion of the treating physician.

Main Outcome Measures.—Overall survival was the primary end point, with a non-inferiority margin of a 1-sided hazard ratio of less than 1.3 indicating that SLND alone is noninferior to ALND. Disease-free survival was a secondary end point.

Results.—Clinical and tumor characteristics were similar between 445 patients randomized to ALND and 446 randomized to SLND alone. However, the median number of nodes removed was 17 with ALND and 2 with SLND alone. At a median follow-up of 6.3 years (last follow-up, March 4, 2010), 5-year overall survival was 91.8% (95% confidence interval [CI], 89.1%-94.5%) with ALND and 92.5% (95% CI, 90.0%-95.1%) with SLND alone; 5-year disease-free survival was 82.2% (95% CI, 78.3%-86.3%) with ALND and 83.9% (95% CI, 80.2%-87.9%) with SLND alone. The hazard ratio for treatment-related overall survival was 0.79 (90% CI, 0.56-1.11) without adjustment and 0.87 (90% CI, 0.62-1.23) after adjusting for age and adjuvant therapy.

Conclusion.—Among patients with limited SLN metastatic breast cancer treated with breast conservation and systemic therapy, the use of SLND alone compared with ALND did not result in inferior survival.

Trial Registration.—clinicaltrials.gov Identifier: NCT00003855.

▶ Previous studies have shown that sentinel node biopsy can accurately identify the presence of nodal involvement without the need for an axillary node dissection. The question has remained, however, as to whether a completion node dissection was indicated in those patients with evidence of lymph node involvement to improve overall and disease-free survival. This article reports the results of a prospective randomized phase III trial addressing precisely this point. The American College of Surgeons Oncology Group randomized 891 patients with clinical T1-T2 breast cancer and positive sentinel nodes to either no further surgery or an axillary node dissection. At a median of 6.3 years of follow-up, 5-year overall and disease-free survivals were virtually identical. This finding that there is no advantage for a follow-up axillary node dissection should not be a surprise. Previous National Surgical Adjuvant Breast and Bowel Project studies have shown no therapeutic advantage for axillary node dissection, and it is difficult to find any advantage for use of node dissection in any solid tumor. The bottom line is that, in the absence of grossly involved residual lymph nodes, axillary node dissection cannot be supported as a useful approach.

J. T. Thigpen, MD

Axillary Dissection Versus No Axillary Dissection in Elderly Patients with Breast Cancer and No Palpable Axillary Nodes: Results After 15 Years of Follow-Up

Martelli G, Miceli R, Daidone MG, et al (Fondazione IRCCS Istituto Nazionale dei Tumori, Milan, Italy; et al)

Ann Surg Oncol 18:125-133, 2011

Objective.—To assess the long-term safety of no axillary clearance in elderly patients with breast cancer and nonpalpable axillary nodes.

Background.—Lymph node evaluation in elderly patients with early breast cancer and clinically negative axillary nodes is controversial. Our randomized trial with 5-year follow-up showed no breast cancer mortality advantage for axillary clearance compared with observation in older patients with T1N0 disease.

Methods.—We further investigated axillary treatment in a retrospective analysis of 671 consecutive patients, aged ≥70 years, with operable breast cancer and a clinically clear axilla, treated between 1987 and 1992; 172 received and 499 did not receive axillary dissection; 20 mg/day tamoxifen was prescribed for at least 2 years. We used multivariable analysis to take account of the lack of randomization.

Results.—After median follow-up of 15 years (interquartile range 14–17 years) there was no significant difference in breast cancer mortality between the axillary and no axillary clearance groups. Crude cumulative 15-year incidence of axillary disease in the no axillary dissection group was low: 5.8% overall and 3.7% for pT1 patients.

Conclusions.—Elderly patients with early breast cancer and clinically negative nodes did not benefit in terms of breast cancer mortality from immediate axillary dissection in this nonrandomized study. Sentinel node biopsy could also be foregone due to the very low cumulative incidence of axillary disease in this age group. Axillary dissection should be restricted to the small number of patients who later develop overt axillary disease.

▶ This landmark trial has already had a significant impact on oncologic practice, in that patients with early stage breast cancer who are found to have limited positive sentinel lymph nodes (SLNs) increasingly will forego completion axillary lymph node dissection (ALND). Although the trial did not reach its accrual goal, it is unlikely that complete accrual would have changed the conclusion that there is no significant difference in the overall survival of patients with SLN-positive disease between those who undergo completion ALND and those who have no further surgery. It is also important to note that the trial demonstrated regional relapse rates of less than 1% in the SLN-positive patients who did not undergo completion ALND.

There are several important points to note about the trial. First, the patient and tumor characteristics were relatively favorable: most patients were older than 50 years with predominantly stage T1, estrogen receptor—positive tumors. Furthermore, in the completion ALND arm, most patients had only 1 positive node, and almost 50% had micrometastasis only. In the completion ALND arm, only 27% had additional positive nodes, and only 13% had 4 or more positive nodes. Thus, the trial primarily comprised patients with a limited burden of axillary disease.

It is also critically important to point out that all patients in this trial received whole-breast irradiation. Although the trial precluded treatment of the regional lymphatics, it is likely that a large component of the level I, and possibly level II, nodes was included in the tangential fields. Patient selection, coincidental irradiation of the level I/II axilla, and the continued use of hormonal therapy and systemic chemotherapy may have contributed to the high regional control rate in the patients who did not undergo completion ALND. It is important to consider these factors when interpreting the results of the trial. Patients who have positive SLNs and are treated with mastectomy but not irradiation or those who are treated with partial-breast irradiation may not experience the same low regional relapse rates without completion ALND; these results do not necessarily apply to those clinical scenarios. The results of this trial clearly demonstrate that patients with limited disease in the SLNs who are treated with breast-conserving surgery and whole-breast irradiation will experience high locoregional control, minimal morbidity, and uncompromised survival by foregoing completion ALND. Despite the selection factors and limitations, this trial clearly has already been practice changing and will likely have a lasting impact on patient care.

B. G. Haffty, MD

Advanced Breast Cancer

Multicenter Phase III Randomized Trial Comparing Docetaxel and Trastuzumab With Docetaxel, Carboplatin, and Trastuzumab As First-Line Chemotherapy for Patients With *HER2*-Gene-Amplified Metastatic Breast Cancer (BCIRG 007 Study): Two Highly Active Therapeutic Regimens

Valero V, Forbes J, Pegram MD, et al (The Univ of Texas M D Anderson Cancer Ctr, Houston; Univ of Newcastle, New South Wales, Australia; Univ of California, Los Angeles; et al)

J Clin Oncol 29:149-156, 2011

Purpose.—Docetaxel-trastuzumab (TH) is effective therapy for *HER2*-amplified metastatic breast cancer (MBC). Preclinical findings of synergy between docetaxel, carboplatin, and trastuzumab (TCH) prompted a phase III randomized trial comparing TCH with TH in patients with *HER2*-amplified MBC.

Patients and Methods.—Two hundred sixty-three patients were randomly assigned to receive eight 3-week cycles of TH (trastuzumab plus docetaxel 100 mg/m^2) or TCH (trastuzumab plus carboplatin at area under the serum concentration-time curve 6 and docetaxel 75 mg/m^2). Trastuzumab was given at 4 mg/kg loading dose followed by a 2 mg/kg dose once per week during chemotherapy, and then 6 mg/kg once every 3 weeks until progression.

Results.—Patient characteristics were balanced between groups. There was no significant difference between TH and TCH in terms of the primary end point, time to progression (medians of 11.1 and 10.4 months, respectively; hazard ratio, 0.914; 95% CI, 0.694 to 1.203; P =.57), response rate (72% for both groups), or overall survival (medians of 37.1 and 37.4 months, respectively; P =.99). Rates of grades 3 or 4 adverse effects for TH and TCH, respectively, were neutropenic-related complications, 29% and 23%; thrombocytopenia, 2% and 15%; anemia, 5% and 11%; sensory neuropathy, 3% and 0.8%; fatigue, 5% and 12%; peripheral edema, 3.8% and 1.5%; and diarrhea, 2% and 10%. Two patients given TCH died of sepsis, and one patient given TH experienced sudden cardiac death. Absolute left ventricular ejection fraction decline > 15% was seen in 5.5% of patients on the TH arm and 6.7% of patients on the TCH arm.

Conclusion.—Adding carboplatin did not enhance TH antitumor activity. TH (docetaxel, 100 mg/m2) and TCH (docetaxel, 75 mg/m^2) demonstrated efficacy with acceptable toxicity in women with *HER2*-amplified MBC.

▶ This trial addresses whether carboplatin should be given with docetaxel and trastuzumab (TH) for *HER2*-overexpressing metastatic breast cancer. The results suggest that the addition of carboplatin is unnecessary because docetaxel, carboplatin, and trastuzumab (TCH) and TH both yield the same response rate, progression-free survival, and overall survival. When one combines this information with the fact that most *HER2*-overexpressing cancers do not benefit from inclusion of an anthracycline (because only 35% have coamplification of *TOP2A* and thus are more sensitive to an anthracycline), it would appear that TH would be a reasonable regimen in most patients with *HER2*-overexpressing metastatic breast cancer. There is one caveat to keep in mind. The dose of the docetaxel in this trial in the arm without carboplatin was 100 mg/m^2, which is substantially more toxic than the more commonly used 75 mg/m^2. This, in fact, is probably the reason that TH was not less toxic than TCH. Whether TH with a docetaxel dose of 75 mg/m^2 would yield the same results is purely speculative; hence, one would need to use the higher dose if this study is to be used as a basis for omitting carboplatin.

J. T. Thigpen, MD

RIBBON-1: Randomized, Double-Blind, Placebo-Controlled, Phase III Trial of Chemotherapy With or Without Bevacizumab for First-Line Treatment of Human Epidermal Growth Factor Receptor 2–Negative, Locally Recurrent or Metastatic Breast Cancer

Robert NJ, Diéras V, Glaspy J, et al (Virginia Cancer Specialists, Fairfax; Univ of California, Los Angeles; Genentech, South San Francisco, CA; et al)

J Clin Oncol 29:1252-1260, 2011

Purpose.—This phase III study compared the efficacy and safety of bevacizumab (BV) when combined with several standard chemotherapy regimens versus those regimens alone for first-line treatment of patients with human epidermal growth factor receptor 2–negative metastatic breast cancer.

Patients and Methods.—Patients were randomly assigned in 2:1 ratio to chemotherapy plus BV or chemotherapy plus placebo. Before random assignment, investigators chose capecitabine (Cape; 2,000 mg/m^2 for 14 days), taxane (Tax) -based (nab-paclitaxel 260 mg/m^2, docetaxel 75 or 100 mg/m^2), or anthracycline (Anthra) -based (doxorubicin or epirubicin combinations [doxorubicin/cyclophosphamide, epirubicin/cyclophosphamide, fluorouracil/epirubicin/cyclophosphamide, or fluorouracil/doxorubicin/cyclophosphamide]) chemotherapy administered every 3 weeks. BV or placebo was administered at 15 mg/kg every 3 weeks. The primary end point was progression-free survival (PFS). Secondary end points included overall survival (OS), 1-year survival rate, objective response rate, duration of objective response, and safety. Two independently powered cohorts defined by the choice of chemotherapy (Cape patients or pooled Tax/Anthra patients) were analyzed in parallel.

Results.—RIBBON-1 (Regimens in Bevacizumab for Breast Oncology) enrolled 1,237 patients (Cape cohort, n = 615; Tax/Anthra cohort, n = 622). Median PFS was longer for each BV combination (Cape cohort: increased from 5.7 months to 8.6 months; hazard ratio [HR], 0.69; 95% CI, 0.56 to 0.84; log-rank $P < .001$; and Tax/Anthra cohort: increased from 8.0 months to 9.2 months; HR, 0.64; 95% CI, 0.52 to 0.80; log-rank $P < .001$). No statistically significant differences in OS between the placebo-and BV-containing arms were observed. Safety was consistent with results of prior BV trials.

Conclusion.—The combination of BV with Cape, Tax, or Anthra improves clinical benefit in terms of increased PFS in first-line treatment of metastatic breast cancer, with a safety profile comparable to prior phase III studies.

▶ This study is 1 of 3 trials looking at the addition of bevacizumab to chemotherapy in the management of patients with HER2-negative metastatic breast cancer. This and the other 2 trials all show benefit for the addition of bevacizumab in terms of the primary end point of each trial, progression-free survival (PFS). The hazard ratios (HR) for each are as follows: E2100 HR, 0.60, $P < .001$; AVADO HR, 0.77, $P = .006$. This trial had 2 hazard ratios: capecitabine cohort HR, 0.69 and taxane/anthracycline cohort HR, 0.64, both $P < .001$. Of particular importance is the consistency of the results. In each instance, the improvement is about a 30% reduction in the hazard of progression. These trials led to accelerated approval of the agent. This approval was withdrawn this year because of the lack of a significant improvement in overall survival, but this lack was not surprising in light of the additional therapy that all of these patients receive after progression. The withdrawal was also inconsistent with other decisions of the US Food and Drug Administration (FDA) such as the approval of lapatinib based on improvement in time to progression without a survival improvement. Ostensibly, the decision was based on the toxicity of bevacizumab, but the only consistently increased toxicity with bevacizumab is hypertension, which is easily managed in most patients. Based on the data rather than the FDA decision, the use of bevacizumab should be considered in metastatic breast cancer because of the clear and consistent improvement in PFS with manageable toxicity.

J. T. Thigpen, MD

Eribulin monotherapy versus treatment of physician's choice in patients with metastatic breast cancer (EMBRACE): a phase 3 open-label randomised study

Cortes J, on behalf of the EMBRACE (Eisai Metastatic Breast Cancer Study Assessing Physician's Choice Versus E7389) investigators (Vall d'Hebron Univ Hosp and Vall d'Hebron Inst of Oncology, Barcelona, Spain; et al)
Lancet 377:914-923, 2011

Background.—Treatments with survival benefit are greatly needed for women with heavily pretreated metastatic breast cancer. Eribulin mesilate is a non-taxane microtubule dynamics inhibitor with a novel mode of action. We aimed to compare overall survival of heavily pretreated patients receiving eribulin versus currently available treatments.

Methods.—In this phase 3 open-label study, women with locally recurrent or metastatic breast cancer were randomly allocated (2:1) to eribulin mesilate (1·4 mg/m^2 administered intravenously during 2–5 min on days 1 and 8 of a 21-day cycle) or treatment of physician's choice (TPC). Patients had received between two and five previous chemotherapy regimens (two or more for advanced disease), including an anthracycline and a taxane, unless contraindicated. Randomisation was stratified by geographical region, previous capecitabine treatment, and human epidermal growth factor receptor 2 status. Patients and investigators were not masked to treatment allocation. The primary endpoint was overall survival in the intention-to-treat population. This study is registered at ClinicalTrials.gov, number NCT00388726.

Findings.—762 women were randomly allocated to treatment groups (508 eribulin, 254 TPC). Overall survival was significantly improved in women assigned to eribulin (median 13·1 months, 95% CI 11·8–14·3) compared with TPC (10·6 months, 9·3–12·5; hazard ratio 0·81, 95% CI 0·66–0·99; $p = 0 \cdot 041$). The most common adverse events in both groups were asthenia or fatigue (270 [54%] of 503 patients on eribulin and 98 [40%] of 247 patients on TPC at all grades) and neutropenia (260 [52%] patients receiving eribulin and 73 [30%] of those on TPC at all grades). Peripheral neuropathy was the most common adverse event leading to discontinuation from eribulin, occurring in 24 (5%) of 503 patients.

Interpretation.—Eribulin showed a significant and clinically meaningful improvement in overall survival compared with TPC in women with heavily pretreated metastatic breast cancer. This finding challenges the notion that improved overall survival is an unrealistic expectation during evaluation of new anticancer therapies in the refractory setting.

► Eribulin mesylate is a nontaxane antimicrotubule agent with activity in breast cancer. In this trial, the investigators randomly assigned patients with 2 to 5 prior treatment regimens to either eribulin mesylate or physician's choice. Analysis of the intention-to-treat population for overall survival was the primary goal of the trial. The study demonstrated a survival advantage for those patients assigned to eribulin; the investigators enthusiastically note that this proves that attaining a survival advantage in this heavily pretreated patient population is thus feasible, contrary to what some have claimed and what all previous trials looking at overall survival as a primary end point have suggested, since none were positive. There are several considerations, however, that suggest that one should draw this conclusion with caution. Firstly, the potential confounding effect of postprogression therapy, a concern cited in trials of breast cancer, cannot be assessed adequately in this trial. Secondly, to quote an old expression, "even a blind hog finds an acorn every now and then," this is 1 trial, and there will occasionally, by chance alone, be positive trials that do not reflect reality. The trial does demonstrate that eribulin is active in heavily pretreated metastatic breast cancer, but it does not prove that overall survival is the best end point for a study in a setting in which multiple additional treatments will be given following progression.

J. T. Thigpen, MD

Human Epidermal Growth Factor Receptor 2–Positive Breast Cancer and Central Nervous System Metastases

Leyland-Jones B (Emory Univ, Atlanta, GA)

J Clin Oncol 27:5278-5286, 2009

Purpose.—To determine the incidence, outcomes, and current strategies for management of brain metastases in patients with human epidermal growth factor receptor 2 (HER2)–positive breast cancer.

Methods.—A literature review was performed to obtain data on central nervous system metastases in patients with breast cancer.

Results.—HER2 amplification/overexpression is a prognostic and predictive factor for the development of CNS metastases. Autopsy data show that the incidence rate for CNS metastases in patients with breast cancer is approximately 30%; this may be higher (ie, 30% to 50%) in patients with HER2-positive disease. Treatment with trastuzumab is not associated with an increased incidence of CNS metastases. Data from three phase III adjuvant trials showed the incidence was similar between patients who received trastuzumab and those who did not. Furthermore, trastuzumab can significantly improve overall survival in HER2-positive patients who already have CNS metastases compared with patients who do not receive trastuzumab or those who have HER2-negative brain metastases. This survival advantage is conferred via systemic control of the disease. The current standard of care for patients with CNS metastases is whole-brain radiotherapy (WBRT), with or without surgery, or stereotactic radiosurgery. In the future, novel therapies or combinations of therapies may additionally improve survival in these patients.

Conclusion.—The incidence of CNS metastases in trastuzumab-treated patients is similar to that in all patients with HER2-positive disease. Trastuzumab can improve survival in patients with HER2-positive disease with CNS metastases.

▶ Patients with human epidermal growth factor receptor 2 (HER2)+ breast cancer generally have more aggressive disease with shorter survival times. The success of trastuzumab added to chemotherapy has resulted in longer survival of these patients. The possibility that this might result in a higher incidence of central nervous system (CNS) metastases has been of concern. This study examines CNS metastases in patients with HER2+ breast cancer treated with trastuzumab.

The study basically was a literature review. Important observations from this review include the following: (1) Trastuzumab treatment of HER2+ breast cancer does not appear to be associated with a higher incidence of CNS metastases; (2) Trastuzumab significantly improves survival in those who have CNS metastases, and it is believed that the mechanism is improved control of systemic disease rather than an effect on the CNS metastases per se; and (3) Currently, management of the CNS metastases consists of surgery and radiation. The investigators also speculate that in the future, novel approaches to control of the CNS metastases will become increasingly more important.

Of note, at least one targeted agent has shown some promise in the management of CNS metastases. Lapatinib has been used in 242 patients with HER2+ breast carcinoma and CNS metastases.[1] Objective responses defined as a 50% reduction in the volume of CNS disease occurred in 6% of the patients, and 21 of the patients achieved at least a 20% reduction in the volume of CNS lesions. Lapatinib may well be one of those novel agents with a future role in the management of CNS metastases.

J. T. Thigpen, MD

Reference

1. Lin NU, Diéras V, Paul D, et al. Multicenter phase II study of lapatinib in patients with brain metastases from HER2-positive breast cancer. *Clin Cancer Res*. 2009; 15:1452-1459.

Iniparib plus Chemotherapy in Metastatic Triple-Negative Breast Cancer

O'Shaughnessy J, Osborne C, Pippen JE, et al (Baylor Charles A. Sammons Cancer Ctr, Dallas, TX; et al)

N Engl J Med 364:205-214, 2011

Background.—Triple-negative breast cancers have inherent defects in DNA repair, making this cancer a rational target for therapy based on poly (adenosine diphosphate–ribose) polymerase (PARP) inhibition.

Methods.—We conducted an open-label, phase 2 study to compare the efficacy and safety of gemcitabine and carboplatin with or without iniparib, a small molecule with PARP-inhibitory activity, in patients with metastatic triple-negative breast cancer. A total of 123 patients were randomly assigned to receive gemcitabine (1000 mg per square meter of body-surface area) and carboplatin (at a dose equivalent to an area under the concentration–time curve of 2) on days 1 and 8 — with or without iniparib (at a dose of 5.6 mg per kilogram of body weight) on days 1, 4, 8, and 11 — every 21 days. Primary end points were the rate of clinical benefit (i.e., the rate of objective response [complete or partial response] plus the rate of stable disease for ≥6 months) and safety. Additional end points included the rate of objective response, progression-free survival, and overall survival.

Results.—The addition of iniparib to gemcitabine and carboplatin improved the rate of clinical benefit from 34% to 56% (P = 0.01) and the rate of overall response from 32% to 52% (P = 0.02). The addition of iniparib also prolonged the median progression-free survival from 3.6 months to 5.9 months (hazard ratio for progression, 0.59; P = 0.01) and the median overall survival from 7.7 months to 12.3 months (hazard ratio for death, 0.57; P = 0.01). The most frequent grade 3 or 4 adverse events in either treatment group included neutropenia, thrombocytopenia, anemia, fatigue or asthenia, leukopenia, and increased alanine aminotransferase level. No significant difference was seen between the two groups in the rate of adverse events.

Conclusions.—The addition of iniparib to chemotherapy improved the clinical benefit and survival of patients with metastatic triple-negative breast cancer without significantly increased toxic effects. On the basis of these results, a phase 3 trial adequately powered to evaluate overall survival and progression-free survival is being conducted.(Funded by BiPar Sciences [now owned by Sanofi-Aventis]; ClinicalTrials.gov number, NCT00540358.)

▶ Poly(adenosine diphosphate–ribose) polymerase (PARP) inhibitors have attracted major interest because of early trials that indicated significant activity for these agents in *BRCA* mutation–associated breast and ovarian cancers. Cancers associated with *BRCA* mutations exhibit deficiencies of usual DNA repair mechanisms. This brings into play pathways such as PARP inhibitors, which are not thought normally to play a major role. More recently, attention has been focused on other DNA repair deficiencies that might expand the patient population amenable to treatment with PARP inhibitors. This particular study focuses on triple-negative breast cancers (estrogen negative, progesterone negative, and human epidermal growth factor receptor type 2 negative), which have inherent defects in DNA repair. The PARP inhibitor is iniparib, which some now think may actually exert its effect through mechanisms other than PARP inhibition. The study randomized patients to gemcitabine/carboplatin ± iniparib. The study is a randomized phase II study that is not sufficiently powered to provide a definitive answer as to the proper role for iniparib, but the results do suggest that the addition of iniparib improved both progression-free and overall survival as well as the primary end point of clinical benefit (complete response + partial response + stable disease). As the investigators indicate in their conclusions, this should trigger a phase III trial to define whether the agent has a defined role in the management of triple-negative breast carcinoma. Similar studies of gemcitabine/carboplatin plus iniparib were reported at the American Society of Clinical Oncology 2011 meeting in June 2011 at Chicago, but the uncontrolled phase II design of these trials makes it impossible to comment on activity in recurrent ovarian carcinoma without further studies.

J. T. Thigpen, MD

Oral poly(ADP-ribose) polymerase inhibitor olaparib in patients with *BRCA1* or *BRCA2* mutations and advanced breast cancer: a proof-of-concept trial

Tutt A, Robson M, Garber JE, et al (King's College London School of Medicine, UK; Memorial Sloan-Kettering Cancer Ctr, NY; Dana-Farber Cancer Inst, Boston, MA; et al)

Lancet 376:235-244, 2010

Background.—Olaparib, a novel, orally active poly(ADP-ribose) polymerase (PARP) inhibitor, induced synthetic lethality in *BRCA*-deficient cells. A maximum tolerated dose and initial signal of efficacy in *BRCA*-deficient ovarian cancers have been reported. We therefore assessed the efficacy, safety, and tolerability of olaparib alone in women with *BRCA1* or *BRCA2* mutations and advanced breast cancer.

Methods.—Women (aged ≥18 years) with confirmed *BRCA1* or *BRCA2* mutations and recurrent, advanced breast cancer were assigned to two sequential cohorts in a phase 2 study undertaken in 16 centres in Australia, Germany, Spain, Sweden, the UK, and the USA. The first cohort (n=27) was given continuous oral olaparib at the maximum tolerated dose (400 mg twice daily), and the second (n=27) was given a lower dose (100 mg twice daily). The primary efficacy endpoint was objective response rate (ORR). This study is registered with ClinicalTrials.gov, number NCT00494234.

Findings.—Patients had been given a median of three previous chemotherapy regimens (range 1–5 in cohort 1, and 2–4 in cohort 2). ORR was 11 (41%) of 27 patients (95% CI 25–59) in the cohort assigned to 400 mg twice daily, and six (22%) of 27 (11–41) in the cohort assigned to 100 mg twice daily. Toxicities were mainly at low grades. The most frequent causally related adverse events in the cohort given 400 mg twice daily were fatigue (grade 1 or 2, 11 [41%]; grade 3 or 4, four [15%]), nausea (grade 1 or 2, 11 [41%]; grade 3 or 4, four [15%]), vomiting (grade 1 or 2, three [11%]; grade 3 or 4, three [11%]), and anaemia (grade 1 or 2, one [4%]; grade 3 or 4, three [11%]). The most frequent causally related adverse events in the cohort given 100 mg twice daily were nausea (grade 1 or 2, 11 [41%]; none grade 3 or 4) and fatigue (grade 1 or 2, seven [26%]; grade 3 or 4, one [4%]).

Interpretation.—The results of this study provide positive proof of concept for PARP inhibition in *BRCA*-deficient breast cancers and shows a favourable therapeutic index for a novel targeted treatment strategy in patients with tumours that have genetic loss of function of *BRCA1*-associated or *BRCA2*-associated DNA repair. Toxicity in women with *BRCA1* and *BRCA2* mutations was similar to that reported previously in those without such mutations (Fig 2).

▶ Since the identification of the roles of *BRCA1* and *BRCA2* mutations in breast and other cancers, there has been interest in deciphering how these mutations can be targeted therapeutically. Preclinical experiments revealed that single-strand breaks in *BRCA* mutant models were dependent on the enzyme PARP and that these breaks resulted in highly selective cell killing. A number of poly(adenosine diphosphateribose) polymerase (PARP) inhibitors were developed and shown in the laboratory to have activity in models with *BRCA* mutations.[1] One of these agents, the oral PARP inhibitor olaparib, was evaluated in a phase I trial, and its activity was confirmed in *BRCA* mutation carriers.[2]

The trial conducted by Tutt and colleagues compared 2 doses of olaparib in 54 women with advanced *BRCA* breast cancer and showed single-agent activity in this cohort; more efficacy was seen in the higher, 400-mg twice-daily dose. Toxicity with this regimen was generally mild. This article is of great significance, as it opens up a new area of treatment for a specific group of patients. What is most exciting is the demonstration of activity, good tolerance, and ease of administration. As this was not a randomized trial, I would

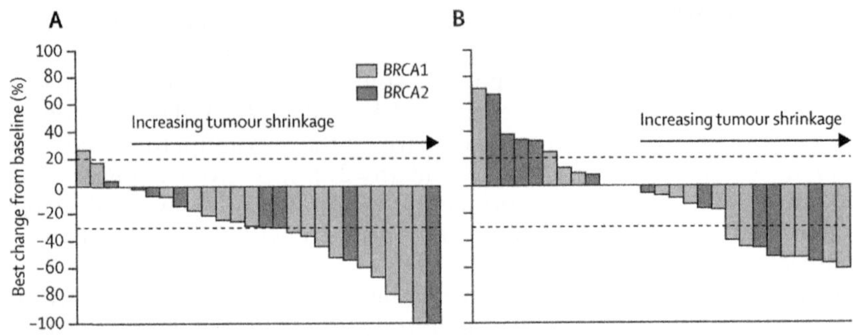

FIGURE 2.—Best percentage change from baseline in target lesion size by *BRCA* mutation genotype in the intention-to-treat population. (A) Olaparib 400 mg twice daily. (B) Olaparib 100 mg twice daily. Reference lines indicate boundaries for progressive disease (20%) and partial response (−30%). (Reprinted from The Lancet, Tutt A, Robson M, Garber JE, et al. Oral poly(ADP-ribose) polymerase inhibitor olaparib in patients with *BRCA1* or *BRCA2* mutations and advanced breast cancer: a proof-of-concept trial. *Lancet.* 2010;376:235-244. Copyright 2010, with permission from Elsevier.)

rate it as level-B evidence. However, I think it is important to realize that a randomized trial would not be feasible in this population because of the small number of patients and because it would be difficult to find a control arm; thus, level-A evidence is unlikely to be reported.

Further studies are being done with olaparib in *BRCA* mutation carriers to confirm these results, but this is indeed a top article. Although *BRCA* mutation-associated breast cancers are in the minority, they are often aggressive and occur in young women. These results open up a new avenue for treating both advanced and possibly early disease in *BRCA* mutation carriers with breast cancer. The study also shows the power of translational medicine, as this is an excellent demonstration of the basic science that leads to a powerful therapeutic target.

K. A. Gelmon, MD, FRCPC

References

1. Bryant HE, Schultz N, Thomas HD, et al. Specific killing of BRCA2 deficient tumours with inhibitors of poly(ADP-ribose) polymerase. *Nature.* 2005;434: 913-917.
2. Fong PC, Boss DS, Yap TA, et al. Inhibition of poly(ADP-ribose) polymerase in tumors from BRCA mutation carriers. *N Engl J Med.* 2009;361:123-134.

Diagnostic Imaging

Breast MRI Screening of Women With a Personal History of Breast Cancer

Brennan S, Liberman L, Dershaw DD, et al (Memorial Sloan-Kettering Cancer Ctr, NY)

AJR Am J Roentgenol 195:510-516, 2010

Objective.—The purpose of this article is to determine the cancer detection and biopsy rate among women who have breast MRI screening solely on the basis of a personal history of breast cancer.

Materials and Methods.—This retrospective review of 1,699 breast MRI examinations performed from 1999 to 2001 yielded 144 women with prior breast cancer but no family history who commenced breast MRI screening during that time. Minimal breast cancer was defined as ductal carcinoma in situ (DCIS) or node-negative invasive breast cancer < 1 cm in size.

Results.—Of 144 women, 44 (31% [95% CI, 15–29%]) underwent biopsies prompted by MRI examination. Biopsies revealed malignancies in 17 women (12% [95% CI, 7–18%]) and benign findings only in 27 women (19% [95% CI, 13–26%]). Of the 17 women in whom cancer was detected, seven also had benign biopsy results. In total, 18 malignancies were found. One woman had two metachronous cancers. MRI screening resulted in a total of 61 biopsies, with a positive predictive value (PPV) of 39% (95% CI, 27–53%). The malignancies found included 17 carcinomas and one myxoid liposarcoma. Of the 17 cancers, 12 (71%) were invasive, five (29%) were DCIS, and 10 (59%) were minimal breast cancers. Of 17 cancers, 10 were detected by MRI only. The 10 cancers detected by MRI only, versus seven cancers later found by other means, were more likely to be DCIS (4/10 [40%] vs 1/7 [14%]; $p = 0.25$) or minimal breast cancers (7/10 [70%] vs 3/7 [43%]; $p = 0.26$).

Conclusion.—We found that breast MRI screening of women with only a personal history of breast cancer was clinically valuable finding malignancies in 12%, with a reasonable biopsy rate (PPV, 39%).

▶ The diagnosis of recurrent breast cancer using mammography and ultrasound is difficult due to complicating features such as scar and fat necrosis.[1] When recurrent cancer is discovered, it is usually larger than in women with comparable characteristics without a history of prior treatment.

In this article by Brennan and colleagues, the percentage of malignancies detected by MRI in women with a history of breast cancer (12%) was substantially higher than that in the major breast MRI screening trials for women at high genetic risk of breast cancer (1%-4%).[2-8] This was achieved with a very acceptable positive predictive value of 39% compared to that in the high-risk trials (7%-43%).[2-8]

These data are significant in that they provide supporting evidence for routine MRI screening of women with a personal history of breast cancer. This group was identified in the American Cancer Society 2007 screening guidelines as having significant risk but classified as "no recommendation for or against" screening on the basis of a lack of evidence. Perhaps more great work such as the current study will lead the American Cancer Society to expand the indications for MRI screening to include women with a personal history of breast cancer.

S. E. Harms, MD

References

1. Houssami N, Abraham LA, Miglioretti DL, et al. Accuracy and outcomes of screening mammography in women with a personal history of early-stage breast cancer. *JAMA*. 2011;305:790-799.

2. Kuhl CK, Schmutzler RK, Leutner CC, et al. Breast MR imaging screening in 192 women proved or suspected to be carriers of a breast cancer susceptibility gene: preliminary results. *Radiology.* 2000;215:267-279.
3. Kriege M, Brekelmans CT, Boetes C, et al. Magnetic Resonance Imaging Screening Study Group. Efficacy of MRI and mammography for breast-cancer screening in women with a familial or genetic predisposition. *N Engl J Med.* 2004;351: 427-437.
4. Warner E, Plewes DB, Hill KA, et al. Surveillance of *BRCA1* and *BRCA2* mutation carriers with magnetic resonance imaging, ultrasound, mammography and clinical breast examination. *JAMA.* 2004;292:1317-1325.
5. Leach MO, Boggis CR, Dixon AK, et al. MARIBS Study Group. Screening with magnetic resonance imaging and mammography of a UK population at high familial risk of breast cancer: a prospective multicentre cohort study (MARIBS). *Lancet.* 2005;365:1769-1778.
6. Lehman CD, Isaacs C, Schnall MD, et al. Cancer yield of mammography, MR, and US in high-risk women: prospective multi-institution breast cancer screening study. *Radiology.* 2007;244:381-388.
7. Lehman CD, Blume JD, Weatherall P, et al. International Breast MRI Consortium Working Group. Screening women at high risk for breast cancer with mammography and magnetic resonance imaging. *Cancer.* 2005;103:1898-1905.
8. Sardanelli F, Podo F, D'Agnolo G, et al. Multicenter comparative multimodality surveillance of women at genetic-familial high risk for breast cancer (HIBCRIT study): interim results. *Radiology.* 2007;242:698-715.

Breast MRI After Conservation Therapy: Usual Findings in Routine Follow-Up Examinations

Li J, Dershaw DD, Lee CF, et al (Memorial Sloan-Kettering Cancer Ctr, NY)
AJR Am J Roentgenol 195:799-807, 2010

Objective.—The objective of our study was to define the usual alterations in the ipsilateral and contralateral breast on MRI of women who have undergone surgery and radiation for the treatment of primary breast cancer.

Materials and Methods.—Database searches identified 744 breast MR examinations of 248 women with newly diagnosed primary breast cancer who had undergone standard breast conservation therapy (BCT) and who had undergone MRI before radiotherapy and at least twice after BCT; these MR examinations were reviewed retrospectively. In each MR study, both breasts were evaluated for background enhancement and cystic alteration. In the treated breast, edema, skin thickening, seroma, and enhancement at the lumpectomy site were assessed.

Results.—Background enhancement and cystic alteration decreased bilaterally on MRI after completion of surgery and radiation. Edema, skin thickening, seroma, and enhancement at the lumpectomy site progressively decreased over time. These changes never resolved in some women, with edema present in 25.9% of women at 6 or more years after BCT and seroma present in 3.7%. Lumpectomy site enhancement was seen in 37% of studies obtained in the first 12 months after treatment and persisted in 15% of women at 5 or more years. Rim enhancement was seen in women with seromas, whereas focal enhancement was typically seen in those without seromas. The persistence of lumpectomy site enhancement was seen in 12 of 16 women with fat necrosis, indicated by fat signal in the seroma and was seen in only five of 19 patients without fat seen in the surgery cavity ($p = 0.007$).

Conclusion.—After a patient has undergone BCT, MRI shows changes in both breasts. Although the changes in our study population were greatest in the treated breast, parenchymal enhancement and cystic alteration decrease bilaterally indicating a systemic influence. Edematous changes, seroma, focal enhancement, and skin thickening were seen only in the treated breast. All posttreatment MRI findings decrease progressively, and all may persist. Lumpectomy site enhancement is most persistent in women with fat necrosis (Figs 7 and 8).

▶ There are several studies that demonstrate the effectiveness of MRI in the diagnostic setting in helping to confirm the presence of recurrent cancer in patients suspected of having recurrent cancer but for whom the findings on mammography, ultrasonography, and/or physical examination are equivocal.[1-4] However, false-positive enhancement leading to the unnecessary biopsy of benign lesions remains a major downside of using MRI in this clinical setting. An understanding of normal expected post-treatment changes identified on MRI following breast conservation is critical for minimizing the number of biopsy recommendations based solely on enhancement in and around the lumpectomy site. The differentiation of enhancing recurrent disease from enhancing benign post-treatment changes, especially enhancement in fat necrosis, can be very difficult. Early studies reported that enhancement of the lumpectomy site should resolve by 18-24 months.[1-4] However, it has become clear that post-lumpectomy site enhancement can last for several years.[5]

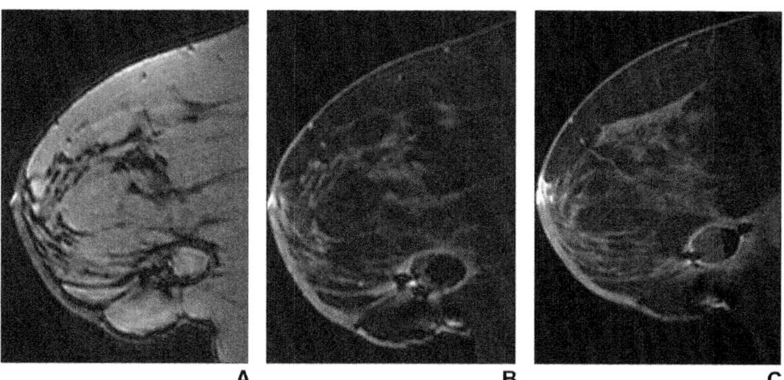

FIGURE 7.—Rim enhancement with fat necrosis in 44-year-old woman with right breast invasive ductal carcinoma. **A** and **B**, Obtained 9 months after breast conservation therapy (BCT), T1-weighted image without fat suppression (**A**) and contrast-enhanced T1-weighted image (**B**) show seroma contains mixed fat and minimal water signal and shows homogeneous rim enhancement. **C**, Obtained 21 months after BCT, contrast-enhanced T1-weighted image shows homogeneous rim enhancement persists in fat-containing seroma. Fat—water fluid level is now present in seroma cavity. (Reprinted from Li J, Dershaw DD, Lee CF, et al. Breast MRI after conservation therapy: usual findings in routine follow-up examinations. *AJR Am J Roentgenol.* 2010;195:799-807, with permission from the American Journal of Roentgenology.)

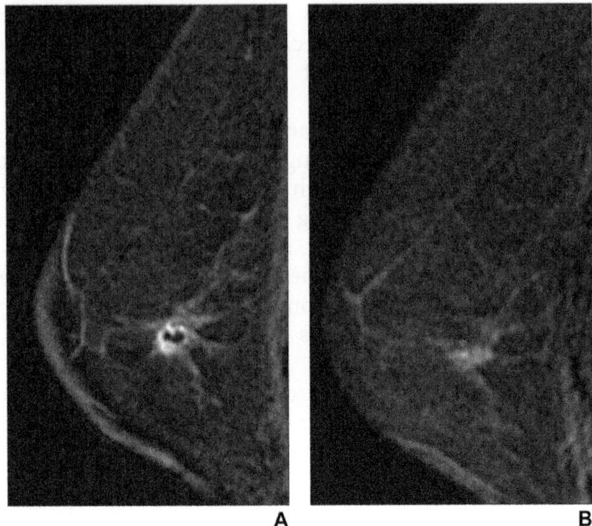

FIGURE 8.—Focal enhancement in 58-year-old woman with left breast invasive ductal carcinoma. **A**, Obtained 10 months after breast conservation therapy (BCT), contrast-enhanced T1-weighted image with fat saturation shows focal enhancement at lumpectomy site without any associated seroma or other mass. **B**, Obtained 36 months after BCT, image from same sequence as that shown in **A** shows enhancement of lumpectomy bed persists but is diminished. (Reprinted from Li J, Dershaw DD, Lee CF, et al. Breast MRI after conservation therapy: usual findings in routine follow-up examinations. *AJR Am J Roentgenol.* 2010;195:799-807, with permission from the American Journal of Roentgenology.)

In the current article, Li and colleagues found that lumpectomy site enhancement persisted for 5 or more years in 15% of patients. Enhancement at 5 or more years was most often secondary to fat necrosis. As the authors state, the mere presence of enhancement at the surgical site should not lead to biopsy. Stability or a decrease in enhancement over serial MRI examinations is a normal finding, while progression of enhancement should be viewed as suspicious. The difficulty comes when MRI is ordered years after breast conservation in an asymptomatic patient and there are no previous MRI examinations for comparison. In this setting, when enhancement is identified at the surgical site in an asymptomatic patient with normal mammography and clinical examination results, short-term follow-up MRI in 6 months should be strongly considered as an alternative to biopsy.

S. G. Orel Roth, MD

References

1. Heywang-Köbrunner SH, Schlegel A, Beck R, et al. Contrast-enhanced MRI of the breast after limited surgery and radiation therapy. *J Comput Assist Tomogr.* 1993; 17:891-900.
2. Whitehouse GH, Moore NR. MR imaging of the breast after surgery for breast cancer. *Magn Reson Imaging Clin N Am.* 1994;2:591-603.
3. Dao TH, Rahmouni A, Campana F, Laurent M, Asselain B, Fourquet A. Tumor recurrence versus fibrosis in the irradiated breast: differentiation with dynamic gadolinium-enhanced MR imaging. *Radiology.* 1993;187:751-755.

4. Morakkabati N, Leutner CC, Schmiedel A, Schild HH, Kuhl CK. Breast MR imaging during or soon after radiation therapy. *Radiology*. 2003;229:893-901.
5. Solomon B, Orel S, Reynolds C, Schnall M. Delayed development of enhancement in fat necrosis after breast conservation therapy: a potential pitfall of MR imaging of the breast. *AJR Am J Roentgenol*. 1998;170:966-968.

Axillary Ultrasound and Fine-Needle Aspiration in the Preoperative Evaluation of the Breast Cancer Patient: An Algorithm Based on Tumor Size and Lymph Node Appearance

Mainiero MB, Cinelli CM, Koelliker SL, et al (The Warren Alpert Med School of Brown Univ, Providence, RI; The Johns Hopkins Hosp, Baltimore, MD; et al)
AJR Am J Roentgenol 195:1261-1267, 2010

Objective.—The objective of our study was to evaluate the utility of ultrasound-guided fine-needle aspiration (FNA) of the axillary lymph nodes in breast cancer patients depending on the size of the primary tumor and the appearance of the lymph nodes.

Subjects and Methods.—Data were collected about tumor size, lymph node appearance, and the results of ultrasound-guided FNA and axillary surgery of 224 patients with breast cancer undergoing 226 ultrasound-guided FNA. Lymph nodes were classified as benign if the cortex was even and measured < 3 mm, indeterminate if the cortex was even but measured ≥ 3 mm or measured < 3 mm but was focally thickened, and suspicious if the cortex was focally thickened and measured ≥ 3 mm or the fatty hilum was absent. The results of ultrasound-guided FNAs were analyzed by the sonographic appearance of the axillary lymph nodes and by the size of the primary tumor. The sensitivity and specificity of ultrasound-guided FNA were calculated with axillary surgery as the reference standard. The sensitivity and specificity of axillary ultrasound to predict the ultrasound-guided FNA result were calculated.

Results.—Of the 224 patients, 51 patients (23%) had a positive ultrasound-guided FNA result, which yields an overall sensitivity of 59% and specificity of 100%. The sensitivity of ultrasound-guided FNA was 29% in patients with primary tumors ≤ 1 cm, 50% in patients with tumors > 1 to ≤ 2 cm, 69% in patients with tumors >2 to ≤5 cm, and 100% in patients with tumors > 5 cm. The sensitivity of ultrasound-guided FNA in patients with normal-appearing lymph nodes was 11%; indeterminate lymph nodes, 44%; and suspicious lymph nodes, 93%. Sonographic characterization of lymph nodes as suspicious or indeterminate was 94% sensitive and 72% specific in predicting positive findings at ultrasound-guided FNA.

Conclusion.—Ultrasound-guided FNA of the axillary lymph nodes is most useful in the preoperative assessment of patients with large tumors (>2 cm) or lymph nodes that appear abnormal.

▶ In this article by Mainiero and colleagues, the authors evaluated the utility of ultrasound-guided axillary lymph node FNA in patients with breast cancer according to the size of the primary breast cancers and the sonographic appearance of the axillary lymph nodes. In this study, 226 ultrasound-guided FNAs were performed in 222 women and 2 men. The authors showed that ultrasound-guided axillary lymph node FNA was most useful in the preoperative assessment of patients with large tumors (> 2 cm) and/or axillary lymph nodes that appeared abnormal on sonography.

In recent years, the use of sonography to evaluate the axillary lymph node basins of patients with known or suspected breast cancer has increased. Axillary sonography has been coupled with ultrasound-guided axillary lymph node FNA in practices with strong cytology support[1] and ultrasound-guided axillary lymph node core biopsy in practices without good cytology support. If ultrasound-guided axillary lymph node biopsy is negative for metastatic disease, the patient then undergoes sentinel lymph node biopsy. A positive ultrasound-guided axillary lymph node biopsy obviates sentinel lymph node biopsy, and the patient then undergoes axillary lymph node dissection. At several institutions, patients with metastatic disease proven by axillary lymph node biopsy are treated with neoadjuvant chemotherapy prior to axillary lymph node dissection.

In this prospective study, patients with newly diagnosed breast cancer who were considered to be candidates for sentinel lymph node biopsy underwent ultrasound-guided axillary lymph node FNA regardless of whether the lymph nodes were suspicious clinically or on ultrasound evaluation. Of the 226 ultrasound-guided FNAs, 161 (71%) were negative for malignancy and 14 (6%) were insufficient for cytologic evaluation. Of the 226 FNA results, there were 51 (23%) true positives, 139 (62%) true negatives, 36 (16%) false negatives, and no false positives.

The pathology reports from the sentinel lymphadenectomies and axillary lymph node dissections were the gold standards in this study. Of the 226 axillae examined, 87 (38%) were positive for metastatic disease. Ultrasound-guided FNA correctly identified 51 (59%) of the 87 cases with metastatic disease. Of the patients with positive ultrasound-guided FNA results, 27 underwent neoadjuvant chemotherapy, and in 9 patients, there was no evidence of metastatic disease at axillary lymph node dissection. These 9 patients were classified as having true-positive ultrasound-guided FNA results, as the negative findings at axillary lymph node dissection were thought to be due to the preoperative chemotherapy.

The sensitivity of ultrasound-guided FNA for detecting metastatic disease in the axilla increased with increasing breast tumor size and with increased prevalence of metastatic disease in the axilla on pathologic evaluation. The sensitivity of ultrasound-guided FNA was highest (93%) in lymph nodes with suspicious sonographic features. The sonographic feature most predictive of a positive ultrasound-guided axillary lymph node FNA result was the absence of a fatty hilum. A fatty hilum was absent in 15 (7%) of the 226 axillae evaluated, and in all 15 cases, cytology was positive for malignancy on ultrasound-guided FNA.

This article by Mainiero and colleagues was well organized and easy to read. It shows the value of axillary sonography and ultrasound-guided axillary lymph node FNA in the evaluation of patients with newly diagnosed breast cancer.

Institutions lacking adequate cytology support are likely to achieve similar results with ultrasound-guided core biopsy instead of ultrasound-guided FNA.

More studies like this one are needed to show the value, as well as the limitations, of ultrasound-guided biopsy of axillary lymph nodes in patients with newly diagnosed breast cancer. I believe that this study by Mainiero and colleagues and future studies will be critical as axillary ultrasonography and ultrasound-guided axillary lymph node biopsy undergo a metamorphosis from research endeavors to components of standard practice.[2]

G. J. Whitman, MD

References

1. Krishnamurthy S, Sneige N, Bedi DG, et al. Role of ultrasound-guided fine-needle aspiration of indeterminate and suspicious axillary lymph nodes in the initial staging of breast carcinoma. *Cancer.* 2002;95:982-988.
2. American College of Radiology. ACR Practice Guideline for the Performance of a Breast Ultrasound Examination. Revised 2007. http://www.acr.org/SecondaryMainMenuCategories/quality_safety/guidelines/breast/us_breast.aspx. Accessed May 25, 2011.

Effect of Screening Mammography on Breast-Cancer Mortality in Norway

Kalager M, Zelen M, Langmark F, et al (Cancer Registry of Norway, Oslo; Harvard School of Public Health, Boston, MA)

N Engl J Med 363:1203-1210, 2010

Background.—A challenge in quantifying the effect of screening mammography on breast-cancer mortality is to provide valid comparison groups. The use of historical control subjects does not take into account chronologic trends associated with advances in breast-cancer awareness and treatment.

Methods.—The Norwegian breast-cancer screening program was started in 1996 and expanded geographically during the subsequent 9 years. Women between the ages of 50 and 69 years were offered screening mammography every 2 years. We compared the incidence-based rates of death from breast cancer in four groups: two groups of women who from 1996 through 2005 were living in counties with screening (screening group) or without screening (nonscreening group); and two historical-comparison groups that from 1986 through 1995 mirrored the current groups.

Results.—We analyzed data from 40,075 women with breast cancer. The rate of death was reduced by 7.2 deaths per 100,000 person-years in the screening group as compared with the historical screening group (rate ratio, 0.72; 95% confidence interval [CI], 0.63 to 0.81) and by 4.8 deaths per 100,000 person-years in the nonscreening group as compared with the historical nonscreening group (rate ratio, 0.82; 95% CI, 0.71 to 0.93; $P<0.001$ for both comparisons), for a relative reduction in mortality of 10% in the screening group ($P=0.13$). Thus, the difference in the reduction in mortality between the current and historical groups that could be attributed to screening alone was 2.4 deaths per 100,000 person-years, or a third of the total reduction of 7.2 deaths.

Conclusions.—The availability of screening mammography was associated with a reduction in the rate of death from breast cancer, but the screening itself accounted for only about a third of the total reduction. (Funded by the Cancer Registry of Norway and the Research Council of Norway.)

▶ One would think that after decades of successful randomized screening mammography trials, the benefit from screening would be acknowledged by everyone. After all, nearly every trial has shown substantial statistically significant benefits.[1,2] The best-conducted trials, such as the 2-county Swedish trial, found a 33% reduction in the breast cancer mortality rate in women offered screening between ages 40 and 75 years.[1,2] Even in the controversial 40- to 49-year-old age group, combined meta-analyses of all 5 Swedish trials found a 30% mortality reduction.[1] Service screening studies as well as advances in mammography technology suggest that annual screening might reduce breast cancer deaths by as much as 50%.[2,3]

Yet every time the efficacy of screening appears to be validated, some study appears to offer a new reason to cast doubt on the value of early detection. This study by Kalager and colleagues reported on the follow-up of Norwegian women aged 50 to 69 years who were offered screening every 2 years along with advanced treatment for detected cancers. These women had a 28% mortality rate reduction compared with historical breast cancer death rates.[4] Women not offered screening but who received identical advanced treatment showed an 18% breast cancer mortality rate reduction compared with the same historical death rates.[4] The authors concluded that screening accounted for only a 10% mortality rate reduction (28%-18%) or about one-third (10/28) of the benefit. Thus, they surmised that about two-thirds of the benefit seen in studies such as the Swedish 2-county trial, conducted in the 1980s, could now be attained in the absence of screening by means of advances in chemotherapy, surgery, and radiotherapy.

As expected in our media-driven society, this article by Kalager and colleagues was quickly publicized in newspaper headlines and television news shows, a flagrant example of the power of sound bites based on a superficial analysis that failed to recognize the study's flaws.

The main flaw in Kalager and colleagues' study is the mean follow-up period of only 2.2 years, which is insufficient to support their conclusions. This extremely short follow-up would be more than adequate for evaluating the treatment of an acute disease, such as the effect of antibiotic agents on pneumonia, but it is completely premature for studying the effect of early detection or treatment on a chronic disease such as breast cancer. Indeed, no prior screening mammography trial has ever shown any significant separation of mortality curves between study and control groups in a time period shorter than 4 to 5 years after the initiation of screening. Since the maximum length of follow-up for the Norwegian women was 8.9 years, Kalager and colleagues could have analyzed results for the subset of the population that had a mean follow-up of 4 to 5 years, but they did not report any such results.

Moreover, the actual mean follow-up per patient was shorter than 2.2 years. Screening in each Norwegian county was implemented gradually over a 2-year period. However, the authors considered the beginning of the follow-up period as the date that countywide screening began rather than the date that full or even partial screening was implemented. This gradual introduction of screening in a county also allowed late-stage cancers among screening group women not yet offered screening to be included in the study group merely because of their residence in the county. This problem could have been ameliorated by offering all women in the study group a greater number of screening rounds so that any pollution of the screening group by cancers detected either prior to the patients' screening or only very shortly prior to reaching the clinical threshold would be minimal.

Curiously, the Kalager and colleagues article did not include any follow-up data after 2005, even though it was published in late 2010. By that time, the Norwegian Cancer Registry could have provided follow-up data through 2008. Unfortunately, the authors did not avail themselves of that opportunity for a longer, more robust follow-up sample.

Another weakness in the Norwegian study is that only 77% of women offered screening accepted the invitation to be screened, whereas presumably 100% of patients with cancer accepted some form of ad-vanced treatment. A related limitation of this study is that an unknown number of women in the control group obtained screening on their own, outside the program. Although the authors are unsure how often this happened, the comparatively low 12% breast cancer mortality rate in the control group suggests that such control group contamination may have been significant.

The article by Kalager and colleagues, along with the accompanying editorial by Welch,[4] mistakenly argues that substantial mortality reduction found in earlier mammography service screening studies conducted throughout Scandinavia are no longer valid because mortality reduction was calculated with reference to historical data from the prescreening era, with insufficient adjustment for advances in treatment. I strongly disagree with that conclusion. Several recent service screening studies have compared contemporaneous mortality rates from adjacent screened versus nonscreened counties that otherwise had identical medical care. Other recent service screening studies have compared mortality rates from a single county where screening was initiated on a near-contemporaneous staggered basis according to odd or even birth dates. Although women in each arm had access to the same modern medical care, the breast cancer mortality rates of those offered screening were as much as 30% to 40% lower than those of women in the control group.[2,3,5]

S. A. Feig, MD

References

1. Smith RA, Duffy SW, Gabe R, Tabar L, Yen AM, Chen TH. The randomized trials of breast cancer screening: what have we learned? *Radiol Clin North Am.* 2004; 42:793-806.

2. Feig SA, Duffy SW. Screening results, controversies, and guidelines. In: Bassett LW, Mahoney M, Apple SK, D'Orsi CJ, eds. *Diagnosis of Diseases of the Breast*. 3rd ed. Philadelphia: Saunders; 2010:56-78.
3. Hellquist BN, Duffy SW, Abdsaleh S, et al. Effectiveness of population-based service screening with mammography for women ages 40–49 years: evaluation of the Swedish Mammography Screening in Young Women (SCRY) cohort. *Cancer*. 2011;117:714-722.
4. Welch HG. Screening mammography—a long run for a short slide? *N Engl J Med*. 2010;363:1276-1278.
5. Feig SA. Effect of service screening mammography on population mortality from breast carcinoma. *Cancer*. 2002;95:451-457.

Noninvasive Cancer

Update on DCIS Outcomes from the American Society of Breast Surgeons Accelerated Partial Breast Irradiation Registry Trial

Jeruss JS, Kuerer HM, Beitsch PD, et al (Northwestern Univ Feinberg School of Medicine, Chicago, IL; Univ of Texas M D Anderson Cancer Ctr, Houston; Dallas Breast Ctr, TX; et al)
Ann Surg Oncol 18:65-71, 2011

Background.—Since the initial reports on use of MammoSite accelerated partial breast irradiation (APBI) for treatment of ductal carcinoma in situ (DCIS), additional follow-up data were collected. We hypothesized that APBI delivered via MammoSite would continue to be well tolerated, associated with a good cosmetic outcome, and carry a low risk for recurrence in patients with DCIS.

Materials and Methods.—From 2002–2004, 194 patients with DCIS were enrolled in a registry trial to assess the MammoSite. Follow-up data were available for all 194 patients. Median follow-up was 54.4 months; 63 patients had at least 5 years of follow-up. Data obtained included patient-, tumor-, and treatment-related factors, and recurrence incidence.

Results.—Of the 194 patients, 87 (45%) had the MammoSite placed at lumpectomy; 107 patients (55%) had the device placed postlumpectomy. In the first year of follow-up, 16 patients developed a breast infection, though the method of device placement was not associated with infection risk. Also, 46 patients developed a seroma that was associated with applicator placement at the time of lumpectomy ($P = 0.001$). For patients with at least 5 years of follow-up, 92% had favorable cosmetic results. There were 6 patients (3.1%) who had an ipsilateral breast recurrence, with 1 (0.5%) experiencing recurrence in the breast and axilla, for a 5-year actuarial local recurrence rate of 3.39%.

Conclusions.—During an extended follow-up period, APBI delivered via MammoSite continued to be well tolerated for patients with DCIS. Use of this device may make lumpectomy possible for patients who would otherwise choose mastectomy because of barriers associated with standard radiation therapy.

▶ This article by Jeruss and colleagues on the 5-year results for patients with DCIS treated in the American Society of Breast Surgeons (ASBS) MammoSite registry trial is an important addition to the literature on the safety and efficacy of APBI for patients with DCIS. Currently, the American Society for Therapeutic Radiology and Oncology (ASTRO) consensus guidelines place patients aged 50 years or older with DCIS in the cautionary group because of limited data on patients in this population who have been treated with APBI.[1] However, the Radiation Therapy Oncology Group 0413 trial has prohibited the enrollment of these patients since January 2007.[2] Additional single-institution studies with early follow-up have reported excellent local control rates in patients treated with either balloon-based brachytherapy or 3-dimensional conformal external-beam APBI in the setting of DCIS.[3,4] Goyal and colleagues performed a matched-pair analysis of patients with DCIS treated in the ASBS registry trial who would have met the eligibility criteria for the Eastern Cooperative Oncology Group 5194 trial, in which patients with DCIS were treated with breast-conserving surgery without postoperative radiation therapy. The analysis demonstrated a significant reduction in in-breast tumor recurrence with the use of APBI in patients with low- to intermediate-grade DCIS smaller than 2.5 cm and in patients with high-grade DCIS smaller than 1 cm.[5] It is an exciting prospect that, with further maturation of the data, DCIS will also be placed in the suitable category of the ASTRO consensus guidelines, thereby allowing more women to receive treatment to the volume of breast tissue that remains at the highest risk of recurrence in a time-efficient manner with low toxicity.

The article of Jeruss and colleagues also reinforces several important points regarding the use of APBI with a single-entry breast brachytherapy device. Closed-cavity placement reduces the risk of persistent seroma and prevents the unnecessary placement of a device if the pathology is not consistent with APBI. The distance of the skin from the periphery of the balloon, in the case of a single-lumen MammoSite, is a surrogate for the dose to the skin. The higher the dose delivered to the skin, the higher the risk of acute and late skin toxicity and poorer cosmetic results. Several multilumen breast brachytherapy devices are now available for APBI. As the skin is not our target in early stage breast cancer, we need to use these multilumen devices to optimize dosimetric coverage of the targeted breast tissue, while limiting the dose to normal structures such as the skin and ribs. This will also make APBI available to more patients whose clinical and pathologic presentation is compatible with APBI.

E. S. Bloom, MD

References

1. Smith BD, Arthur DW, Buchholz TA, et al. Accelerated partial breast irradiation consensus statement from the American Society for Radiation Oncology (ASTRO). *Int J Radiat Oncol Biol Phys.* 2009;74:987-1001.
2. NSABP B-39/RTOG 0413: a randomized phase III study of conventional whole breast irradiation (WBI) versus partial breast irradiation (PBI) for women with

stage 0, I, or II breast cancer. http://www.sjchs.org/body.cfm?id=604&action=detail&ref=242. Accessed May 6, 2011.
3. Israel PZ, Vicini F, Robbins AB, et al. Ductal carcinoma in situ of the breast treated with accelerated partial breast irradiation using balloon-based brachytherapy. *Ann Surg Oncol.* 2010;17:2940-2944.
4. Park SS, Grills IS, Chen PY, et al. Accelerated Partial Breast Irradiation for Pure Ductal Carcinoma in Situ. *Int J Radiat Oncol Biol Phys.* 2010 Aug 26 [Epub ahead of print].
5. Goyal S, Vicini F, Beitsch PD, et al. Ductal carcinoma in situ treated with breast-conserving surgery and accelerated partial breast irradiation: comparison of the Mammosite registry trial with intergroup study E5194. *Cancer.* 2011;117:1149-1155.

Effect of Radiotherapy Boost and Hypofractionation on Outcomes in Ductal Carcinoma In Situ

Wai ES, Lesperance ML, Alexander CS, et al (Vancouver Island Ctr, Victoria, British Columbia, Canada; Univ of Victoria, British Columbia, Canada; BC Cancer Agency, Victoria, Canada; et al)

Cancer 117:54-62, 2011

Background.—Boost radiotherapy (RT) improves outcomes for patients with invasive breast cancer, but whether this is applicable to patients with pure ductal carcinoma in situ (DCIS) is unclear. This study examined outcomes from whole breast RT, with or without a boost, and the impact of different dose-fractionation schedules in a population-based cohort of women with pure DCIS treated with breast-conserving surgery (BCS).

Methods.—Data was analyzed for 957 subjects diagnosed between 1985 and 1999. RT use was analyzed over time. Ten-year Kaplan-Meier local control (LC), breast cancer specific survival (BCSS), and overall survival (OS) were compared using the log-rank test. Cox regression modeling of LC was performed.

Results.—Median follow-up was 9.3 years. Of the patient cohort 475 (50%) had no RT (NoRT) after BCS, 338 (35%) had RT without a partial breast boost (RTNoB), and 144 (15%) had RT with boost (RT + B). Subjects with risk factors of local recurrence were more likely to receive RT. Subjects receiving adjuvant RT had a trend toward improved LC (15-year LC: NoRT 87%; RTNoB 94%; RT + B 91%; $P = .065$). Multivariable analysis showed that RT with or without a boost was significantly associated with improved LC (HR, 0.29 and 0.38, respectively, compared with NoRT, $P = .025$), with no difference associated with a boost or different dose-fractionation schedules.

Conclusions.—Adjuvant RT improves local control in patients with DCIS treated with BCS. Hypofractionation is as effective as standard fractionation schedules. Boost RT was not associated with improved LC compared with whole breast RT alone.

▶ Level I evidence supports the use of whole-breast RT after BCS to reduce local failure rates in patients with DCIS.[1-4] However, randomized data that address the optimal dose and fractionation schedule are lacking. The ongoing Trans Tasman Radiation Oncology Group randomized trial will test the impact of hypofractionation and a lumpectomy cavity boost on disease control, but the findings of this study will not be known for many years. Until these data are available, the recent report by Wai and colleagues may help guide treatment decisions in the radiotherapeutic management of DCIS.

In line with the large randomized studies that have compared lumpectomy with or without whole-breast RT, this population-based study demonstrates the impact of adjuvant RT on reducing local recurrence. However, the authors also report an overall survival (OS) advantage in the irradiated group that is not corroborated by any of the randomized studies.[1-4] One potential explanation for this finding is the significant imbalance in patients and tumor characteristics between the irradiated and nonirradiated groups. Most notably, patients in the nonirradiated group were significantly older than those in the irradiated group, and this factor increased the likelihood of death due to intercurrent illness. Furthermore, there was no significant benefit of radiation in terms of breast cancer—specific survival; therefore, it is unlikely that the 6% to 8% absolute OS improvement seen in the irradiated group was because of a therapeutic effect. This study suggests that whole-breast RT improves local control (LC) after BCS but is unlikely to impact OS.

Although randomized data demonstrate the benefit of a lumpectomy cavity boost of 10 to 16 Gy following whole-breast RT in patients with invasive breast cancer, data regarding the utility of a boost in patients with DCIS are limited to retrospective series and subset analyses of randomized trials.[5,6] In this study, there was no LC improvement with a boost; however, the typical caveats of a retrospective analysis remain. Further investigation of higher risk patients in a randomized setting is required to definitely determine the effect of dose escalation at the lumpectomy bed.

Wai and colleagues have reported the largest known series supporting the use of hypofractionated RT in patients with DCIS. Recently published randomized data revealed equivalent long-term cosmetic and oncologic results in patients with early stage invasive breast cancer treated with hypofractionated RT compared with those treated with a standard course.[7] However, prior to this study, only smaller retrospective series have described the results of shorter course RT in patients with DCIS.[8,9] The efficacy of a hypo-fractionated regimen in patients with DCIS will eventually be clarified by the results of randomized trials, but this population-based analysis is a major contribution in support of the feasibility and efficacy of extending eligibility for hypofractionated RT to patients with DCIS.

Currently, DCIS represents more than 20% of new breast cancer diagnoses.[10] The option of a hypofractionated RT regimen promises improved patient convenience and decreased resource utilization.[11,12] As adjuvant RT after BCS remains underused in certain geographic areas, the opportunity to provide shorter course RT may help extend the application of risk-reducing adjuvant therapy.[13] Routine use of hypofractionated RT techniques could have a widespread impact on patients and providers by increasing access to care and decreasing costs with, potentially, no measurable loss in LC, cosmesis, or survival.[11-13]

P. L. Dorn, MD
S. J. Chmura, MD, PhD

References

1. Fisher B, Land S, Mamounas E, Dignam J, Fisher ER, Wolmark N. Prevention of invasive breast cancer in women with ductal carcinoma in situ: an update of the National Surgical Adjuvant Breast and Bowel Project experience. *Semin Oncol.* 2001;28:400-418.
2. Holmberg L, Garmo H, Granstrand B, et al. Absolute risk reductions for local recurrence after postoperative radiotherapy after sector resection for ductal carcinoma in situ of the breast. *J Clin Oncol.* 2008;26:1247-1252.
3. Houghton J, George WD, Cuzick J, et al. Radiotherapy and tamoxifen in women with completely excised ductal carcinoma in situ of the breast in the UK, Australia, and New Zealand: randomised controlled trial. *Lancet.* 2003;362:95-102.
4. Bijker N, Meijnen P, Peterse JL, et al. EORTC Radiotherapy Group. EORTC Breast Cancer Cooperative Group. Breast-conserving treatment with or without radiotherapy in ductal carcinoma-in-situ: ten-year results of European Organisation for Research and Treatment of Cancer randomized phase III trial 10853—a study by the EORTC Breast Cancer Cooperative Group and EORTC Radiotherapy Group. *J Clin Oncol.* 2006;24:3381-3387.
5. Julian TB, Land SR, Wang Y, et al. Is boost therapy necessary in the treatment of DCIS [abstract]? *J Clin Oncol.* 2008;26:537.
6. Omlin A, Amichetti M, Azria D, et al. Boost radiotherapy in young women with ductal carcinoma in situ: a multicentre, retrospective study of the Rare Cancer Network. *Lancet Oncol.* 2006;7:652-656.
7. Whelan TJ, Pignol JP, Levine MN, et al. Long-term results of hypofractionated radiation therapy for breast cancer. *N Engl J Med.* 2010;362:513-520.
8. Williamson D, Dinniwell R, Fung S, Pintilie M, Done SJ, Fyles AW. Local control with conventional and hypofractionated adjuvant radiotherapy after breast-conserving surgery for ductal carcinoma in-situ. *Radiother Oncol.* 2010;95: 317-320.
9. Constantine C, Parhar P, Lymberis S, et al. Feasibility of accelerated whole-breast radiation in the treatment of patients with ductal carcinoma in situ of the breast. *Clin Breast Cancer.* 2008;8:269-274.
10. Allegra CJ, Aberle DR, Granschow P, et al. National Institutes of Health State-of-the-Science Conference statement: Diagnosis and Management of Ductal Carcinoma In Situ September 22—24, 2009. *J Natl Cancer Inst.* 2010;102:161-169.
11. Dwyer P, Hickey B, Burmeister E, Burmeister B. Hypofractionated whole-breast radiotherapy: impact on departmental waiting times and cost. *J Med Imaging Radiat Oncol.* 2010;54:229-234.
12. Hoopes DJ, Kaziska D, Weed D, Smith BD, Hale ER, Johnstone PA. Patient preferences and physician practice patterns regarding breast radiotherapy (abstract 165). Presented at: The 2009 annual meeting of the American Society for Therapeutic Radiology and Oncology. http://www.abstractsonline.com/Plan/ViewAbstract.aspx?mID=2375&sKey=1a2a0c46—61ed-446b-a034—3fbafe0797cc&cKey=267c0eee-3190—4e33-b527-b18ac20e0052&mKey=6A222D27-F999—46F9-A8FE-B1167C972612. Accessed May 10, 2011.
13. Dragun AE, Huang B, Tucker TC, Spanos WJ. Disparities in the application of adjuvant radiotherapy after breast-conserving surgery for early stage breast cancer: impact on overall survival. *Cancer.* 2011;12:2590-2598.

Radiation Therapy

Systematic review of the effect of external beam radiation therapy to the breast on axillary recurrence after negative sentinel lymph node biopsy

van Wely BJ, Teerenstra S, Schinagl DAX, et al (Radboud Univ, Nijmegen, The Netherlands; et al)

Br J Surg 98:326-333, 2011

Background.—Axillary recurrence after negative sentinel lymph node biopsy (SLNB) in patients with invasive breast carcinoma remains a concern. Previous investigations to identify prognostic factors for axillary recurrence identified that a disproportionate number of patients with an axillary recurrence after negative SLNB were not treated with external beam radiation therapy (EBRT) of the breast as part of initial treatment. This finding prompted a systematic review to test the hypothesis that EBRT to the breast reduces the risk of axillary recurrence after negative SLNB.

Methods.—A literature search was performed in PubMed, the Cochrane Library and the Spanish-language database LILACS to identify articles publishing data regarding follow-up of sentinel lymph node (SLN)-negative patients. Reports and articles lacking information on the initial treatment were excluded.

Results.—Forty-five articles were accepted for review. A total of 23 357 SLN-negative patients were identified with median follow-up ranging from 15 to 102 months. Some 18 878 patients were treated with EBRT to the breast as part of their initial treatment. One hundred and twenty-seven patients with an axillary recurrence were identified, of whom 73 had EBRT as part of their initial treatment. Meta-analysis showed that EBRT was associated with a lower rate of axillary recurrence ($P < 0 \cdot 001$), but this finding was subject to heterogeneity.

Conclusion.—This review and meta-analysis showed that EBRT is associated with a significantly lower axillary recurrence rate after negative SLNB.

► The publication of results from the American College of Surgeons Oncology Group (ACOSOG) Z011 trial has created a great deal of excitement within the breast cancer community of patients and providers.[1] In the trial, patients treated with breast conservation who had 1 or 2 pathologically positive SLNs were randomized to either completion axillary dissection or no further surgical treatment of the axilla. Of the patients who were randomized to completion dissection, 27% had additional axillary disease. This same percentage was predicted in those who underwent no further axillary surgery, but after over 6 years of follow-up, fewer than 1% of these patients had an axillary recurrence.[1] The favorable results of this study have not only led to a change in treatment for many breast cancer patients but have also generated a number of new questions. Foremost in this list of questions is how to explain these favorable results.

There are a number of potential reasons for the discrepancy between the 27% risk of disease versus the less than 1% recurrence rate. High on the hypothesis list is that the radiation that was used to treat the breast also effectively treated a large component of the axillary volume at risk for residual disease. Indeed, a number of previous studies have indicated that a fair percentage of the axillary level I/II nodes are within the tangent fields typically used for whole-breast irradiation.[2] Moreover, minor modifications of the superior and posterior field borders can allow 80% to 90% of the axillary volume to be treated.[2] The ACOSOG breast committee is currently trying to obtain records of the radiation fields used for the patients treated in the Z011 trial to try to retrospectively determine what percentage of the axilla was treated.

Those interested in this important clinical question should carefully read this article by van Wely and colleagues. They report a systematic review of axillary recurrence rates after a negative SLN biopsy. They also correlate recurrences with a variety of factors, including the use of whole-breast irradiation, chemotherapy, and hormone therapy. It would be equally interesting to review data on a large cohort of patients with positive SLNs who did not undergo axillary dissection. However, until the recent publication of results from the Z011 trial, this practice was limited to highly selected individuals. In contrast, SLN surgery without dissection is considered to be the optimal standard for patients with negative SLNs. The 45 studies reviewed in this article, which show low rates of axillary recurrence, provide further evidence of the efficacy of this approach. Specifically, the axillary recurrence rate in the 23 357 patients included in this analysis was only 0.5%.

What is more interesting about this article is the finding that the axillary recurrence rate was 3 times higher in patients who did not receive breast radiation versus those who did (1.2% vs 0.4%). In contrast, neither the use of chemotherapy nor hormone therapy affected the axillary recurrence rate. The less than 1% absolute improvement in the axillary recurrence rate with the use of radiation reported in this study has little clinical relevance, and the small magnitude of the absolute difference gained from radiation use would be expected because of the sensitivity of SLN surgery. A commonly accepted false-negative rate for patients who undergo SLN surgery is less than 10%, and the estimated true-positive rate is only 20% to 30%. This would predict that only 2% to 3% of the population will have axillary disease after negative SLN surgery, which does not leave much room for improvement with radiation therapy. However, if you apply the same degree of benefit for patients with positive SLNs who do not undergo dissection, the relevance may be greater.

In the Z011 trial, the rate of additional axillary disease was 27%, so a reduction to one-third of this rate is a meaningful benefit for patients. Accordingly, I think these data add credence to the hypothesis that breast irradiation made an important contribution to the excellent results of the ACOSOG Z011 trial. It also makes me more cautious about avoiding axillary dissection in patients with positive SLNs treated with either a mastectomy and no radiation or a lumpectomy followed by partial-breast irradiation.

T. A. Buchholz, MD

References

1. Giuliano AE, Hunt KK, Ballman KV, et al. Axillary dissection vs no axillary dissection in women with invasive breast cancer and sentinel node metastasis: a randomized clinical trial. *JAMA*. 2011;305:569-575.
2. Schlembach PJ, Buchholz TA, Ross MI, et al. Relationship of sentinel and axillary level I-II lymph nodes to tangential fields used in breast irradiation. *Int J Radiat Oncol Biol Phys*. 2001;51:671-678.

Breast Cancer Subtypes and the Risk of Local and Regional Relapse

Voduc KD, Cheang MCU, Tyldesley S, et al (British Columbia Cancer Agency, Vancouver, Canada; Univ of British Columbia, Vancouver; Univ of North Carolina at Chapel Hill)

J Clin Oncol 28:1684-1691, 2010

Purpose.—The risk of local and regional relapse associated with each breast cancer molecular subtype was determined in a large cohort of patients with breast cancer. Subtype assignment was accomplished using a validated six-marker immunohistochemical panel applied to tissue microarrays.

Patients and Methods.—Semiquantitative analysis of estrogen receptor (ER), progesterone receptor (PR), Ki-67, human epidermal growth factor receptor 2 (HER2), epidermal growth factor receptor (EGFR), and cytokeratin (CK) 5/6 was performed on tissue microarrays constructed from 2,985 patients with early invasive breast cancer. Patients were classified into the following categories: luminal A, luminal B, luminal-HER2, HER2 enriched, basal-like, or triple-negative phenotype—nonbasal. Multivariable Cox analysis was used to determine the risk of local or regional relapse associated the intrinsic subtypes, adjusting for standard clinicopathologic factors.

Results.—The intrinsic molecular subtype was successfully determined in 2,985 tumors. The median follow-up time was 12 years, and there have been a total of 325 local recurrences and 227 regional lymph node recurrences. Luminal A tumors (ER or PR positive, HER2 negative, Ki-67 < 14%) had the best prognosis and the lowest rate of local or regional relapse. For patients undergoing breast conservation, HER2-enriched and basal subtypes demonstrated an increased risk of regional recurrence, and this was statistically significant on multivariable analysis. After mastectomy, luminal B, luminal-HER2, HER2-enriched, and basal subtypes were all associated with an increased risk of local and regional relapse on multivariable analysis.

Conclusion.—Luminal A tumors are associated with a low risk of local or regional recurrence. Molecular subtyping of breast tumors using a six-marker immunohistochemical panel can identify patients at increased risk of local and regional recurrence.

▶ Locoregional control is of paramount importance in breast cancer, as demonstrated by the landmark Early Breast Cancer Trialists' Collaborative Group

(EBCTCG) meta-analysis, which demonstrated that for every 4 local recurrences prevented, 1 cancer death was prevented.[1] In this study, Voduc and colleagues examined the relationship between the breast cancer intrinsic molecular subtype and locoregional outcome. Six immunohistochemical stains were performed on 2985 invasive breast tumors from the British Columbia Cancer Agency (BCCA) from 1986 to 1992 and used to categorize tumors into 1 of 6 intrinsic subtypes. Of the patients, 42% underwent breast-conserving surgery (BCS) plus radiotherapy, and 58% underwent mastectomy; among those who underwent mastectomy, 25% underwent postmastectomy radiotherapy (PMRT). About 30% of patients received adjuvant cytotoxic chemotherapy, but none received trastuzumab. At a median follow-up of 12 years, the patients in the BCS cohort with luminal A tumors (ie, estrogen receptor [ER] positive or progesterone receptor [PR] positive, human epidermal growth factor receptor 2 [HER2] negative, and Ki-67 negative) had the lowest risk of local relapse (LR) and regional relapse (RR), and the patients with HER2-enriched (ie, ER negative and PR negative, HER2 positive) and basal subtypes (ER negative, PR negative, HER2 negative, and cytokeratin 5/6 positive or epidermal growth factor receptor positive) had the highest rates of LR and RR. In the mastectomy cohort, similar results were found: patients with all other subtypes had greater rates of LR and RR than those with luminal A tumors.

In the setting of BCS, studies have reported conflicting results regarding LR and RR with respect to intrinsic subtype; some have demonstrated no difference in risk,[2-4] and others have shown a higher risk for patients with triple-negative basal-like tumors.[5,6] These differences likely relate to variations in patient populations and in the use of systemic therapy and to the relatively low risk of LR and RR in many patients with early stage breast cancer. In the postmastectomy and/or locally advanced setting, the data more uniformly suggest a higher risk of LR and RR in patients with basal-like and HER2-positive tumors, particularly in those who do not receive modern systemic therapy.[7]

This analysis by Voduc and colleagues has the statistical power to clearly demonstrate significant variation in locoregional outcome with intrinsic subtype, with a higher risk of LR and RR in patients with basal-like and HER2-positive tumors for both patients who undergo BCS and those who undergo mastectomy. The variation in outcome within the triple-negative category is also elucidated, with better locoregional outcomes reported in patients with triple-negative nonbasal tumors than in patients with basal-like tumors. This finding demonstrates that the triple-negative phenotype alone is not sufficient to predict the risk of LR and RR.

The finding that HER2-positive tumors demonstrated a higher risk of LR and RR must be evaluated within the context that no patients received HER2-targeted therapy. Data from more recent series have begun to suggest a lower risk of LR and RR in patients with breast cancer who receive trastuzumab.[8] It is likely that HER2-targeted therapy significantly reduces the risk of LR and RR, and that with further study, HER2 status will emerge as a factor that is predictive of response to treatment but no longer prognostic for LR and RR.

The impact of radiation with respect to intrinsic subtype is difficult to assess based on this analysis and requires further study. In the setting of BCS (inclusive of radiation), the risk of LR and RR was higher in HER2-positive and basal-like tumors. Only 25% of mastectomy patients received PMRT, and statistical analysis with respect to locoregional outcomes and the use of PMRT in relation to intrinsic subtype was not performed, likely because of inadequate statistical power. In a post hoc analysis of the Danish PMRT study, the risk reduction in LR and RR with PMRT was lower in patients with triple-negative, ER-negative, and HER2-positive disease[7]; this suggests that radiotherapy may be less effective in these patients.

Presumably, most patients in this study from the BCCA were non-Hispanic whites, though there is no information on race and ethnicity in the article. Increasingly, data suggest variations in intrinsic subtype and outcome by race and ethnicity,[9] thereby demonstrating the need to study locoregional outcomes in diverse populations.

The separation of LR and RR as end points in this study is particularly helpful. Many studies categorize local and regional outcomes together, but the role and extent of axillary surgery in patients with early stage breast cancer is currently being challenged, and the risk of RR also impacts radiation field selection. Thus, the finding in this study that basal-like and HER2-positive breast cancers were associated with an elevated risk of both LR and RR is useful in the selection of regional therapy, and this is also an area that requires further study.

The finding of differential local and regional outcomes by intrinsic subtype also provides additional data to challenge the consistency of the 4:1 ratio between local control and survival established by the EBCTCG meta-analysis. It has become increasingly clear that there is variation in the risk of local, regional, and distant failure with respect to intrinsic subtype, and this study demonstrates the critical importance of continued study of the relationship between locoregional outcome and survival, which may vary with intrinsic subtype as well.

This analysis by Voduc and colleagues is a well-conducted and important study that clearly demonstrates the elevated risk of LR and RR in patients with basal-like and HER2-positive tumors treated without HER2-targeted therapy and also identifies critical areas for future investigation regarding locoregional outcomes.

J. E. Panoff, MD
J. L. Wright, MD

References

1. Clarke M, Collins R, Darby S, et al. Effects of radiotherapy and of differences in the extent of surgery for early breast cancer on local recurrence and 15-year survival: an overview of the randomised trials. *Lancet.* 2005;366:2087-2106.
2. Dent R, Trudeau M, Pritchard KI, et al. Triple-negative breast cancer: clinical features and patterns of recurrence. *Clin Cancer Res.* 2007;13:4429-4434.
3. Freedman GM, Anderson PR, Li T, Nicolaou N. Locoregional recurrence of triple-negative breast cancer after breast-conserving surgery and radiation. *Cancer.* 2009; 115:946-951.
4. Haffty BG, Yang Q, Reiss M, et al. Locoregional relapse and distant metastasis in conservatively managed triple negative early-stage breast cancer. *J Clin Oncol.* 2006;24:5652-5657.

5. Nguyen PL, Taghian AG, Katz MS, et al. Breast cancer subtype approximated by estrogen receptor, progesterone receptor, and HER-2 is associated with local and distant recurrence after breast-conserving therapy. *J Clin Oncol.* 2008;26: 2373-2378.
6. Voduc KD, Cheang MC, Tyldesley S, Gelmon K, Nielsen TO, Kennecke H. Breast cancer subtypes and the risk of local and regional relapse. *J Clin Oncol.* 2010;28: 1684-1691.
7. Kyndi M, Sørensen FB, Knudsen H, et al. Estrogen receptor, progesterone receptor, HER-2, and response to postmastectomy radiotherapy in high-risk breast cancer: the Danish Breast Cancer Cooperative Group. *J Clin Oncol.* 2008;26:1419-1426.
8. Panoff JE, Hurley J, Takita C, et al. Risk of locoregional recurrence by receptor status in breast cancer patients receiving modern systemic therapy and post-mastectomy radiation. *Breast Cancer Res Treat.* 2011 Apr 8 [Epub ahead of print].
9. O'Brien KM, Cole SR, Tse CK, et al. Intrinsic breast tumor subtypes, race, and long-term survival in the Carolina Breast Cancer Study. *Clin Cancer Res.* 2010; 16:6100-6110.

Symptoms 10–17 years after breast cancer radiotherapy data from the randomised SWEBCG91-RT trial

Lundstedt D, Gustafsson M, Malmström P, et al (Sahlgrenska Univ Hosp, Gothenburg, Sweden; Lund Univ Hosp, Sweden; et al)
Radiother Oncol 97:281-287, 2010

Background.—Postoperative radio-therapy decreases the risk for local recurrence and improves overall survival in women with breast cancer. We have limited information on radiotherapy-induced symptoms 10–17 years after therapy.

Material and Methods.—Between 1991 and 1997, women with lymph node-negative breast cancer were randomised in a Swedish multi-institutional trial to breast conserving surgery with or without postoperative radiotherapy. In 2007, 10–17 years after randomisation, the group included 422 recurrence-free women. We collected data with a study-specific questionnaire on eight pre-selected symptom groups.

Results.—For six symptom groups (oedema in breast or arm, erysipelas, heart symptoms, lung symptoms, rib fractures, and decreased shoulder mobility) we found similar occurrence in both groups. Excess occurrence after radiotherapy was observed for pain in the breast or in the skin, reported to occur "occasionally" by 38.1% of survivors having undergone radiotherapy and surgery versus 24.0% of those with surgery alone (absolute difference 14.1%; $p = 0.004$) and at least once a week by 10.3% of the radiotherapy group versus 1.7% (absolute difference 8.6%; $p = 0.001$). Daily life and analgesic use did not differ between the groups.

Conclusions.—Ten to 17 years after postoperative radiotherapy 1 in 12 women had weekly pain that could be attributed to radiotherapy. The symptoms did not significantly affect daily life and thus the reduced risk for local recurrence seems to outweigh the risk for long-term symptoms for most women.

▶ Multiple randomized trials have demonstrated that whole-breast irradiation after breast-conserving surgery reduces the risk of local recurrence and improves breast cancer—specific survival.[1] Few randomized studies, however, have evaluated the long-term side effects of whole-breast irradiation. In this article, Lundstedt and colleagues evaluated symptoms in women who participated in the prospective randomized Swedish Breast Cancer Group 1991 RadioTherapy trial. At a median follow-up of 14 years (range, 10-17), women randomized to whole-breast irradiation had a higher incidence of breast or skin pain; 38.1% of patients reported occasional pain compared with only 24.0% in the surgery-alone group. The women who underwent radiotherapy also reported a higher incidence of pain occurring at least once a week. This finding is consistent with the findings of other reports that revealed an increased incidence of breast pain after radiotherapy[2] and suggests that chronic breast pain may persist up to 17 years after treatment. As some patients may be concerned that pain may be a symptom of breast cancer recurrence, these data can reassure patients and physicians that pain after breast-conserving therapy is more likely due to posttreatment fibrosis or inflammatory changes associated with radiotherapy.

It is unclear which factors contribute to radiation-associated pain. In the Swedish trial, radiation was administered at either 48 Gy delivered in 2.4-Gy fractions or 50 Gy delivered in 2.0-Gy fractions using 4- to 6-MV photon beams. No boost was given, and the maximum dose was limited to less than 110% of the specified dose. The incidence of pain in the irradiated patients was not analyzed according to the fractionation schedule, dose heterogeneity, or breast size. Although the randomized nature of the study provides strong support for the association between pain and radiotherapy, it is uncertain how treatment planning and patient characteristics may influence the incidence of treatment-related pain. Furthermore, because a boost was not given and only 5% to 6% of the patients received adjuvant chemotherapy, we do not know how these additional treatments might impact pain.

Nonetheless, these results are inconsistent with the results from the Ontario randomized trial, in which increased breast pain was noted in irradiated patients at 6 months, but at 24 months, there was no difference between the 2 treatment arms (~15% incidence of pain in both the surgery-alone and surgery-plus-radiotherapy arms).[3] In the Canadian trial, 40 Gy in 16 fractions were delivered by a cobalt 60 source with a 12.5-Gy boost to the primary site. One possible explanation for this difference is the lower total dose to the whole breast used in the Canadian experience. It is also unclear whether pain in irradiated patients may in fact increase over time as a reflection of late radiation changes, as Lundstedt and colleagues did not evaluate late effects at various time points.

An interesting finding is that although patients in the irradiated arm reported more breast pain, there was no statistically significant difference between the 2 groups in terms of severe pain, difficulty sleeping because of pain, use of analgesics, or discomfort affecting daily activities and overall well-being. These results confirm other quality-of-life data in patients treated with breast-conserving surgery and radiation and support the fact that possible side effects of radiotherapy appear to be an acceptable trade-off for improved outcomes in patients who choose breast conservation.[4,5]

Importantly, Lundstedt and colleagues found no statistically significant difference between the 2 treatment groups with respect to heart symptoms. This may be the result of more modern treatment planning (eg, 3 of the 4 centers used 3-dimensional treatment planning for most of the duration of the study) and the lack of internal mammary node targeting. Although the median follow-up was 14 years, longer follow-up will certainly be important, as cardiac sequelae from breast radiotherapy may continue to appear over time.

These data quantify long-term symptoms after breast-conserving surgery and whole-breast irradiation and provide a valuable baseline for the prospective randomized studies that are comparing whole-breast irradiation with accelerated partial-breast irradiation (APBI). Early data from phase I and II studies suggest that there are low rates of pain in patients treated with various forms of APBI[6,7]; however, longer follow-up and comparison to whole-breast irradiation will be important to determine whether such accelerated treatment courses to the surgical cavity will potentially increase the severity or incidence of symptoms such as breast pain and rib fracture.

K. C. Horst, MD

References

1. Clarke M, Collins R, Darby S, et al. Early Breast Cancer Trialists' Collaborative Group (EBCTCG). Effects of radiotherapy and of differences in the extent of surgery for early breast cancer on local recurrence and 15-year survival: an overview of the randomised trials. *Lancet.* 2005;366:2087-2106.
2. Hopwood P, Haviland JS, Sumo G, Mills J, Bliss JM, Yarnold JR, START Trial Management Group. Comparison of patient-reported breast, arm, and shoulder symptoms and body image after radiotherapy for early breast cancer: 5-year follow-up in the randomised Standardisation of Breast Radiotherapy (START) trials. *Lancet Oncol.* 2010;11:231-240.
3. Whelan TJ, Levine M, Julian J, Kirkbride P, Skingly P. The effects of radiation therapy on quality of life of women with breast carcinoma: results of a randomized trial. Ontario Clinical Oncology Group. *Cancer.* 2000;88:2260-2266.
4. Freedman GM, Li T, Anderson PR, Nicolaou N, Konski A. Health states of women after conservative surgery and radiation for breast cancer. *Breast Cancer Res Treat.* 2010;121:519-526.
5. Hayman JA, Fairclough DL, Harris JR, Weeks JC. Patient preferences con-cerning the trade-off between the risks and benefits of routine radiation therapy after conservative surgery for early-stage breast cancer. *J Clin Oncol.* 1997;15: 1252-1260.
6. Chen PY, Wallace M, Mitchell C, et al. Four-year efficacy, cosmesis, and toxicity using three-dimensional conformal external beam radiation therapy to deliver accelerated partial breast irradiation. *Int J Radiat Oncol Biol Phys.* 2010;76: 991-997.
7. Kuske RR, Winter K, Arthur DW, et al. Phase II trial of brachytherapy alone after lumpectomy for select breast cancer: toxicity analysis of RTOG 95-17. *Int J Radiat Oncol Biol Phys.* 2006;65:45-51.

Long-Term Cardiovascular Mortality After Radiotherapy for Breast Cancer

Bouillon K, Haddy N, Delaloge S, et al (Radiation Epidemiology Group-CESP—Unit 1018 INSERM, Villejuif, France; Institut Gustave Roussy, Villejuif, France; et al)

J Am Coll Cardiol 57:445-452, 2011

Objectives.—This study sought to investigate long-term cardiovascular mortality and its relationship to the use of radiotherapy for breast cancer.

Background.—Cardiovascular diseases are among the main long-term complications of radiotherapy, but knowledge is limited regarding long-term risks because published studies have, on average, <20 years of follow-up.

Methods.—A total of 4,456 women who survived at least 5 years after treatment of a breast cancer at the Institut Gustave Roussy between 1954 and 1984 were followed up for mortality until the end of 2003, for over 28 years on average.

Results.—A total of 421 deaths due to cardiovascular diseases were observed, of which 236 were due to cardiac disease. Women who had received radiotherapy had a 1.76-fold (95% confidence interval [CI]: 1.34 to 2.31) higher risk of dying of cardiac disease and a 1.33-fold (95% CI: 0.99 to 1.80) higher risk of dying of vascular disease than those who had not received radiotherapy. Among women who had received radiotherapy, those who had been treated for a left-sided breast cancer had a 1.56-fold (95% CI: 1.27 to 1.90) higher risk of dying of cardiac disease than those treated for a right-sided breast cancer. This relative risk increased with time since the breast cancer diagnosis ($p = 0.05$).

Conclusions.—This study confirmed that radiotherapy, as delivered until the mid-1980s, increased the long-term risk of dying of cardiovascular diseases. The long-term risk of dying of cardiac disease is a particular concern for women treated for a left-sided breast cancer with contemporary tangential breast or chest wall radiotherapy. This risk may increase with a longer follow-up, even after 20 years following radiotherapy.

▶ This article by Bouillon and colleagues again shows that radiotherapy delivered to the left breast and nodal area can increase the risk of long-term cardiovascular mortality. This study is consistent with several other articles[1,2] but is unique in its relatively long follow-up duration (average, 28 years). These data suggest that the relative risk of long-term cardiovascular mortality continues to increase over time. As the absolute risk of cardiovascular disease increases with age, the increasing relative risk will translate into a larger absolute number of clinical events. Furthermore, as our cardiology colleagues have gotten better at caring for cardiovascular disease, excesses in mortality may underestimate the magnitude of the problem, ie, there are probably even greater excesses in cardiac morbidity. A recent review of studies with long-term follow-up (>15 years) reported a relative risk of cardiac morbidity between 1.2 and 3.1.[1]

One major unknown variable is the degree to which modest tangent-only techniques influence the risk of cardiovascular disease. Several studies[3-5] have suggested that the excess risk is largely due to the use of anterior photon internal mammary node (IMN) fields (a technique that is no longer widely used). Of the patients in the study by Bouillon and colleagues who received left-sided radiotherapy, those most likely to have received IMN radiotherapy had a relative risk of 2.0 for dying from cardiac disease and a relative risk of 2.8 for dying from vascular disease, compared with those most likely to have received radiotherapy to the chest wall and/or breast alone (ie, not to the IMNs). Thus, much, and maybe almost all, of the excess risk associated with radiotherapy can be ascribed to the radiation delivered to the nodes. Additional work is needed to understand the impact of more modern radiotherapy techniques (with minimal cardiac exposure) on the risks of cardiovascular disease.

Preliminary analyses of more recent research are encouraging. Data from studies of patients treated after about 1985 with up to 15 years of follow-up suggest that more modern techniques are safer.[6-9] Similarly, studies of patients treated between 1992 and 2002 did not report an excess risk of radiotherapy-induced cardiac morbidity.[10,11] However, the follow-up in these studies was modest (<10 years), and the study by Bouillon and colleagues illustrates the importance of long-term follow-up.

Time will tell. Until then, radiation oncologists should exploit available tools and techniques to reduce doses to cardiovascular structures (eg, more judicious use of nodal radiotherapy, careful selection of gantry angles that maximally spare the heart, and respiratory maneuvers to increase the physical separation between the breast/chest wall and the heart). Conformal field shaping (ie, a heart block) is an easy way to markedly reduce cardiac exposure when left-sided tangents are used.[12] Intensity-modulated radiotherapy does not provide any additional advantage over a heart block when traditional tangent fields are used. Thus, cardiac avoidance is not typically a justification for intensity-modulated radiotherapy.

S. Demirci, MD
L. B. Marks, MD

References

1. Demirci S, Nam J, Hubbs JL, Nguyen T, Marks LB. Radiation-induced cardiac toxicity after therapy for breast cancer: interaction between treatment era and follow-up duration. *Int J Radiat Oncol Biol Phys.* 2009;73:980-987.
2. Darby SC, McGale P, Taylor CW, Peto R. Long-term mortality from heart disease and lung cancer after radiotherapy for early breast cancer: prospective cohort study of about 300,000 women in US SEER cancer registries. *Lancet Oncol.* 2005;6:557-565.
3. Jones JM, Ribeiro GG. Mortality patterns over 34 years of breast cancer patients in a clinical trial of post-operative radiotherapy. *Clin Radiol.* 1989;40:204-208.
4. Rutqvist LE, Lax I, Fornander T, Johansson H. Cardiovascular mortality in a randomized trial of adjuvant radiation therapy versus surgery alone in primary breast cancer. *Int J Radiat Oncol Biol Phys.* 1992;22:887-896.
5. Rutqvist LE, Johansson H. Mortality by laterality of the primary tumour among 55,000 breast cancer patients from the Swedish Cancer Registry. *Br J Cancer.* 1990;61:866-868.
6. Giordano SH, Kuo YF, Freeman JL, Buchholz TA, Hortobagyi GN, Goodwin JS. Risk of cardiac death after adjuvant radiotherapy for breast cancer. *J Natl Cancer Inst.* 2005;97:419-424.

7. Patt DA, Goodwin JS, Kuo YF, et al. Cardiac morbidity of adjuvant radiotherapy for breast cancer. *J Clin Oncol.* 2005;23:7475-7482.
8. Hooning MJ, Aleman BM, van Rosmalen AJ, Kuenen MA, Klijn JG, van Leeuwen FE. Cause-specific mortality in long-term survivors of breast cancer: a 25-year follow-up study. *Int J Radiat Oncol Biol Phys.* 2006;64:1081-1091.
9. Nixon AJ, Manola J, Gelman R, et al. No long-term increase in cardiac-related mortality after breast-conserving surgery and radiation therapy using modern techniques. *J Clin Oncol.* 1998;16:1374-1379.
10. Pinder MC, Duan Z, Goodwin JS, Hortobagyi GN, Giordano SH. Congestive heart failure in older women treated with adjuvant anthracycline chemotherapy for breast cancer. *J Clin Oncol.* 2007;25:3808-3815.
11. Doyle JJ, Neugut AI, Jacobson JS, et al. Radiation therapy, cardiac risk factors, and cardiac toxicity in early-stage breast cancer patients. *Int J Radiat Oncol Biol Phys.* 2007;68:82-93.
12. Marks LB, Hebert ME, Bentel G, Spencer DP, Sherouse GW, Prosnitz LR. To treat or not to treat the internal mammary nodes: a possible compromise. *Int J Radiat Oncol Biol Phys.* 1994;29:903-909.

Coverage of axillary lymph nodes with high tangential fields in breast radiotherapy

Alço G, Iğdem SI, Ercan T, et al (Florence Nightingale Gayrettepe Hosp, Istanbul, Turkey; Istanbul Bilim Univ, Turkey)
Br J Radiol 83:1072-1076, 2010

The aim of this study is to evaluate the coverage of axillary nodal volumes with high tangent fields (HTF) in breast radiotherapy and to determine the utility of customised blocking. The treatment plans of 30 consecutive patients with early breast cancer were evaluated. The prescription dose was 50 Gy to the whole breast. Axillary level I—II lymph node volumes were delineated and the cranial border of the tangential fields was set just below the humeral head to create HTF. Dose—volume histograms (DVH) were used to calculate the doses received by axillary nodal volumes. In a second planning set, HTF were modified with multileaf collimators (MLC-HTF) to obtain an adequate dose coverage of axillary nodes. The mean doses of the axillary nodes, the ipsilateral lung and heart were compared between the two plans (HTF *vs* MLC-HTF) using a paired sample t-test. The doses received by 95% of the breast volumes were not significantly different for the two plans. The doses received by 95% of the level I and II axillary volumes were 16.79 Gy and 11.59 Gy, respectively, for HTF, increasing to 47.2 Gy and 45.03 Gy, respectively, for MLC-HTF. Mean lung doses and per cent volume of the ipsilateral lung receiving 20 Gy (V20) were also increased from 6.47 Gy and 10.47%, respectively, for HTF, to 9.56 Gy and 16.77%, respectively, for MLC-HTF. Our results suggest that HTF do not adequately cover the level I and II axillary lymph node regions. Modification of HTF with MLC is necessary to obtain an adequate cover-age of axillary levels without compromising healthy tissue in the majority of the patients.

▶ This nicely performed dosimetric study by Alço and colleagues provides a novel yet simple method to ensure adequate coverage of level I-II axillary nodal regions with an MLC-based HTF treatment plan. Thirty consecutive patients who had not undergone axillary node dissection underwent computed tomography (CT) simulation, contouring of level I-II nodal regions, and treatment planning in 1 of 2 ways: (a) with standard HTF (setting the superior field border just below the humeral head) or (b) by extending the posterior (deep) tangential border to adequately cover the nodes, using the MLC to block unnecessary dose to more caudal regions (thus blocking excessive dose to the heart and lung). The authors confirmed what other studies have suggested, that "standard" HTF do not adequately cover level I-II nodes in the vast majority of patients. Furthermore, they provide us with an uncomplicated technique for achieving significantly better coverage of the nodal regions without appreciably increasing heart doses. While it is inevitable that the lung doses would be higher with posterior field edge extension in the MLC-based plans, the authors note that in all but 1 patient, the lung doses remained in the acceptable range based on routinely used lung dose constraints (ie, $V20 \leq 20\%$).

This study provides a useful method to ensure coverage of level I-II nodes without drastically increasing heart dose and allows for maintaining acceptable lung doses in the vast majority of patients. In a setting where adequate nodal coverage is clinically warranted, the importance of contouring the nodal basins and using 3-dimensional treatment techniques is underscored by this very simple but well-conducted investigation. This study brings to light, once again, that in the current era of 3-dimensional treatment planning, using standard field borders for treatment volume delineation is not adequate in the vast majority of patients. Thus, if CT-based simulation is being used, contouring the volumes at risk and using 3-dimensional techniques tailored to the individual patient are warranted. This straightforward technique should be considered in appropriate patients who require level I-II axillary nodal treatment in lieu of the traditional HTF.

M. S. Moran, MD

Surgical Treatment

Association of Risk-Reducing Surgery in *BRCA1* or *BRCA2* Mutation Carriers With Cancer Risk and Mortality

Domchek SM, Friebel TM, Singer CF, et al (Univ of Pennsylvania School of Medicine, Philadelphia; Med Univ of Vienna, Austria; et al)
JAMA 304:967-975, 2010

Context.—Mastectomy and salpingo-oophorectomy are widely used by carriers of *BRCA1* or *BRCA2* mutations to reduce their risks of breast and ovarian cancer.

Objective.—To estimate risk and mortality reduction stratified by mutation and prior cancer status.

Design, Setting, and Participants.—Prospective, multicenter cohort study of 2482 women with *BRCA1* or *BRCA2* mutations ascertained between 1974 and 2008. The study was conducted at 22 clinical and research genetics centers in Europe and North America to assess the relationship of risk-reducing mastectomy or salpingo-oophorectomy with cancer outcomes. The women were followed up until the end of 2009.

Main Outcomes Measures.—Breast and ovarian cancer risk, cancer-specific mortality, and overall mortality.

Results.—No breast cancers were diagnosed in the 247 women with risk-reducing mastectomy compared with 98 women of 1372 diagnosed with breast cancer who did not have risk-reducing mastectomy. Compared with women who did not undergo risk-reducing salpingo-oophorectomy, women who underwent salpingo-oophorectomy had a lower risk of ovarian cancer, including those with prior breast cancer (6% vs 1%, respectively; hazard ratio [HR], 0.14; 95% confidence interval [CI], 0.04-0.59) and those without prior breast cancer (6% vs 2%; HR, 0.28 [95% CI, 0.12-0.69]), and a lower risk of first diagnosis of breast cancer in *BRCA1* mutation carriers (20% vs 14%; HR, 0.63 [95% CI, 0.41-0.96]) and *BRCA2* mutation carriers (23% vs 7%; HR, 0.36 [95% CI, 0.16-0.82]). Compared with women who did not undergo risk-reducing salpingo-oophorectomy, undergoing salpingo-oophorectomy was associated with lower all-cause mortality (10% vs 3%; HR, 0.40 [95% CI, 0.26-0.61]), breast cancer-specific mortality (6% vs 2%; HR, 0.44 [95% CI, 0.26-0.76]), and ovarian cancer-specific mortality (3% vs 0.4%; HR, 0.21 [95% CI, 0.06-0.80]).

Conclusions.—Among a cohort of women with *BRCA1* and *BRCA2* mutations, the use of risk-reducing mastectomy was associated with a lower risk of breast cancer; risk-reducing salpingo-oophorectomy was associated with a lower risk of ovarian cancer, first diagnosis of breast cancer, all-cause mortality, breast cancer–specific mortality, and ovarian cancer–specific mortality.

▶ This study by Domchek and colleagues reports outcomes after risk-reduction surgery in a large international prospective cohort of *BRCA* mutation carriers. It builds on prior articles that demonstrated that bilateral risk-reduction mastectomy (RRM) decreases breast cancer risk and that prophylactic bilateral salpingo-oophorectomy (PSO) reduces both ovarian cancer risk and breast cancer risk. The additional contributions of this report to those of prior studies are its findings on (1) the effects on mortality, (2) the differences between carriers of *BRCA1* and *BRCA2* mutations, and (3) the differences in outcomes associated with these procedures in women with and without prior breast cancer.

Of the women who underwent RRM, none were found to have breast cancer, compared with 98 (7%) of the 1372 women who did not undergo RRM, and results were not different between *BRCA1* and *BRCA2* mutation carriers. Similar to prior published reports, this study showed that PSO was associated with decreased risk of both ovarian and breast cancer in both *BRCA1* and *BRCA2* mutation carriers. As would be expected, PSO was associated with decreased risk of ovarian cancer regardless of a prior diagnosis of breast cancer. However, the decreased risk of breast cancer associated with PSO varied depending on a history of prior breast cancer and the age at which PSO was performed. Although PSO was associated with decreased breast cancer risk in both *BRCA1* and *BRCA2* mutation carriers without prior breast cancer, this effect was restricted in *BRCA1* mutation carriers to women who underwent PSO prior to age 50 years. In mutation carriers who were previously diagnosed with breast cancer, PSO was not associated with reduced risk of a second diagnosis of breast cancer.

The most valuable contribution of this study is the mortality data presented (and made uniquely possible by this large cohort of *BRCA* carriers) that clearly demonstrate a benefit of PSO, which was associated with significantly lower breast cancer–specific mortality, lower ovarian cancer–specific mortality, and lower all-cause mortality rates. Associations of RRM with breast cancer–specific mortality and all-cause mortality were not reported; therefore, the reader is left to assume that probably no significant associations were identified. This is not surprising since these women who were known to be at high risk were recommended for intensive breast cancer screening, such that most breast cancers that were diagnosed were likely early stage disease with good prognosis that would have been unlikely to impact mortality. There is a limitation to the study in that it is not a randomized controlled trial, but that would not be feasible. Despite this caveat, this study represents the largest and most comprehensive evaluation of risk-reduction surgery in *BRCA* carriers.

Although RRM is associated with a dramatic reduction in breast cancer risk in both *BRCA1* and *BRCA2* mutation carriers, this study underscores the greater overall benefit of PSO in these women, with associated reductions in ovarian cancer risk, breast cancer risk, and mortality. When *BRCA* mutation carriers seek information on RRM, they should also be counseled regarding the benefits of PSO.

A. C. Degnim, MD

Locoregional Recurrence After Sentinel Lymph Node Dissection With or Without Axillary Dissection in Patients With Sentinel Lymph Node Metastases: The American College of Surgeons Oncology Group Z0011 Randomized Trial

Giuliano AE, McCall L, Beitsch P, et al (John Wayne Cancer Inst at Saint John's Health Ctr, Santa Monica, CA; American College of Surgeons Oncology Group, Durham, NC; Dallas Surgical Group, TX; et al)
Ann Surg 252:426-432, 2010

Background and Objective.—Sentinel lymph node dissection (SLND) has eliminated the need for axillary dissection (ALND) in patients whose sentinel node (SN) is tumor-free. However, completion ALND for patients with tumor-involved SNs remains the standard to achieve locoregional control. Few studies have examined the outcome of patients who do not undergo ALND for positive SNs. We now report local and regional recurrence information from the American College of Surgeons Oncology Group Z0011 trial.

Methods.—American College of Surgeons Oncology Group Z0011 was a prospective trial examining survival of patients with SN metastases detected by standard H and E, who were randomized to undergo ALND after SLND versus SLND alone without specific axillary treatment. Locoregional recurrence was evaluated.

Results.—There were 446 patients randomized to SLND alone and 445 to SLND + ALND. Patients in the 2 groups were similar with respect to age, Bloom-Richardson score, estrogen receptor status, use of adjuvant systemic therapy, tumor type, T stage, and tumor size. Patients randomized to SLND + ALND had a median of 17 axillary nodes removed compared with a median of only 2 SN removed with SLND alone ($P < 0.001$). ALND also removed more positive lymph nodes ($P < 0.001$). At a median follow-up time of 6.3 years, there were no statistically significant differences in local recurrence ($P = 0.11$) or regional recurrence ($P = 0.45$) between the 2 groups.

Conclusions.—Despite the potential for residual axillary disease after SLND, SLND without ALND can offer excellent regional control and may be reasonable management for selected patients with early-stage breast cancer treated with breast-conserving therapy and adjuvant systemic therapy.

▶ This is the long-awaited randomized clinical trial, albeit smaller than initially designed, to confirm what mounting data have suggested for the past 7 years, namely, that there is no reason to perform axillary lymph node dissection (ALND) for low-burden axillary disease identified by sentinel node (SN) biopsy. Considered a trial before its time, Z0011 was prematurely closed in 2004 because of poor accrual and fewer events than anticipated. While smaller, nonrandomized reports noted axillary recurrence rates consistently lower than 1% upon observation of the remaining axillary lymph nodes,[1-4] American Society of Clinical Oncology[5] and National Comprehensive Cancer Network[6] guidelines recommending completion ALND became widely ignored.[7] In 2010, randomized clinical trial data from the Z0011 study showed results consistent with those from a large retrospective report from the National Cancer Data Base.[8]

In the Z0011 study, Giuliano and colleagues define inclusion criteria and provide important conclusions for patients with T1 and T2 tumors treated with breast conservation therapy who had fewer than 2 positive SNs. What do we recommend for everyone else? Should patients with T3 tumors always undergo ALND? Should a 65-year-old woman with a T1 tumor undergo ALND if she chooses to have a mastectomy? Do we need another randomized trial to help these patients avoid the morbidity of ALND?

These findings can be cautiously extrapolated to other patient populations. We know that ALND does not impact survival. Although we do not have randomized data to confirm these conclusions for other patient populations, data from the National Cancer Data Base show the same low rates of local recurrence for patients undergoing either mastectomy or breast conservation therapy.[8] Most importantly, the regional recurrence rates in this study and others were substantially lower than anticipated. It is time to revise guidelines for managing the positive SN.

D. J. Winchester, MD

References

1. Jeruss JS, Winchester DJ, Sener SF, et al. Axillary recurrence after sentinel node biopsy. *Ann Surg Oncol.* 2005;12:34-40.
2. Naik AM, Fey J, Gemignani M, et al. The risk of axillary relapse after sentinel lymph node biopsy for breast cancer is comparable with that of axillary lymph node dissection: a follow-up study of 4008 procedures. *Ann Surg.* 2004;240: 462-468.
3. Fant JS, Grant MD, Knox SM, et al. Preliminary outcome analysis in patients with breast cancer and a positive sentinel lymph node who declined axillary dissection. *Ann Surg Oncol.* 2003;10:126-130.
4. Guenther JM, Hansen NM, DiFronzo LA, et al. Axillary dissection is not required for all patients with breast cancer and positive sentinel nodes. *Arch Surg.* 2003; 138:52-56.
5. Lyman GH, Giuliano AE, Somerfield MR, et al. American Society of Clinical Oncology. American Society of Clinical Oncology guideline recommendations for sentinel lymph node biopsy in early-stage breast cancer. *J Clin Oncol.* 2005; 23:7703-7720.
6. National Comprehensive Cancer Network. NCCN Clinical Practice Guidelines in Oncology: Breast Cancer. Version 2.2011, http://www.nccn.org/professionals/physician_gls/PDF/breast.pdf. Accessed December 28, 2010.
7. Wasif N, Ye X, Giuliano AE. Survey of ASCO members on management of sentinel node micrometastases in breast cancer: variation in treatment recommendations according to specialty. *Ann Surg Oncol.* 2009;16:2442-2449.
8. Bilimoria KY, Bentrem DJ, Hansen NM, et al. Comparison of sentinel lymph node biopsy alone and completion axillary lymph node dissection for node-positive breast cancer. *J Clin Oncol.* 2009;27:2946-2953.

Tumor Biology

Intrinsic Breast Tumor Subtypes, Race, and Long-Term Survival in the Carolina Breast Cancer Study

O'Brien KM, Cole SR, Tse C-K, et al (Univ of North Carolina, Chapel Hill; et al)
Clin Cancer Res 16:6100-6110, 2010

Purpose.—Previous research identified differences in breast cancer–specific mortality across 4 intrinsic tumor subtypes: luminal A, luminal B, basal-like, and human epidermal growth factor receptor 2 positive/estrogen receptor negative ($HER2^+/ER^-$).

Experimental Design.—We used immunohistochemical markers to subtype 1,149 invasive breast cancer patients (518 African American, 631 white) in the Carolina Breast Cancer Study, a population-based study of women diagnosed with breast cancer. Vital status was determined through 2006 using the National Death Index, with median follow-up of 9 years.

Results.—Cancer subtypes luminal A, luminal B, basal-like, and $HER2^+/ER^-$ were distributed as 64%, 11%, 11%, and 5% for whites, and 48%, 8%, 22%, and 7% for African Americans, respectively. Breast cancer mortality was higher for participants with HER2$^+$/ER$^-$ and basal-like breast cancer compared with luminal A and B. African Americans had higher breast cancer-specific mortality than whites, but the effect of race was statistically significant only among women with luminal A breast cancer. However, when compared with the luminal A subtype within racial categories, mortality for participants with basal-like breast cancer was higher among whites (HR = 2.0, 95% CI: 1.2–3.4) than African Americans (HR = 1.5, 95% CI: 1.0–2.4), with the strongest effect seen in postmenopausal white women (HR = 3.9, 95% CI: 1.5–10.0).

Conclusions.—Our results confirm the association of basal-like breast cancer with poor prognosis and suggest that basal-like breast cancer is not an inherently more aggressive disease in African American women compared with whites. Additional analyses are needed in populations with known treatment profiles to understand the role of tumor subtypes and race in breast cancer mortality, and in particular our finding that among women with luminal A breast cancer, African Americans have higher mortality than whites.

▶ Over the last 10 years, various molecular tests, especially gene expression profiling, have been used to help refine breast cancer subtypes and to evaluate breast cancer prognoses and response to therapy. Recently, immuno-phenotyping using immunohistochemical (IHC) analysis to approximate molecular subtype as determined by gene expression profiling has become increasingly popular because of its ease of use and cost effectiveness. In this study, O'Brien and colleagues focused on the relationships among race, menopausal status, IHC-based subtypes, and survival.

This study confirmed previously published results by demonstrating that most basal-like and HER2$^+$/ER$^-$ breast cancers had poorer prognosis than luminal A and B breast cancers, regardless of the source population; African American women had higher rates of breast cancer–specific mortality than whites.[1-3] The study is valuable in that it was a large multiracial, population-based study in which the investigators used flexible models in addition to standard statistical techniques to examine racial differences in survival by IHC subtype. Although it is not surprising that basal-like breast cancer was seen more frequently in African American women (especially young African American women) than in white women, it is important to note that basal-like breast cancer does not appear to be inherently more aggressive in African American women than in white women. Specifically, when survival of the patients with different subtypes of breast cancer was analyzed by race, African Americans were shown to have significantly higher mortality rates than whites in luminal A breast cancer only. In addition, the hazard ratios of basal-like breast cancer compared to luminal A breast cancer were slightly higher in whites (especially postmenopausal white women) than in African American women. These findings allow us to better understand the significance of intrinsic subtypes and race in breast cancer mortality. Because intrinsic subtype is more important than racial category in terms of prognosis, efforts should be made to accurately classify tumors.

Although the racial differences in breast cancer mortality could result from differences in treatment and in the availability of care for ER$^+$ breast cancer in the African American population, it is also possible that variations in IHC testing and interpretation might be contributory. Over the past decade, various testing methods and scoring criteria for ER, progesterone receptor, and HER2 have been used, especially before the latest guidelines from the American Society of Clinical Oncology and the College of American Pathologists were published.[4,5] On the other hand, an accurate IHC-based subtype may not necessarily reflect the intrinsic breast cancer subtype defined by genomic tests and therefore can intrinsically lead to misclassification. Another limitation of this study is that the investigators were unable to generate precise hazard ratios in subgroups defined by race and menopausal status owing to the small within-strata sample size. Larger studies that take treatment profiles into consideration are needed to further confirm the findings.

Y. Gong, MD

References

1. Huo D, Ikpatt F, Khramtsov A, et al. Population differences in breast cancer: survey in indigenous African women reveals over-representation of triple-negative breast cancer. *J Clin Oncol.* 2009;27:4515-4521.
2. Lund MJ, Trivers KF, Porter PL, et al. Race and triple negative threats to breast cancer survival: a population-based study in Atlanta, GA. *Breast Cancer Res Treat.* 2009;113:357-370.
3. Spitale A, Mazzola P, Soldini D, Mazzucchelli L, Bordoni A. Breast cancer classification according to immunohistochemical markers: clinicopathologic features and short-term survival analysis in a population-based study from the South of Switzerland. *Ann Oncol.* 2009;20:628-635.
4. Hammond ME, Hayes DF, Dowsett M, et al. American Society of Clinical Oncology/College of American Pathologists guideline recommendations for immunohistochemical testing of estrogen and progesterone receptors in breast cancer. *J Clin Oncol.* 2010;28:2784-2795.
5. Wolff AC, Hammond ME, Schwartz JN, et al. American Society of Clinical Oncology, College of American Pathologists. American Society of Clinical Oncology/College of American Pathologists guideline recommendations for human epidermal growth factor receptor 2 testing in breast cancer. *J Clin Oncol.* 2007;25:118-145.

3 Gynecology

Ovarian

"Primary peritoneal" high-grade serous carcinoma is very likely metastatic from serous tubal intraepithelial carcinoma: Assessing the new paradigm of ovarian and pelvic serous carcinogenesis and its implications for screening for ovarian cancer

Seidman JD, Zhao P, Yemelyanova A (Washington Hosp Ctr, DC; Georgetown Univ Med Ctr, Washington, DC; Johns Hopkins Hosp, Baltimore, MD)

Gynecol Oncol 120:470-473, 2011

Objective.—Primary peritoneal high-grade serous carcinoma is thought to arise from the peritoneum, but recent data suggest that the fallopian tube may be an occult source of many of these tumors. This study was performed to evaluate this hypothesis in an unselected series of cases.

Methods.—Fallopian tubes from 51 consecutive cases meeting the GOG criteria for primary peritoneal high-grade serous carcinoma, FIGO stages II-IV, were analyzed.

Results.—Serous tubal intraepithelial carcinoma (STIC) was identified in 19 patients (37%). When the fimbriae were examined, STIC was identified in 46%, and when all tubal tissue was examined, 56%. STIC was confined to the fimbriae in 53%, involved fimbriae and nonfimbrial mucosa in 20%, and was confined to nonfimbrial mucosa in 20%. Patients with STIC were significantly older than those without STIC (75 years vs. 67 years, respectively; $p = 0.007$). Patients with STIC were significantly more likely to have FIGO stage IV disease as compared to those without STIC (42% vs. 12.5%, respectively; $p = 0.037$).

Conclusions.—At least half the cases of primary peritoneal high-grade serous carcinoma are associated with intraepithelial carcinoma of the fallopian tube, usually involving the fimbriae. These findings support the view that, like "primary ovarian carcinoma," what has been traditionally classified as "primary peritoneal carcinoma" is probably derived from occult high-grade serous carcinoma in the fallopian tube. These findings have important implications for ultrasound screening trials for ovarian cancer which are based on the assumption that an enlarged ovary is a very early manifestation of disease.

▶ This article proposes a new perspective on the origin of serous carcinomas in the peritoneal cavity. Prior to these considerations, the working hypothesis has been that serous carcinomas originated from celomic epithelium, which surrounded the ovary during development and also lined the entire peritoneal cavity. Studies had suggested that, regardless of site of origin, these neoplasms all responded similarly to systemic therapy and could therefore be managed in a similar fashion. This small series of 51 consecutive cases of primary peritoneal high-grade serous carcinomas suggests that as many as half of these lesions thought to originate from peritoneal epithelial tissue actually may originate in the fallopian tube, and thus attention is directed to the fallopian tube as a potential site of origin. However, before this information can be incorporated into considerations for screening for early ovarian cancer, additional pieces of information will be needed. First, the actual overall frequency of tubal origin will need to be determined. Even if we assume that half of the primary peritoneal neoplasms arise in the tube, this may still constitute only 5% to 10% of all of these neoplasms. Second, we need a screening approach that actually works to detect disease early and reduce mortality, and no evidence to date proves that any approach reduces mortality. Third, we need a larger study to confirm these observations.

J. T. Thigpen, MD

A phase II study of two topotecan regimens evaluated in recurrent platinum-sensitive ovarian, fallopian tube or primary peritoneal cancer: A Gynecologic Oncology Group Study (GOG 146Q)

Herzog TJ, Sill MW, Walker JL, et al (Columbia Univ, NY; Roswell Park Cancer Inst, Buffalo, NY; Univ of Oklahoma; et al)

Gynecol Oncol 120:454-458, 2011

Objective.—To evaluate the efficacy and safety of topotecan in patients with recurrent ovarian, primary peritoneal, and fallopian tube carcinomas.

Methods.—A randomized phase II analysis of platinum-sensitive patients with measurable disease was performed independently assessing intravenous topotecan 1.25 mg/m^2 daily × 5 every 21 days (regimen I) and topotecan 4.0 mg/m^2/day on days 1, 8, and 15 of a 28-day cycle (regimen II). All patients were treated until disease progression, unmanageable toxicity, or patient refusal. Insufficient accrual related to regimen I resulted in a redesign of the study as a single arm phase II trial assessing only regimen II. More complete efficacy data is presented for regimen II as enrollment on regimen I was insufficient for some analyses.

Results.—A total of 81 patients were enrolled. One patient was ineligible. Fifteen patients received regimen I, while 65 patients were treated with regimen II. The response rate on regimen I (daily × 5) was 27% (90% CI: 10–51%) and 12% (90% CI: 6–21%) on regimen II (weekly). The median PFS and OS were 4.8 and 27.8 months, respectively, for regimen II. Grade 3/4 neutropenia rate was 93% with daily × 5 dosing and 28% for weekly treatment. Febrile neutropenia was very low in both groups.

Conclusion.—The weekly regimen of topotecan appeared less active but resulted in less toxicity than the daily regimen in platinum-sensitive recurrent ovarian cancer patients.

▶ This study is an attempt to determine whether the commonly used weekly schedule of topotecan yields efficacy similar to that of the Food and Drug Administration–approved 5-day schedule. As with most studies involving the 5-day schedule, the Gynecology Oncology Group (GOG) had trouble accruing to the study and finished the trial as a phase II study of the weekly schedule. The results, however, are sufficiently interesting to cause hesitation in opting for the weekly schedule. Only 27 patients were administered the 5-day schedule before closure of that arm, but the response rate of 27% is essentially identical to the 33% seen in an earlier GOG trial of the 5-day schedule in platinum-sensitive patients. The 12% response rate seen with the weekly schedule is consistent with reported phase II trials in the literature and is only half as effective in inducing objective responses as the 5-day schedule. These observations are consistent with preclinical data on the topoisomerase inhibitors, which show that duration of exposure to these agents is the predominant determinant of efficacy. While patient and physician convenience is certainly important, efficacy should be our primary consideration; hence the 5-day schedule should still be the preferred schedule unless toxicity considerations prevent its use.

J. T. Thigpen, MD

Addition of bevacizumab to weekly paclitaxel significantly improves progression-free survival in heavily pretreated recurrent epithelial ovarian cancer

O'Malley DM, Richardson DL, Rheaume PS, et al (The Ohio State Univ College of Medicine, Columbus)

Gynecol Oncol 121:269-272, 2011

Objective.—Weekly paclitaxel has been shown to be an effective cytotoxic regimen for recurrent epithelial ovarian cancer (EOC), and may act through inhibition of angiogenesis. Bevacizumab, a potent angiogenesis inhibitor, has also been shown to have activity in patients with EOC. Therefore, we sought to determine if the addition of bevacizumab to weekly paclitaxel led to an increased survival compared to weekly paclitaxel alone.

Methods.—A single institutional review was conducted for patients with recurrent EOC treated with weekly paclitaxel (60–70 mg/m^2) on days 1, 8, 15, and 22 of a 28 day cycle and those treated with weekly paclitaxel and bevacizumab (10–15 mg/kg on day 1 and 15). Response rates (RR) were calculated, and progression-free survival (PFS), and overall survival (OS) were compared using Kaplan–Meier survival analysis.

Results.—Twenty-nine patients treated with weekly paclitaxel and 41 patients treated with paclitaxel/bevacizumab were identified. The groups were similar in demographics, initial optimal cytoreduction, stage, histology, grade, platinum sensitivity, and median number of previous regimens (4 vs. 4, p=0.69).The overall response rate (ORR) was 63% (complete response (CR) 34% and partial response (PR) 29%) for paclitaxel/bevacizumab and 48% (CR 17% and PR 31%) for weekly paclitaxel (p=0.23). Improvement in PFS was seen in those treated with paclitaxel/bevacizumab in comparison to weekly paclitaxel alone (median PFS 13.2 vs. 6.2 months, p<.01). There was a trend towards improved OS for paclitaxel/bevacizumab (median OS 20.6 vs. 9.1 months; p=0.12). Toxicities were similar between the two regimens although more bowel perforations (2 vs. 0) were seen in the paclitaxel/bevacizumab group.

Conclusion.—A significant increase in PFS with a trend towards improved OS was demonstrated in this heavily pretreated population treated with paclitaxel/bevacizumab as compared to weekly paclitaxel alone. This data should be helpful in guiding future trials to determine the optimal care for women with recurrent EOC.

▶ Bevacizumab had been evaluated extensively in ovarian carcinoma. Initial phase II data from the Gynecologic Oncology Group showed a 21% objective response rate and 40% of patients progression free at 6 months. These data led to the initiation of 2 large phase III trials in newly diagnosed disease, GOG 218 (Unites States) and ICON7 (United Kingdom). These studies were both reported in the summer of 2010 as showing a significant improvement in progression-free survival (PFS) and a trend toward improved overall survival (OS) in those patients who received bevacizumab with paclitaxel/carboplatin up front followed by bevacizumab maintenance (15 total months in GOG 218 and 12 total months in ICON 7). In June 2011, a phase III of gemcitabine/carboplatin bevacizumab showed the same thing: significantly improved PFS and a trend toward improved OS. These studies all support the conclusion that bevacizumab is a very active agent in ovarian carcinoma. This trial looks at bevacizumab in combination with weekly paclitaxel in patients with recurrent disease. The sample size is relatively small, so no definitive conclusions can be reached. However, the trends toward improvements in PFS and OS strongly support the use of the drug in this setting. The burning question that remains is whether a patient who received bevacizumab frontline would, when progression of disease occurs, still benefit from the drug in the recurrent disease setting. There is no definitive answer as of yet, but it would be reasonable to consider using bevacizumab in combination with chemotherapy in the recurrent disease setting.

J. T. Thigpen, MD

CA125 surveillance increases optimal resectability at secondary cytoreductive surgery for recurrent epithelial ovarian cancer

Fleming ND, Cass I, Walsh CS, et al (Cedars-Sinai Women's Cancer Res Inst, Los Angeles, CA)

Gynecol Oncol 121:249-252, 2011

Objective.—Recent data suggest that serial CA125 surveillance following remission in asymptomatic patients with epithelial ovarian cancer (EOC) does not impact overall survival. However, earlier detection of recurrence may influence resectability at secondary cytoreductive surgery (SCS). We hypothesized that a shorter time interval between CA125 elevation and SCS correlates with a higher likelihood of optimal resection among eligible patients.

Methods.—We identified patients with recurrent epithelial ovarian cancer who underwent SCS from 1995 to 2009 at our institution. All patients initially underwent primary cytoreductive surgery followed by platinum-based chemotherapy. CA125 elevation was considered the first value two-times the patient's nadir level. Our "study interval" was the time between CA125 elevation and SCS. Optimal SCS was defined as microscopic residual disease (≤0.5 cm). Our analysis compared patients who underwent optimal vs. suboptimal SCS.

Results.—Seventy-four patients who underwent SCS for recurrent EOC met inclusion criteria. Median disease-free interval prior to SCS was 19 vs. 12 months for the optimal and suboptimal SCS groups. More patients undergoing suboptimal SCS had ascites (21% vs. 2%, p = 0.01) and carcinomatosis (42% vs. 5%, p<0.0001). Patients who underwent optimal SCS went to the operating room 5.3 vs. 16.4 weeks (HR 1.03, 95% CI 1.01-1.06, p = 0.04) from the time of their CA125 elevation. Optimal SCS was associated with a longer overall survival (47 vs. 23 months, p<0.0001).

Conclusions.—Each week delay after first CA125 elevation correlated with a 3% increased chance of suboptimal resection at SCS. Serial CA125 surveillance for early detection of recurrence may increase rates of optimal SCS and potentially influence overall survival.

▶ In ovarian cancer patients who achieve a complete response to initial chemotherapy, common practice in the United States follows these patients with serial CA125 measurements. CA125 increases in the absence of recurrence and a median of 3 months before evidence of other disease appears. Whether immediate treatment based solely on the rising CA125 offers a therapeutic advantage has been hotly debated, but a recent European trial showed that patients treated early based on a rising CA125 not only did not show a survival advantage but also incurred an earlier deterioration of quality of life. This trial, however, did not address the issue of secondary cytoreductive surgery. Current literature suggests, based on uncontrolled retrospective studies, that patients who achieve a state free of gross residual disease as a result of secondary cytoreduction experience an improved survival. This study examined outcome in 74 patients who underwent secondary surgical cytoreduction. Those who underwent earlier surgical cytoreduction based solely on a rising CA125 demonstrated a lower frequency of factors predictive of unsuccessful surgical cytoreduction and also an improved overall survival. These data are provocative and suggest a major flaw in the European trial of CA125 monitoring of patients in complete remission after initial therapy, the failure to consider the role of secondary surgical cytoreduction. For a definitive evaluation of this issue, a prospective randomized trial of secondary surgical cytoreduction is needed and is underway as Gynecologic Oncology Group Protocol 213.

J. T. Thigpen, MD

Clinical Activity of Gemcitabine Plus Pertuzumab in Platinum-Resistant Ovarian Cancer, Fallopian Tube Cancer, or Primary Peritoneal Cancer

Makhija S, Amler LC, Glenn D, et al (Emory Univ, Atlanta, GA; Genentech, South San Francisco, CA; Sharp Rees-Stealy Med Group, San Diego, CA; et al)

J Clin Oncol 28:1215-1223, 2010

Purpose.—Pertuzumab is a humanized monoclonal antibody that inhibits human epidermal growth factor receptor 2 (HER2) heterodimerization and has single-agent activity in recurrent epithelial ovarian cancer. The primary objective of this phase II study was to characterize the safety and estimate progression-free survival (PFS) of pertuzumab with gemcitabine in patients with platinum-resistant ovarian cancer.

Patients and Methods.—Patients with advanced, platinum-resistant epithelial ovarian, fallopian tube, or primary peritoneal cancer who had received a maximum of one prior treatment for recurrent cancer were randomly assigned to gemcitabine plus either pertuzumab or placebo. Collection of archival tissue was mandatory to permit exploration of biomarkers that would predict benefit from pertuzumab in this setting.

Results.—One hundred thirty patients (65 per arm) were treated. Baseline characteristics were similar between arms. The adjusted hazard ratio (HR) for PFS was 0.66 (95% CI, 0.43 to 1.03; $P = .07$) in favor of gemcitabine + pertuzumab. The objective response rate was 13.8% in patients who received gemcitabine + pertuzumab compared with 4.6% in patients who received gemcitabine + placebo. In patients whose tumors had low HER3 mRNA expression (< median, $n = 61$), an increased treatment benefit was observed in the gemcitabine + pertuzumab arm compared with the gemcitabine alone arm (PFS HR = 0.32; 95% CI, 0.17 to 0.59; $P = .0002$). Grade 3 to 4 neutropenia, diarrhea, and back pain were increased in patients treated with gemcitabine + pertuzumab. Symptomatic congestive heart failure was reported in one patient in the gemcitabine + pertuzumab arm.

Conclusion.—Pertuzumab may add activity to gemcitabine for the treatment of platinum-resistant ovarian cancer. Low HER3 mRNA expression may predict pertuzumab clinical benefit and be a valuable prognostic marker.

▶ Patients with ovarian cancer who either have failed to achieve a complete response with prior platinum-based therapy or who relapse within 6 months of achieving a complete response are categorized as clinically platinum resistant. These patients are treated with active agents other than a platinum compound. This patient population is the focus of this trial. Gemcitabine is an active agent in this setting with an objective response rate reportedly in the midteens. This study assigned all patients to treatment with gemcitabine and randomly assigned half of the patients to receive concurrent pertuzumab, a monoclonal antibody that inhibits human epidermal growth factor (HER) 2 dimerization. Patients receiving pertuzumab exhibited a superior response rate in this randomized phase II trial. The trial included an exploration of biomarkers, and this aspect of the study revealed that those whose tumors exhibited low levels of HER3 expression benefited most from the addition of pertuzumab (hazard ratio = 0.32). These data suggest that HER3 might be a valuable prognostic marker for response to pertuzumab. Phase III trials are planned.

J. T. Thigpen, MD

Clinical Outcome of Tertiary Surgical Cytoreduction in Patients with Recurrent Epithelial Ovarian Cancer

Fotopoulou C, Richter R, Braicu IE, et al (Charité Univ Med Ctr Berlin, Germany)

Ann Surg Oncol 18:49-57, 2011

Background.—The value of tertiary cytoreductive surgery (TCS) on overall survival (OS) of patients with relapsed epithelial ovarian cancer (ROC) is not well defined. Aim of the present study was to evaluate the operative and clinical outcome after TCS.

Methods.—We systematically evaluated all consecutive patients undergoing TCS. Tumor dissemination pattern, operative morbidity, residual tumor, and survival are described based on a validated intraoperative documentation tool. Predictors of survival and complete tumor resection are analyzed with Cox regression or logistic regression models.

Results.—Between October 2000 and December 2008, 135 patients (median age, 51 years; range, 22–80 years) of mainly initial FIGO stage ≤III (106 patients, 78.5%) were evaluated. In 53 patients (39.3%) a complete tumor-resection was obtained. The 1-month operative mortality was 6%. During a median follow-up period of 9.6 months (range, 0.1–75 months), 78 patients (57.8%) died, while 52 patients (38.5%) experienced a further relapse. Median OS was 19.1 months for the total collective (95% confidence interval [95% CI], 14.84–23.35). Median OS was 37.8 months (95% CI, 12.7–62.7) for patients without residual tumor; versus 19.0 months (95% CI, 9.8–28.2) for residual tumor ≤1 cm and 6.9 months (95% CI, 3.05–10.7) for residual tumor >1 cm ($P < .001$). The presence of peritoneal carcinomatosis did not seem to significantly affect OS. Complete tumor resection was identified as the strongest predictor of OS. Other independent predictors of OS were interval to primary diagnosis ≤3 years (hazard ratio [HR], 0.28; 95% CI, 0.14–0.59) and serous papillary histology (HR, 0.23; 95% CI, 0.09–0.56). A total of 42 patients (31.1%) presented at least 1 major complication. Multivariate analysis identified tumor involvement of the middle abdomen and peritoneal carcinomatosis as independent predictors of complete tumor resection.

Conclusions.—Postoperative tumor residual disease remains the strongest predictor of survival even in TCS setting. To identify the optimal candidates for TCS, the predictive value of ascites and peritoneal carcinomatosis should be confirmed by future prospective trials.

▶ Bulk reductive surgery has been a part of the standard approach to newly diagnosed advanced ovarian carcinoma for at least the last 35 years in the United States. Although evidence was initially based on retrospective data, at least 1 randomized trial has now shown a survival advantage for bulk reductive surgery as opposed to no bulk reductive surgery (a study of interval bulk reduction in Europe). Based on the success of initial bulk reductive surgery, use of secondary surgical debulking in the recurrent disease setting has also been proposed and studied in retrospective series. These studies suggest that secondary bulk reduction is of significant benefit in those patients in whom all gross disease can be removed at secondary debulking. Although no prospective study has yet been published, one is currently ongoing to attempt to confirm the retrospective data in a prospective trial. This study evaluates the role of tertiary surgical bulk reduction in a retrospective evaluation of 135 patients undergoing such a procedure. Based on the analysis, it would appear that the same criteria apply here as in secondary surgical bulk reduction. Those patients who achieve a status of no gross residual disease with tertiary bulk reduction clearly benefit. A second important criterion should also be remembered: those with platinum-sensitive recurrent disease have the best chance to benefit.

J. T. Thigpen, MD

Clinical predictors of bevacizumab-associated gastrointestinal perforation

Tanyi JL, McCann G, Hagemann AR, et al (Univ of Pennsylvania Health System, Philadelphia)

Gynecol Oncol 120:464-469, 2011

Objectives.—Bevacizumab is a generally well-tolerated drug, but bevacizumab-associated gastrointestinal perforations (BAP) occur in 0 to 15% of patients with ovarian carcinoma. Our goal was to evaluate the clinical predictors of BAP in order to identify factors, which may preclude patients from receiving treatment.

Methods.—We conducted a review of patients with recurrent epithelial ovarian carcinoma treated with bevacizumab between 2006 and 2009. Demographic and treatment data were collected for statistical analysis.

Results.—Eighty-two patients were identified; perforation occurred in 8 (9.76%). Among patients with perforation, a significantly higher incidence of prior bowel surgeries ($p = 0.0008$) and prior bowel obstruction or ileus ($p < 0.0001$) were found compared to non-perforated patients. The median age at onset of bevacizumab in the perforated group was 3 years younger (60 vs. 63 years, $p = 0.61$). The incidence of thromboembolic events, GI comorbidities, number of prior chemotherapies, and body mass index were similar between the groups. None of the patients in the perforated group developed grade 3 or 4 hypertension, compared to a 32.4% incidence among the non-perforated patients ($p = 0.09$). Upon multivariate analysis, when controlled for age greater or less than 60, prior bowel surgery, obstruction/ileus, and grade 3 or 4 hypertension, only the presence of obstruction/ileus was noted to be a significant predictor of perforation ($p = 0.04$).

Conclusions.—Predicting BAP remains a challenge. Bowel obstruction or ileus appears to be associated with increased risk of BAP.

▶ Gastrointestinal perforation is one of the most substantial adverse effects associated with bevacizumab in patients with ovarian carcinoma. Although not definitive, early phase II data on bevacizumab in ovarian carcinoma suggested that patients with multiple prior treatments for recurrent disease were more likely to develop the problem. The highest reported frequency was in a study that permitted 3 or more prior lines of therapy. Whether this higher frequency reflected the number of prior lines of chemotherapy or other management approaches was not clear. This article reviews results in a series of 82 patients with 8 episodes of bowel perforation. Two factors were significantly related to the occurrence of bowel perforation: prior bowel surgeries and prior episodes of bowel obstruction or ileus. Particularly in patients with recurrent ovarian carcinoma who may have had multiple prior surgeries, use of bevacizumab should be considered earlier in the disease course (frontline or first recurrence) to avoid a clinical setting in which the likelihood of this complication is increased.

J. T. Thigpen, MD

Decreased hypersensitivity reactions with carboplatin-pegylated liposomal doxorubicin compared to carboplatin-paclitaxel combination: Analysis from the GCIG CALYPSO relapsing ovarian cancer trial

Joly F, Ray-Coquard I, Fabbro M, et al (Centre François Baclesse, Caen, France; Centre Leon Bérard, Lyon, France; CRLC Val d'Aurelle, Montpellier, France; et al)

Gynecol Oncol 122:226-232, 2011

Objective.—To describe and analyze observed hypersensitivity reactions (HSR) from the randomized, multicenter phase III CALYPSO trial that evaluated the efficacy and safety of the combination of carboplatin and pegylated liposomal doxorubicin (CD) compared with standard carboplatin-paclitaxel (CP) in patients with platinum–sensitive relapsed ovarian cancer (ROC).

Methods.—HSR documented within case report forms and SAE reports were specifically analyzed. Analyses were based on the population with allergy of any grade and for grade >2 allergy.

Results.—Overall 976 patients were recruited to this phase III trial, with toxicity data available for 466 and 502 on the CD and CP arms, respectively. There was a 15.5% HSR rate associated with CD (2.4% grade >2) versus 33.1% with CP (8.8% grade >2), $p<0.001$. HSRs occurred more often during first cycle in the CD (46%) arm than in the CP arm (16%). Multivariate predictors of allergy were chemotherapy regimen and age; patients randomized to CD and patients ≥70 years old on CP had less allergy. Few patients (<6%) stopped treatment due to allergy. Allergy rates were higher in patients who did not receive prior supportive treatment; however there was no relationship between allergy and the type of carboplatin product received, or response rate.

Conclusions.—Use of PLD with carboplatin instead of paclitaxel and older age were the only 2 factors predicting a low rate of HSRs in patients with ROC. CD has previously demonstrated superior progression-free survival and therapeutic index than CP. Taken together these data support the use of CD as a safe and effective therapeutic option for platinum-sensitive ROC.

▶ The paradigm in place for the management of recurrent ovarian cancer for the past 20 years has been to categorize patients as platinum sensitive or platinum resistant based on response to prior platinum-based therapy. Those who achieve a complete response that lasts at least 6 months are categorized as platinum sensitive, whereas the rest are considered platinum resistant. Patients categorized as platinum sensitive have generally been recommended to receive platinum-based therapy at relapse. Three large phase III trials in the past 8 years have shown platinum-based doublets to be superior to single-agent platinum: paclitaxel/carboplatin, gemcitabine/carboplatin, and now pegylated liposomal doxorubicin (PLD)/carboplatin. The last doublet was actually compared with another doublet, paclitaxel/carboplatin, and demonstrated a superior progression-free survival (PFS) (the CALYPSO trial). This particular ancillary study looks at the patients who experienced a carboplatin hypersensitivity reaction on the CALYPSO trial. The number of patients involved was not insignificant (15.5% on the PLD/carboplatin regimen versus 33.1% on the paclitaxel/carboplatin regimen). The data suggest that significantly fewer hypersensitivity reactions were observed among those patients receiving PLD/carboplatin, although the mechanism responsible for this decrease is not clear. This observation, combined with the PFS advantage with PLD/carboplatin, suggests that this doublet should be the regimen of choice in the patient with platinum-sensitive disease.

J. T. Thigpen, MD

Development of a Multimarker Assay for Early Detection of Ovarian Cancer

Yurkovetsky Z, Skates S, Lomakin A, et al (Univ of Pittsburgh Cancer Inst, PA; Univ of Pittsburgh, PA; Fox Chase Cancer Ctr, Philadelphia, PA; et al)

J Clin Oncol 28:2159-2166, 2010

Purpose.—Early detection of ovarian cancer has great promise to improve clinical outcome.

Patients and Methods.—Ninety-six serum biomarkers were analyzed in sera from healthy women and from patients with ovarian cancer, benign pelvic tumors, and breast, colorectal, and lung cancers, using multiplex xMAP bead-based immunoassays. A Metropolis algorithm with Monte Carlo simulation (MMC) was used for analysis of the data.

Results.—A training set, including sera from 139 patients with early-stage ovarian cancer, 149 patients with late-stage ovarian cancer, and 1,102 healthy women, was analyzed with MMC algorithm and cross validation to identify an optimal biomarker panel discriminating early-stage cancer from healthy controls. The four-biomarker panel providing the highest diagnostic power of 86% sensitivity (SN) for early-stage and 93% SN for late-stage ovarian cancer at 98% specificity (SP) was comprised of CA-125, HE4, CEA, and VCAM-1. This model was applied to an independent blinded validation set consisting of sera from 44 patients with early-stage ovarian cancer, 124 patients with late-stage ovarian cancer, and 929 healthy women, providing unbiased estimates of 86% SN for stage I and II and 95% SN for stage III and IV disease at 98% SP. This panel was selective for ovarian cancer showing SN of 33% for benign pelvic disease, SN of 6% for breast cancer, SN of 0% for colorectal cancer, and SN of 36% for lung cancer.

Conclusion.—A panel of CA-125, HE4, CEA, and VCAM-1, after additional validation, could serve as an initial stage in a screening strategy for epithelial ovarian cancer.

► Ovarian carcinoma is the second most common invasive cancer of the female genital tract, but it is by far the most common cause of death from gynecologic cancer. Some have assumed that this is because ovarian cancer is not responsive to current treatment modalities, but trials in advanced ovarian cancer report that essentially 75% of patients achieve a clinical complete response, far higher than any other solid tumor other than germ cell tumors. The problem rather lies in that fact that 75% to 80% of patients present with stage III to IV disease because of the lack of an effective early diagnostic test (compare this to 92% of breast cancers presenting as stage I to II and 88% of endometrial cancers presenting as stage I to II). Numerous studies have been reported to evaluate the use of serial CA-125 and transvaginal sonography as a screening approach. The most recent US trial, the Prostate, Lung, Colorectal, and Ovarian Cancer Screening Trial, involving more than 78 000 women screened for ovarian cancer in this fashion, produced a positive predictive value of 1.3% and no change in the mortality rate. The key to any screening test is its ability to reduce mortality related to the disease. This article presents the results of early studies of a panel of 4 markers and suggests that this panel is promising as a potential screening approach for ovarian cancer. The data presented, however, do not support the use of this approach as a screening test. The total number of women in the study is far too small for any conclusion that the approach is effective, and the results to date do not address the issue of mortality reduction. Other attempts at such an approach, including the use of proteomic profiling, have also failed. The authors are correct to conclude that further studies of a randomized design including much larger numbers of women will be required before any conclusions can be drawn. We remain without a confirmed screening approach for ovarian cancer.

J. T. Thigpen, MD

Docetaxel plus trabectedin appears active in recurrent or persistent ovarian and primary peritoneal cancer after up to three prior regimens: A phase II study of the Gynecologic Oncology Group

Monk BJ, Sill MW, Hanjani P, et al (Creighton Univ School of Medicine at St Joseph's Hosp and Med Ctr, Phoenix, AZ; Univ at Buffalo, NY; Abington Memorial Hosp, PA; et al)

Gynecol Oncol 120:459-463, 2011

Objective.—This study aims to estimate the activity of docetaxel 60 mg/m^2 IV over 1 h followed by trabectedin 1.1 mg/m^2 over 3 h with filgrastim, pegfilgrastim, or sargramostim every 3 weeks (one cycle).

Methods.—Patients with recurrent and measurable disease, acceptable organ function, PS≤2, and ≤3 prior regimens were eligible. A two-stage design was utilized with a target sample size of 35 subjects per stage. Another Gynecologic Oncology Group study within the same protocol queue involving a single agent taxane showed a response rate (RR) of (16%) (90% CI 8.6–28.5%) and served as a historical control for direct comparison. The present study was designed to determine if the current regimen had an RR of ≥36% with 90% power.

Results.—Seventy-one patients were eligible and evaluable (prior regimens: 1 = 28%, 2 = 52%, 3 = 20%). The median number of cycles was 6 (438 total cycles, range 1–22). The number of patients responding was 21 (30%; 90% CI 21–40%). The odds ratio for responding was 2.2 (90% 1-sided CI 1.07–Infinity). The median progression-free survival and overall survival were 4.5 months and 16.9 months, respectively. The median response duration was 6.2 months. Numbers of subjects with grade 3/4 toxicity included neutropenia 7/14; constitutional 8/0; GI (excluding nausea/vomiting) 11/0; metabolic 9/1; pain 6/0. There were no treatment-related deaths nor cases of liver failure.

Conclusions.—This combination was well tolerated and appears more active than the historical control of single agent taxane therapy in those with recurrent ovarian and peritoneal cancer after failing multiple lines of chemotherapy. Further study is warranted.

▶ Trabectedin is an agent derived from the sea squirt. In a prior phase III trial comparing pegylated liposomal doxorubicin trabectedin, the combination produced a significantly longer progression-free survival (PFS) and a trend toward improved overall survival. The Food and Drug Administration (FDA) refused to approve the drug in ovarian carcinoma because the FDA does not accept PFS as a valid end point in ovarian carcinoma contrary to what the proceedings of an FDA/ASCO/AACR conference on end points in ovarian carcinoma state on the FDA Web site (the conference concluded that PFS was a surrogate for survival unless extensive postprogression therapy blurred the correlation). This Gynecologic Oncology Group (GOG) study of trabectedin combined with another active agent in platinum-resistant ovarian carcinoma suggests, based on comparison with a historical GOG control of docetaxel alone in this setting, that the addition of trabectedin to this agent in a recurrent disease population improved response rate (30% vs 16%). Since this is not a randomized comparison, no definitive conclusions can be drawn, but the results do support the conclusions of the phase III trial with pegylated liposomal doxorubicin that adding trabectedin to other active drugs improves the efficacy of the regimen.

J. T. Thigpen, MD

Effect of Screening on Ovarian Cancer Mortality: The Prostate, Lung, Colorectal and Ovarian (PLCO) Cancer Screening Randomized Controlled Trial

Buys SS, for the PLCO Project Team (Univ of Utah Health Sciences Ctr, Salt Lake City; et al)

JAMA 305:2295-2303, 2011

Context.—Screening for ovarian cancer with cancer antigen 125 (CA-125) and transvaginal ultrasound has an unknown effect on mortality.

Objective.—To evaluate the effect of screening for ovarian cancer on mortality in the Prostate, Lung, Colorectal and Ovarian (PLCO) Cancer Screening Trial.

Design, Setting, and Participants.—Randomized controlled trial of 78 216 women aged 55 to 74 years assigned to undergo either annual screening (n = 39 105) or usual care (n = 39 111) at 10 screening centers across the United States between November 1993 and July 2001.

Intervention.—The intervention group was offered annual screening with CA-125 for 6 years and transvaginal ultrasound for 4 years. Participants and their health care practitioners received the screening test results and managed evaluation of abnormal results. The usual care group was not offered annual screening with CA-125 for 6 years or transvaginal ultrasound but received their usual medical care. Participants were followed up for a maximum of 13 years (median [range], 12.4 years [10.9-13.0 years]) for cancer diagnoses and death until February 28, 2010.

Main Outcome Measures.—Mortality from ovarian cancer, including primary peritoneal and fallopian tube cancers. Secondary outcomes included ovarian cancer incidence and complications associated with screening examinations and diagnostic procedures.

Results.—Ovarian cancer was diagnosed in 212 women (5.7 per 10 000 person-years) in the intervention group and 176 (4.7 per 10 000 person-years) in the usual care group (rate ratio [RR], 1.21; 95% confidence interval [CI], 0.99-1.48). There were 118 deaths caused by ovarian cancer (3.1 per 10 000 person-years) in the intervention group and 100 deaths

(2.6 per 10 000 person-years) in the usual care group (mortality RR, 1.18; 95% CI, 0.82-1.71). Of 3285 women with false-positive results, 1080 underwent surgical follow-up; of whom, 163 women experienced at least 1 serious complication (15%). There were 2924 deaths due to other causes (excluding ovarian, colorectal, and lung cancer) (76.6 per 10 000 person-years) in the intervention group and 2914 deaths (76.2 per 10 000 person-years) in the usual care group (RR, 1.01; 95% CI, 0.96-1.06).

Conclusions.—Among women in the general US population, simultaneous screening with CA-125 and transvaginal ultrasound compared with usual care did not reduce ovarian cancer mortality. Diagnostic evaluation following a false-positive screening test result was associated with complications.

Trial Registration.—clinicaltrials.gov Identifier: NCT00002540.

▶ This article reports the results of a trial evaluating annual cancer antigen 125 (CA-125) and transvaginal sonography as a screening tool for the detection of early ovarian cancer in 78 216 women randomized to screening or no screening. The primary end point of the study was overall mortality. The trial showed no overall reduction in mortality as a result of screening, and there were numerous complications among the women who underwent surgery for a positive screen result. The results of this study must be taken in the context of a British trial reported in *The Lancet*, which showed a positive predictive value of 35% for a screening approach that analyzed the CA-125 data with a mathematical algorithm (ROCA). Mortality is awaited from this trial, but the positive predictive value is strikingly better than the 1.3% seen in the study reported here. The bottom line is that no approach as yet has demonstrated the ability to reduce mortality from ovarian cancer, and all approaches have resulted in surgeries for false-positive findings with associated morbidity.

J. T. Thigpen, MD

Effects of bevacizumab and pegylated liposomal doxorubicin for the patients with recurrent or refractory ovarian cancers

Kudoh K, Takano M, Kouta H, et al (Ohki Memorial Kikuchi Cancer Clinic for Women, Tokorozawa, Saitama, Japan; et al)

Gynecol Oncol 122:233-237, 2011

Objectives.—Currently, pegylated liposomal doxorubicin (PLD) is regarded as one of the standard treatment options in recurrent ovarian cancers (ROC). Bevacizumab has shown significant antitumor activity for ROC in single-agent or in combination with cytotoxic agents. We have conducted a preliminary study to investigate effects of combination of bevacizumab and PLD for heavily pretreated patients with ROC.

Methods.—Thirty patients with ROC were treated with combination therapy with weekly bevacizumab and PLD, 2 mg/kg of continuous weekly bevacizumab and 10 mg/m^2 of PLD (3 weeks on, 1 week off). The treatment was continued until development of disease progression, or unmanageable adverse effects. Response evaluation was based upon Response Evaluation Criteria in Solid Tumors (RECIST) version 1.0, and Gynecologic Cancer Intergroup (GCIG) CA125 response criteria. Adverse effects were analyzed according to Common Terminology Criteria for Adverse Events (CTCAE) version 3.0.

Results.—Overall response rate was 33%, and clinical benefit rate (CR+PD+SD) was 73%. Median progression-free survival was 6 months (range: 2–20 months), and a 6-months progression-free survival was 47%. Any hematological toxicities more than grade 3 were not observed. Two cases developed non-hematologic toxicities more than grade 2; a case with grade 3 hand-foot syndrome, another with grade 3 gastrointestinal perforation (GIP). The case with GIP was conservatively treated and recovered after 2 months, and there was no case with treatment-related death.

Conclusion.—The present investigation suggested that combination therapy with bevacizumab and PLD was active and well tolerated for patients with ROC. We recommend the regimen be evaluated in further clinical studies.

▶ Patients with platinum-resistant recurrent ovarian cancer are generally treated with single agents with demonstrated activity in this patient population. There are now some 21 different agents with reported activity in the platinum-resistant setting. To date, no study has demonstrated a superior outcome for patients treated with combinations of agents as opposed to single agent therapy. The demonstration of activity for bevacizumab and the success of front-line trials combining chemotherapy and bevacizumab for newly diagnosed ovarian cancer suggests that combinations of cytotoxic agents with bevacizumab might offer an advantage in the platinum-resistant population. This phase II study is noteworthy for evaluating the combination of pegylated liposomal doxorubicin (PLD) and bevacizumab in a heavily pretreated ovarian cancer population. What the study tells us is primarily that PLD can be combined safely with bevacizumab. What it does not tell us is whether the combination offers any advantage over either agent alone. Firstly, the study is not randomized and thus cannot give an accurate read on whether the combination is better than PLD or bevacizumab alone. Secondly, the patient population is not sufficiently well described to allow conclusions from such a small series. For example, one of the patients had platinum-sensitive disease. Of the other 29, all we know is that they were classified as platinum-resistant. Were any of them actually refractory (no response and no treatment-free interval) or were they all responders with progression at 5-6 months (a much better population with a greater likelihood of response)? In all likelihood, combinations of a cytotoxic agent with bevacizumab will yield better results in platinum-resistant disease than a single agent, and other agents can be logically combined with bevacizumab (eg, weekly paclitaxel). We need further study in controlled settings to determine this definitively.

J. T. Thigpen, MD

Ovarian cancer patient surveillance after curative-intent initial treatment

Harmandayan GZ, Gao F, Mutch DG, et al (Saint Louis Univ Med Ctr, MO; Washington Univ School of Medicine, St Louis, MO; et al)

Gynecol Oncol 120:205-208, 2011

Objective.—Patient surveillance after potentially curative treatment of ovarian carcinoma has important clinical and financial implications for patients and society. The optimal intensity of surveillance for these patients is unknown. We aimed to document the current follow-up practice patterns of gynecologic oncologists.

Methods.—We created four idealized vignettes describing patients with stages I–III ovarian cancer. We mailed a custom-designed survey instrument based on the vignettes to the members of the Society of Gynecologic Oncologists (SGO). SGO members were asked, via this instrument, how often they requested 11 discrete follow-up evaluations for their patients for the first 10 postoperative years after treatment with curative intent.

Results.—We received 283 evaluable responses (30%) from the 943 SGO members and candidate members. The most frequently performed items for each year were office visit, pelvic examination, and serum CA-125 level. Imaging studies such as chest X-ray, abdominal–pelvic CT, chest CT, abdominal–pelvic MRI, and transvaginal ultrasound were rarely recommended. There was marked variation in the frequency of use of most tests. There was a decrease in the frequency of testing over time for all modalities.

Conclusion.—This dataset provides detailed documentation of the self-reported surveillance practices of highly credentialed experts who manage patients with ovarian cancer in the 21st century. The optimal follow-up strategy remains unknown and controversial. Our survey showed marked variation in surveillance intensity. Identifying the sources of this variation warrants further research.

▶ The optimal follow-up for patients in clinical complete remission after initial management of ovarian carcinoma is not known. This study attempted to determine what gynecologic oncologists actually do in practice. Although no definitive conclusions can be drawn from the data, several interesting observations can be made. First of all, the number of patient visits per year declines as the time since initial diagnosis increases. The data basically show that the most intense follow-up focuses on the first 3 years. Reference to any survival curve for advanced ovarian carcinoma confirms the validity of this approach, as the fall-off of the survival curve is steep during the first 3 years and thus indicates that most recurrences take place during this period. Three to 4 visits per year for the first 3 years are thus reasonable with 2 visits per year for the next 2 years and 1 per year after that. Secondly, the data reflect a surprisingly low number of CT scans ordered in follow-up. This is not so surprising if one considers that the majority of advanced ovarian cancers produce CA-125 and that, in these patients, CA-125 is a reasonable predictor for recurrence. A recent European trial suggested that increasing CA-125 should not be used as an indicator for therapeutic intervention because there is no advantage to earlier treatment in that setting and because earlier intervention based solely on increasing CA-125 is associated with an earlier deterioration of quality of life. However, it is reasonable to use CA-125 as an indicator for ordering CT scans and other imaging to determine recurrence status, and such a use is associated with tremendous savings in the number of scans done.

J. T. Thigpen, MD

Pathologic findings following false-positive screening tests for ovarian cancer in the Prostate, Lung, Colorectal and Ovarian (PLCO) cancer screening trial

Nyante SJ, Black A, Kreimer AR, et al (Natl Cancer Inst, Rockville, MD; et al)
Gynecol Oncol 120:474-479, 2011

Objective.—In the Prostate, Lung, Colorectal and Ovarian Cancer Screening Trial (PLCO), ovarian cancer screening with transvaginal ultrasound (TVU) and CA-125 produced a large number of false-positive tests. We examined relationships between histopathologic diagnoses, false-positive test group, and participant and screening test characteristics.

Methods.—The PLCO ovarian cancer screening arm included 39,105 women aged 55–74 years assigned to annual CA-125 and TVU. Histopathologic diagnoses from women with false-positive tests and subsequent surgery were reviewed in this analysis: all CA125+ (n=121); all CA125+/TVU+ (n=46); and a random sample of TVU+ (n=373). Demographic and ovarian cancer risk factor data were self-reported. Pathologic diagnoses were abstracted from surgical pathology reports. We compared participant characteristics and pathologic diagnoses by category of false-positive using Pearson χ^2, Fisher's exact, or Wilcoxon-Mann-Whitney tests.

Results.—Women with a false-positive TVU were younger (P<0.001), heavier (P<0.001), and reported a higher frequency of prior hysterectomy (P<0.001). Serous cystadenoma, the most common benign ovarian diagnosis, was more frequent among women with TVU+ compared to CA-125+ and CA-125+/TVU+ (P<0.001). Benign non-ovarian findings were commonly associated with all false-positives, although more frequently with CA-125+ than TVU+ or CA-125+/TVU+ groups (P=0.019). Non-ovarian cancers were diagnosed most frequently among CA-125+ (P<0.001).

Conclusions.—False-positive ovarian cancer screening tests were associated with a range of histopathologic diagnoses, some of which may be related to patient and screening test characteristics. Further research into the predictors of false-positive ovarian cancer screening tests may aid efforts to reduce false-positive results.

▶ The ovarian portion of the Prostate, Lung, Colorectal and Ovarian Cancer Screening Trial was reported 2 years ago and showed a positive predictive value of 1.3%. This means that of 100 women with positive screening results, 98 did not have ovarian cancer. Most of these patients with false-positive results underwent exploratory laparotomies or laparoscopies (a major invasive procedure). While the conclusion of the investigators in this article is that further research needs to be done to reduce the number of false-positive results, the very low positive predictive value and the significant price for a patient to pay for a false-positive test (a major invasive procedure) suggest that an entirely different approach might be in order. It should be noted, however, that there is 1 trial that presents some hope for the use of CA-125 and transvaginal sonography. Investigators in the United Kingdom conducted a trial that included more than 200 000 women randomly assigned to no screening, screening with transvaginal sonography, or screening with serial CA-125s analyzed by an algorithm (ROCA), which triggers the use of transvaginal sonography. The last option, ROCA-analyzed CA-125 followed by transvaginal ultrasound, yielded a positive predictive value of 35%. If this number holds and leads to a reduction in ovarian cancer mortality, such an approach would then constitute a valid screening test for ovarian cancer. No other approach has to date shown evidence of accomplishing the goal of reduced mortality due to ovarian cancer.

J. T. Thigpen, MD

The Use of Recombinant Erythropoietin for the Treatment of Chemotherapy-Induced Anemia in Patients With Ovarian Cancer Does Not Affect Progression-Free or Overall Survival

Cantrell LA, Westin SN, Van Le L (Univ of Virginia, Charlottesville; The Univ of Texas M D Anderson Cancer Ctr, Houston; University of North Carolina, Chapel Hill)

Cancer 117:1220-1226, 2011

Background.—Studies have suggested that erythropoietin-stimulating agents (ESAs) may affect progression-free survival (PFS) and overall survival (OS) in a variety of cancer types. Because this finding had not been explored previously in ovarian or primary peritoneal carcinoma, the authors of this report analyzed their ovarian cancer population to determine whether ESA treatment for chemotherapy-induced anemia affected PFS or OS.

Methods.—A retrospective review was conducted of women who were treated for ovarian cancer at the corresponding author's institution over a 10-year period (from January 1994 to May 2004). Treatment groups were formed based on the use of an ESA. Two analyses of survival were conducted to determine the effect of ESA therapy on PFS and OS. Disease status was modeled as a function of treatment group using a logistic regression model. Kaplan-Meier curves were generated to compare the groups, and a Cox proportional hazards model was fit to the data.

Results.—In total, 343 women were identified. The median age was 57 (interquartile range, 48-68 years). The majority of women were Caucasian (n = 255; 74%) and were diagnosed with stage III (n = 210; 61%), epithelial (n = 268; 78%) ovarian cancer. Although the disease stage at diagnosis and surgical staging significantly affected the rates of disease recurrence and OS, the receipt of an ESA had no effect on PFS ($P = .9$) or OS ($P = .25$).

Conclusions.—The current results indicated that there was no difference in cancer-related PFS or OS with use of ESA in this cohort of women treated for ovarian cancer.

► The use of erythropoietic agents in the management of patients with cancer was based on 3 phase III trials showing a significant improvement in quality of life in those who responded to such treatment. In addition, several retrospective studies, particularly in carcinoma of the cervix, suggested an improvement in survival coincident with an increase in hemoglobin to 12 g/dL. Use of these was widespread until the reports of studies in head and neck cancer suggesting that use of erythropoietin-stimulating agents (ESAs) was associated with a decrease in survival, the opposite of what had been reported in retrospective studies. The Food and Drug Administration subsequently issued a black box warning, suggesting that such use was associated with a decrease in survival, although, at least in the case of cervix cancer, the cited study did not show a significant decrease in survival, although the trials showing decreased survival occurred in the setting in which ESAs were being used well beyond the increase in hemoglobin to 12 g/dL. As a result of the black box warning, the use of ESAs has been sharply curtailed. This study looks at ovarian carcinoma to determine whether there was any evidence of a decrease in survival associated with the use of ESAs. As is noted in the abstract, no such decrease can be detected. The issue of whether there is an associated improvement in quality of life with improvement in hemoglobin was not addressed in the trial, although prior studies as noted above are associated with a significant improvement in quality of life. Should we therefore be using ESAs to improve quality of life despite the black box warning? Under current circumstances, which require that the patient sign a detailed and onerous consent, it is very difficult to use the ESAs—a shame, given the improvement in quality of life associated with their use.

J. T. Thigpen, MD

Cervix

Ifosfamide, paclitaxel, and carboplatin, a novel triplet regimen for advanced, recurrent, or persistent carcinoma of the cervix: A phase II trial

Downs LS Jr, Chura JC, Argenta PA, et al (Univ of Minnesota, Minneapolis)

Gynecol Oncol 120:265-269, 2011

Objectives.—(1) To determine the response rate of advanced, recurrent, or persistent carcinoma of the cervix to ifosfamide, paclitaxel, and carboplatin chemotherapy; (2) to determine the progression free interval and survival rate in patients treated with this regimen; (3) to describe the toxicities associated with this regimen; and (4) to evaluate the quality of life of patients while on treatment.

Methods.—Eligible patients had histologically proven stage IVB, recurrent, or persistent carcinoma of the cervix not amenable to curative treatment with surgery and/or radiation therapy. Chemotherapy was given on day 1 of a 28-day cycle: mesna (600 mg/m^2) prior to ifosfamide (2 g/m^2), paclitaxel (175 mg/m^2), carboplatin (AUC 5). Response rates were determined according to RECIST criteria. Toxicity was graded according the National Cancer Institute's common toxicity criteria. Quality of life measurements were obtained using the FACT-Cx.

Results.—Twenty-eight patients participated in this study, with 21 evaluable for response rate. Overall, 7 patients (33%) had a demonstrated objective response (4 complete responses, 3 partial responses). Stable disease was documented in 3 patients. The overall median survival for all patients was 10 months. Median progression free survival for evaluable patients was 5.0 months. Bone marrow suppression was the most common toxicity. There were no negative effects of this treatment regimen on quality of life assessments.

Conclusion.—Ifosfamide, paclitaxel, and carboplatin is an effective regimen in treating advanced or recurrent carcinoma of the cervix and has an acceptable toxicity profile.

▶ This relatively small phase II trial of the combination of paclitaxel, ifosfamide, and carboplatin raises several issues in the use of systemic therapy for patients with recurrent carcinoma of the cervix. The current evidence-based standard of care for carcinoma of the cervix is a 2-drug combination of paclitaxel and cisplatin based on a series of Gynecologic Oncology Group (GOG) trials, the last of which showed an advantage for paclitaxel and cisplatin compared with topotecan and cisplatin, gemcitabine and cisplatin, and vinorelbine and cisplatin in regard to both progression-free survival and overall survival. The continued use of cisplatin as opposed to carboplatin in the GOG trials is based on earlier trials involving the 2 agents. Although not directly comparing these 2 platinum agents, the studies strongly suggest that cisplatin is the better of the 2 agents in carcinoma of the cervix. Studies outside of the GOG have suggested that ifosfamide is an active agent against cervix carcinoma. Creating a triplet regimen of paclitaxel plus a platinum agent plus ifosfamide thus makes sense. Based on prior studies, the preferred platinum agent would have been cisplatin, not carboplatin. The results of this small study, however, do not suggest that adding the third agent enhances the activity of the combination. The response rate of 33% is similar to the response rates of the 4 doublets tested in GOG 204 (all around 30%) and similar to the response rates for doublets in previous GOG trials comparing single-agent cisplatin with cisplatin-based doublets. The investigators claim that the triplet is less neurotoxic than cisplatin-based doublets, but the prior experience of the GOG with paclitaxel and cisplatin in ovarian carcinoma suggests that as long as the paclitaxel is given as a 24-hour infusion with cisplatin, there is little problem with neurotoxicity (see GOG 211). There is, therefore, little reason to proceed with further testing of the triplet and abundant reason to substitute carboplatin for cisplatin cautiously, if at all, in cervix carcinoma.

J. T. Thigpen, MD

Phase II study of cisplatin plus cetuximab in advanced, recurrent, and previously treated cancers of the cervix and evaluation of epidermal growth factor receptor immunohistochemical expression: A Gynecologic Oncology Group study

Farley J, Sill MW, Birrer M, et al (Uniformed Services Univ of the Health Sciences, Bethesda, MD; Roswell Park Cancer Inst, Buffalo, NY; Massachusetts General Hosp, Boston, MA; et al)

Gynecol Oncol 121:303-308, 2011

Background.—The purpose of this study was to evaluate the safety and efficacy of cetuximab (C225), an antibody that inhibits epidermal growth factor receptor (EGFR) activity, with cisplatin and to explore associations between EGFR protein expression with patient demographics or clinical outcome.

Methods.—Women with advanced, persistent, or recurrent carcinoma of the cervix were eligible. The women received cisplatin at 30 mg/m^2 on days 1 and 8 with a loading dose of cetuximab at 400 mg/m^2 followed by 250 mg/m^2 on days 1, 8, and 15 in a 21 day cycle. Adverse events were assessed with CTCAE v 3.0. Primary measure of efficacy was tumor response by RECIST. The study was stratified by prior chemotherapy (CT). EGFR protein expression in pre-treatment tumor was analyzed by immunohistochemistry.

Results.—Between September 2004 and March 2008, 76 patients were enrolled. Of these, 69 were eligible and evaluable; 44 (64%) received prior chemotherapy. There were 4 responses in each group, prior chemotherapy and no chemotherapy, 9% and 16%, respectively. Grade 4 toxicities included anemia (1), allergy (1), metabolic (1), and vascular (1). The most common grade 3 toxicities were metabolic (15), dermatologic (8), fatigue (6), and gastrointestinal (6). EGFR protein was expressed in 47/48 (98%) of tumors analyzed with a median cellular expression of 81%. Exploratory analyses revealed a trend between the percentage of cells expressing EGFR protein and PFS (hazard ratio = 1.76, 95% confidence interval = 0.96–3.21).

Conclusions.—The combination of cetuximab with cisplatin was adequately tolerated but did not indicate additional benefit beyond cisplatin therapy.

► The current standard of care for the treatment of advanced or recurrent carcinoma of the cervix is a combination of paclitaxel plus cisplatin based on the results of Gynecologic Oncology Group (GOG) 240, which compared 4 doublets (paclitaxel/cisplatin, topotecan/cisplatin, gemcitabine/cisplatin, and vinorelbine/cisplatin). The GOG has in place a concerted program to evaluate the potential role of new agents in combination with cisplatin. This program consists of a series of phase II studies of new agents and doublets with a bar that the new combination must reach to justify a phase III trial in comparison to paclitaxel/cisplatin. This study is one of this series that evaluates the combination of cisplatin plus cetuximab. The justification for evaluating cetuximab relates to its activities in squamous cell carcinomas of other sites such as the head and neck and positive phase II studies of cetuximab as a single agent in cervix carcinoma. The study treated 76 patients with cisplatin plus cetuximab and observed response rates of 9% in those with prior chemotherapy and 16% in those with prior chemotherapy. These response rates were consistent with response rates seen with cisplatin alone (in fact actually slightly worse), so the conclusion of the study was that there was no further interest in the combination of cisplatin plus cetuximab. The one interesting positive finding was a correlation between the level of epidermal growth factor receptor expression and likelihood of response to treatment. The take-home message is that paclitaxel/cisplatin remains the treatment of choice in recurrent carcinoma of the cervix.

J. T. Thigpen, MD

Phase III, Open-Label, Randomized Study Comparing Concurrent Gemcitabine Plus Cisplatin and Radiation Followed by Adjuvant Gemcitabine and Cisplatin Versus Concurrent Cisplatin and Radiation in Patients With Stage IIB to IVA Carcinoma of the Cervix

Dueñas-González A, Zarbá JJ, Patel F, et al (Universidad Nacional Autónoma de México; Med Ctr, San Roque, Tucumán, Argentina; Eli Lilly Interamerica, Buenos Aires, Argentina; et al)

J Clin Oncol 29:1678-1685, 2011

Purpose.—To determine whether addition of gemcitabine to concurrent cisplatin chemoradiotherapy and as adjuvant chemotherapy with cisplatin improves progression-free survival (PFS) at 3 years compared with current standard of care in locally advanced cervical cancer.

Patients and Methods.—Eligible chemotherapy- and radiotherapy-naive patients with stage IIB to IVA disease and Karnofsky performance score ≥70 were randomly assigned to arm A (cisplatin 40 mg/m^2 and gemcitabine 125 mg/m^2 weekly for 6 weeks with concurrent external-beam radiotherapy [XRT] 50.4 Gy in 28 fractions, followed by brachytherapy [BCT] 30 to 35 Gy in 96 hours, and then two adjuvant 21-day cycles of cisplatin, 50 mg/m^2 on day 1, plus gemcitabine, 1,000 mg/m^2 on days 1 and 8) or to arm B (cisplatin and concurrent XRT followed by BCT only; dosing same as for arm A).

Results.—Between May 2002 and March 2004, 515 patients were enrolled (arm A, n = 259; arm B, n = 256). PFS at 3 years was significantly improved in arm A versus arm B (74.4% *v* 65.0%, respectively; P = .029), as were overall PFS (log-rank P = .0227; hazard ratio [HR], 0.68; 95% CI, 0.49 to 0.95), overall survival (log-rank P = .0224; HR, 0.68; 95% CI, 0.49 to 0.95), and time to progressive disease (log-rank P = .0012; HR, 0.54; 95% CI, 0.37 to 0.79). Grade 3 and 4 toxicities were more frequent in arm A than in arm B (86.5% *v* 46.3%, respectively; $P < .001$), including two deaths possibly related to treatment toxicity in arm A.

Conclusion.—Gemcitabine plus cisplatin chemoradiotherapy followed by BCT and adjuvant gemcitabine/cisplatin chemotherapy improved survival outcomes with increased but clinically manageable toxicity when compared with standard treatment.

► In February 1999, the National Cancer Institute of the United States released a clinical alert to notify all oncologists that 5 randomized trials including 6 comparisons showed that the concurrent use of cisplatin-based chemotherapy with radiation in the treatment of stages IB to IVA carcinoma of the cervix resulted in a significant reduction in mortality ranging from 24% to 51%. Since then, the standard of care for patients with stages IB to IVA carcinoma of the cervix has been the concurrent use of radiation plus weekly cisplatin, 40 mg/m^2. This trial reports the use of combination chemotherapy (gemcitabine plus cisplatin) concurrently with chemotherapy followed by 2 additional cycles of chemotherapy (gemcitabine plus cisplatin). This regimen was compared with weekly cisplatin plus radiation and showed a superior progression-free and overall survival at the expense of some increase in toxicity of tolerable magnitude. These results suggest that combination chemotherapy might yield superior results to the use of single-agent cisplatin. At least in the hands of the Gynecologic Oncology Group (GOG), the combination of paclitaxel/cisplatin is superior to gemcitabine/cisplatin, and these results have now become the basis for an international study using the paclitaxel/cisplatin combination in place of gemcitabine/cisplatin in a randomized trial similar to that reported here. For now, the standard remains weekly cisplatin plus radiation for stages IB to IVA carcinoma of the cervix.

J. T. Thigpen, MD

Endometrial

A feasibility study of carboplatin and weekly paclitaxel combination chemotherapy in endometrial cancer: A Kansai Clinical Oncology Group study (KCOG0015 trial)

Ito K, Tsubamoto H, Itani Y, et al (Kansai Rosai Hosp, Amagasaki, Hyogo, Japan; Hyogo College of Medicine, Nishinomiya, Hyogo, Japan; Nara Prefectural Nara Hosp, Hiramatsu, Japan; et al)
Gynecol Oncol 120:193-197, 2011

Objectives.—The optimal chemotherapy regimen for women with endometrial cancer has not been established. We assessed the feasibility, toxicity and clinical efficacy of combination triweekly carboplatin and weekly paclitaxel in women with endometrial cancer.

Methods.—Eligible patients had histologically confirmed primary advanced or recurrent endometrial cancer (Group A), or had localized high-risk features (Group B). All were treated with paclitaxel 80 mg/m^2 (days 1, 8 and 15) and carboplatin AUC 5 (day 1) each 21-day cycle. A minimum of 3 cycles was planned; if 75% or more of patients were able to receive at least 3 cycles with acceptable toxicity, the regimen was declared "feasible."

Results.—Forty patients were enrolled and administered 163 cycles of therapy; 38 (95%) were chemo-naive. No patients received radiation previously. Group A (measurable disease) contained 15 patients (5 with recurrent disease, 7 receiving neo-adjuvant chemotherapy, and 3 treated adjuvantly following suboptimal cytoreduction). Group B (non-measurable disease) contained 25 patients (primary stage I:10, II:5, III:8, IV:1 and relapse 1). Hematological toxicities(G3/G4) were neutropenia (31%/33%) and thrombocytopenia (6%/0%). Reversible G3 hypersensitivity (5%) and G2 cardiotoxicity (3%) was uncommon. Thirty-one patients (78%) completed ≥ 3 cycles (median 4, range: 1–9). Thirteen of 15 (87%) measurable patients responded (3CR, 10PR). Eighty-seven percent of measurable patients were not progressive at 6 months. In Group A, QOL scores were significantly improved after 3 cycles of chemotherapy (p=0.037), and at the completion of chemotherapy (p=0.045). QOL scores in Group B did not change during therapy.

Conclusions.—This combination chemotherapy is feasible and effective for endometrial cancer patients.

▶ Studies of weekly paclitaxel in breast cancer and in ovarian cancer have suggested that weekly paclitaxel is superior to every-3-week paclitaxel. In the case of ovarian cancer, this observation was based on a large Japanese phase III trial in which paclitaxel was combined with carboplatin. Currently, 3 phase III trials, 2 in Europe and 1 in the United States, are seeking to confirm or refute the results in ovarian cancer. These investigators have taken the Japanese regimen and have applied it to patients who have endometrial cancer with results that suggest that this approach may also work in endometrial cancer. Three words of caution, however, should be noted. First, this study is very small and uncontrolled and, therefore, should not be taken as establishing the value of this approach in endometrial cancer until confirmed in a phase III trial. Second, the evidence-based standard of care for patients with endometrial cancer is a 3-drug combination of paclitaxel, doxorubicin, and cisplatin based on a previously reported phase III trial by the Gynecologic Oncology Group (GOG). The GOG has completed a study comparing the 3-drug regimen with paclitaxel plus carboplatin, but until results are available, paclitaxel plus carboplatin is not the evidence-based standard of care. Third, in patients with ovarian cancer, neurotoxicity has been a major problem with the weekly regimen, but this small trial in endometrial cancer does not show that. A larger trial is needed to assess this issue. For now, the standard of care should remain paclitaxel, doxorubicin, and cisplatin.

J. T. Thigpen, MD

CA 125 normalization with chemotherapy is independently predictive of survival in advanced endometrial cancer

Hoskins PJ, Le N, Correa R (BC Cancer Agency, Vancouver, Canada)

Gynecol Oncol 120:52-55, 2011

Objective.—Changes in CA 125 with chemotherapy predict outcome for epithelial ovarian cancer. There is no such data for advanced endometrial cancer.

Method.—Retrospective review of all women receiving carboplatin and paclitaxel for advanced endometrial cancer at any of the institutions of the British Columbia Cancer Agency between September 1995 and September 2006.

Results.—185 newly diagnosed women were treated. Univariable analysis for progression-free survival identified as adverse predictors: grade 3, positive residual, age >60, deep myometrial invasion, increasing stage/substage, papillary serous subtype, presence of cervical involvement, ECOG 1 or greater, CA 125 above 35 either preoperatively or at start of cycle 1 and CA 125 greater than 24 at the start of cycle 3. Upon multivariate analysis, CA 125 above 24 at cycle 3, grade 3 and positive residual remained as independent predictors. The single most important factor identified by decision tree analysis was CA 125 level at cycle 3.

Conclusion.—As with epithelial ovarian cancer, changes in CA 125 are highly predictive of outcome for advanced, chemotherapy treated endometrial cancer.

▶ CA-125 is the most commonly used marker to determine status of disease in patients with ovarian carcinoma. While CA-125 is not an effective early diagnostic tool, the increase and decrease of marker levels during treatment provides an excellent guide as to whether the disease is responding and whether scans need to be considered. It has been known for some time that CA-125 can also be elevated in patients with endometrial carcinoma, but there is a lack of data evaluating CA-125 as a marker of disease status. This study evaluated CA-125 in 185 patients treated with chemotherapy in British Columbia, Canada. The data demonstrate that CA-125 is a reasonable marker for disease recurrence and for likelihood of recurrence as treatment proceeds. As with ovarian carcinoma, the rate of decrease of CA-125 appears to be an indicator of both response and the durability of that response with a rapid fall marking an excellent response. Based on the data from this patient set, the CA-125 level at the time of cycle 3 provides the best indicator of risk of progression (less than or greater than 24). This should provide the physician with a reliable and inexpensive method for following the progress of chemotherapy treatment of patients with endometrial carcinoma. This is particularly important, as the role of chemotherapy in the disease is expanding.

J. T. Thigpen, MD

Phase II study of fulvestrant in recurrent/metastatic endometrial carcinoma: A Gynecologic Oncology Group Study

Covens AL, Filiaci V, Gersell D, et al (Univ of Toronto, Ontario, Canada; Roswell Park Cancer Inst, Buffalo, NY; et al)

Gynecol Oncol 120:185-188, 2011

Objectives.—To evaluate the activity and toxicity of fulvestrant in advanced, recurrent, or persistent endometrial carcinoma.

Methods.—Eligible patients with advanced, recurrent or persistent endometrial carcinoma not amenable to curative therapy were treated with fulvestrant at a dose of 250 mg by IM injection every 4 weeks for at least 8 weeks. Therapy was continued until evidence of progressive disease, or adverse effects prohibited further therapy. Response was assessed in patients with at least one target lesion as defined by Response Evaluation Criteria in Solid Tumors (RECIST) v1.0. Immunohistochemical analysis of tumor tissue (histology or cytology) for estrogen and progesterone receptors was required from the metastatic or recurrent site.

Results.—Sixty-seven patients were enrolled in this study. Upon review, 14 patients were excluded. In the 22 estrogen receptor (ER) negative patients, no patients demonstrated either a complete or partial response, and 4 (18%) demonstrated stable disease (as best response). In the 31 ER positive patients, 1 (3%), 4 (13%) and 9 (29%) patients demonstrated a complete, partial response, and stable disease (as best response), respectively. The median progression free survival and overall survival in the ER negative patients were 2 and 3 months and in the ER positive patients 10 and 26 months. Treatment was well tolerated, and no patient discontinued therapy due to toxicity.

Conclusions.—Fulvestrant has minimal activity in advanced, recurrent, or persistent endometrial carcinoma.

▶ Endometrial carcinoma is the most common invasive malignancy of the female genital tract (~40 000 cases per year in the United States). Because 88% of cases present as stage I or II disease and are managed with surgery with or without radiation, the role of systemic therapy has been limited. Prior to 2003 and the demonstration that endometrial carcinoma was actually very responsive to combination chemotherapy (Gynecologic Oncology Group [GOG] 122 and 177), hormonal therapy was the mainstay of systemic therapy with the only active agents being progestins. In patients with recurrent disease, response rates to progestin ranged from 16% to 25%. Hormonal therapy is still a valid option that is used at some point in most patients with advanced or recurrent disease. The GOG has conducted a series of phase II trials of hormonal agents to identify other active options. Fulvestrant, the most recent agent in this line of studies, actually shows activity that is not substantially different from that of progestins (16%) in those patients with estrogen receptor (ER)-positive disease. Despite the conclusion that this agent has minimal activity, one could justify its use in patients who have exhausted other chemotherapeutic and hormonal options if the cancer is either known ER positive or grade 1 (84% ER+).

J. T. Thigpen, MD

4 Genitourinary

Prostate

Active Surveillance Compared With Initial Treatment for Men With Low-Risk Prostate Cancer: A Decision Analysis

Hayes JH, Ollendorf DA, Pearson SD, et al (Harvard Med School, Boston, MA; et al)

JAMA 304:2373-2380, 2010

Context.—In the United States, 192 000 men were diagnosed as having prostate cancer in 2009, the majority with low-risk, clinically localized disease. Treatment of these cancers is associated with substantial morbidity. Active surveillance is an alternative to initial treatment, but long-term outcomes and effect on quality of life have not been well characterized.

Objective.—To examine the quality-of-life benefits and risks of active surveillance compared with initial treatment for men with low-risk, clinically localized prostate cancer.

Design and Setting.—Decision analysis using a simulation model was performed: men were treated at diagnosis with brachytherapy, intensity-modulated radiation therapy (IMRT), or radical prostatectomy or followed up by active surveillance (a strategy of close monitoring of newly diagnosed patients with serial prostate-specific antigen measurements, digital rectal examinations, and biopsies, with treatment at disease progression or patient choice). Probabilities and utilities were derived from previous studies and literature review. In the base case, the relative risk of prostate cancer–specific death for initial treatment vs active surveillance was assumed to be 0.83. Men incurred short- and long-term adverse effects of treatment.

Patients.—Hypothetical cohorts of 65-year-old men newly diagnosed as having clinically localized, low-risk prostate cancer (prostate-specific antigen level <10 ng/mL, stage ≤T2a disease, and Gleason score ≤6).

Main Outcome Measure.—Quality-adjusted life expectancy (QALE).

Results.—Active surveillance was associated with the greatest QALE (11.07 quality-adjusted life-years [QALYs]), followed by brachytherapy (10.57 QALYs), IMRT (10.51 QALYs), and radical prostatectomy (10.23 QALYs). Active surveillance remained associated with the highest QALE even if the relative risk of prostate cancer–specific death for initial treatment vs active surveillance was as low as 0.6. However, the QALE gains and the optimal strategy were highly dependent on individual preferences for living under active surveillance and for having been treated.

Conclusions.—Under a wide range of assumptions, for a 65-year-old man, active surveillance is a reasonable approach to low-risk prostate cancer based on QALE compared with initial treatment. However, individual preferences play a central role in the decision whether to treat or to pursue active surveillance.

▶ Prostate cancer remains a challenge for the patients it afflicts as well as the physicians who guide the patient's decision after diagnosis. On one hand there are data that support the use of prostate-specific antigen (PSA) screening and treatment to reduce prostate cancer mortality. Yet the majority of patients diagnosed with prostate cancer fall into the "low-risk" category (PSA < 10, GS < 6, T-stage < T2a), where the risk of death related to the disease is very low.

Given the low risk of prostate cancer—related death in these patients, quality of life among the different forms of treatment and active surveillance is very important. These authors have looked at the quality-adjusted life expectancy (QALE) for patients treated for their prostate cancer with surgery, brachytherapy, intensity-modulated radiation therapy (IMRT), or active surveillance. QALE was superior for active surveillance patients as opposed to those who received upfront treatment. Yet this was highly dependent on the patient's preferences for the upfront treatment versus active surveillance. These data are important as they once again emphasize the need for all urologists and radiation oncologists to offer active surveillance as an excellent alternative and support patients who choose active surveillance as a way to address their localized prostate cancer.

C. A. Lawton, MD

Clinical Results of Long-Term Follow-Up of a Large, Active Surveillance Cohort With Localized Prostate Cancer

Klotz L, Zhang L, Lam A, et al (Univ of Toronto, Ontario, Canada)

J Clin Oncol 28:126-131, 2010

Purpose.—We assessed the outcome of a watchful-waiting protocol with selective delayed intervention by using clinical prostate-specific antigen (PSA), or histologic progression as treatment indications for clinically localized prostate cancer.

Patients and Methods.—This was a prospective, single-arm, cohort study. Patients were managed with an initial expectant approach. Definitive intervention was offered to those patients with a PSA doubling time of less than 3 years, Gleason score progression (to 4 + 3 or greater), or unequivocal clinical progression. Survival analysis and Cox proportional hazard model were applied to the data.

Results.—A total of 450 patients have been observed with active surveillance. Median follow-up was 6.8 years (range, 1 to 13 years). Overall survival was 78.6%. The 10-year prostate cancer actuarial survival was 97.2%. Overall, 30% of patients have been reclassified as higher risk and have been offered definitive therapy. Of 117 patients treated radically, the PSA failure rate was 50%, which was 13% of the total cohort. PSA doubling time of 3 years or less was associated with an 8.5-times higher risk of biochemical failure after definitive treatment compared with a doubling time of more than 3 years ($P < .0001$). The hazard ratio for nonprostate cancer to prostate cancer mortality was 18.6 at 10 years.

Conclusion.—We observed a low rate of prostate cancer mortality. Among the patients who were reclassified as higher risk and who were treated, PSA failure was relatively common. Other-cause mortality accounted for almost all of the deaths. Additional studies are warranted to improve the identification of patients who harbor more aggressive disease despite favorable clinical parameters at diagnosis.

▶ Prostate cancer claims the lives of over 25 000 American men annually. Yet many groups such as the American Cancer Society do not support routine prostate-specific antigen (PSA) screening to detect prostate cancer. The major concern for not supporting routine screening is not overdiagnosis but overtreatment. Active surveillance is the obvious answer for those patients diagnosed with prostate cancer with low-risk features. Active surveillance if done correctly as in this trial, requires regular PSAs, digital rectal examinations, and rebiopsies. If this is done as the trial shows, the risk of death from prostate cancer does not appear to go up, and it saves many patients from overtreatment.

Active surveillance as performed in this trial requires:

1. PSA values every 3 months for 2 years then every 6 months if stable.
2. Digital rectal examination done annually at a minimum.
3. Rebiopsy within 6 to 12 months of initial diagnosis then every 3 to 4 years to age 80 years.

Patients whose Gleason scores increase, whose digital rectal examination confirms progression, or whose PSA doubling time is less than 3 years are offered treatment (ie, reclassified to high risk). Once treated, these patients' outcomes were not significantly different from historical controls of up front treatment for similar PSA, Gleason score, and T-stage patients.

These data reinforce the need to treat or actively surveil patients based on the factors they present with (ie, PSA, Gleason score, and T-stage). It further helps to support the use of PSA screening in an effort to diagnosis some of these American men who will likely die of this disease, as PSA doubling time of less than 3 years was associated with the worse outcome.

C. A. Lawton, MD

Development of RTOG consensus guidelines for the definition of the clinical target volume for postoperative conformal radiation therapy for prostate cancer

Michalski JM, Lawton C, El Naqa I, et al (Washington Univ School of Medicine, St Louis, MO; Med College of Wisconsin, Milwaukee; et al)

Int J Radiat Oncol Biol Phys 76:361-368, 2010

Purpose.—To define a prostate fossa clinical target volume (PF-CTV) for Radiation Therapy Oncology Group (RTOG) trials using postoperative radiotherapy for prostate cancer.

Methods and Materials.—An RTOG-sponsored meeting was held to define an appropriate PF-CTV after radical prostatectomy. Data were presented describing radiographic failure patterns after surgery. Target volumes used in previous trials were reviewed. Using contours independently submitted by 13 radiation oncologists, a statistical imputation method derived a preliminary "consensus" PF-CTV.

Results.—Starting from the model-derived CTV, consensus was reached for a CT image–based PF-CTV. The PFCTV should extend superiorly from the level of the caudal vas deferens remnant to >8–12 mm inferior to vesicourethral anastomosis (VUA). Below the superior border of the pubic symphysis, the anterior border extends to the posterior aspect of the pubis and posteriorly to the rectum, where it may be concave at the level of the VUA. At this level, the lateral border extends to the levator ani. Above the pubic symphysis, the anterior border should encompass the posterior 1–2 cm of the bladder wall; posteriorly, it is bounded by the mesorectal fascia. At this level, the lateral border is the sacrorectogenitopubic fascia. Seminal vesicle remnants, if present, should be included in the CTV if there is pathologic evidence of their involvement.

Conclusions.—Consensus on postoperative PF-CTV for RT after prostatectomy was reached and is available as a CT image atlas on the RTOG website. This will allow uniformity in defining PF-CTV for clinical trials that include postprostatectomy RT.

▶ The appropriate target volume for postoperative radiation therapy in prostate cancer seems to be straightforward. Obviously the radiation oncologist needs to treat the prostate bed with attention to the location of any extracapsular extension or positive margins and, of course, whether the seminal vesicles were involved or not. That said, when Radiation Therapy Oncology Group (RTOG) genitourinary (GU) radiation oncologists outlined their definition of this volume, there was major disagreement. Volumes ranged from very small "prostate only" to "mini pelvis" volumes.

RTOG GU radiation oncologists reviewed the literature, studied the appropriate volumes, and came to a consensus that is outlined in this article. They are to be commended for this work, as it was well researched and the consensus guidelines are clear (and the volumes take into account whether the seminal vesicles are involved or not).

As more and more radiation oncologists consider transitioning from 3-dimensional to intensity-modulated radiation therapy for postoperative radiation therapy in prostate cancer, it is imperative that the volumes as outlined in these guidelines are followed. This will ensure that the target is treated and should still allow for proper protection of organs at risk, in particular bladder and rectum.

C. A. Lawton, MD

Do Anxiety and Distress Increase During Active Surveillance for Low Risk Prostate Cancer?

van den Bergh RCN, Essink-Bot M-L, Roobol MJ, et al (Erasmus Med Ctr, Rotterdam, The Netherlands)

J Urol 183:1786-1791, 2010

Purpose.—Anxiety and distress may be present in patients with low risk prostate cancer who are on active surveillance. This may be a reason to discontinue active surveillance.

Materials and Methods.—A total of 150 Dutch patients with prostate cancer on active surveillance in a prospective active surveillance study received questionnaires at study inclusion and 9 months after diagnosis. We assessed changes in scores on decisional conflict with the decisional conflict scale, depression with the Center for Epidemiologic Studies Depression Scale, generic anxiety with the State Trait Anxiety Inventory, prostate cancer specific anxiety with the Memorial Anxiety Scale for Prostate Cancer and the self-estimated risk of progression. We explored scores 9 months after diagnosis vs those at study inclusion for physical health (SF-12® physical component summary), personality (Eysenck Personality Questionnaire), shared decision making, prostate cancer knowledge, demographics, medical parameters and prostate specific antigen doubling time during followup.

Results.—Questionnaires at study inclusion and 9 months after diagnosis were completed by 129 of 150 (86%) and 108 of 120 participants (90%) a median of 2.4 and 9.2 months after diagnosis, respectively. Anxiety and distress at study inclusion were previously found to be generally favorable. Significant but clinically irrelevant decreases were seen in mean scores of the State Trait Anxiety Inventory ($p = 0.016$), Memorial Anxiety Scale for Prostate Cancer fear of progression subscale ($p = 0.005$) and the self-estimated risk of progression ($p = 0.049$). Anxiety and distress 9 months after diagnosis were mainly predicted by scores at study inclusion. Higher Eysenck Personality Questionnaire neuroticism score and an important role of the physician in the treatment decision had additionally unfavorable effects. Good physical health, palpable disease and older age had favorable effects. No association was seen for prostate specific antigen doubling time. Nine men discontinued active surveillance, including 2 due to nonmedical reasons.

Conclusions.—Anxiety and distress generally remain favorably low during the first 9 months of surveillance.

▶ Active surveillance for patients with low-risk prostate cancer is a reasonable option to consider and is supported by the National Comprehensive Cancer Network guidelines. It allows patients to avoid the toxicities of definitive surgery or radiation, both acute and long term. But the other potential toxicity of active surveillance may come in the form of increased anxiety regarding untreated cancer in one's body, which could be growing.

These authors have tried to assess this potential toxicity in 150 Dutch patients performing active surveillance with their prostate cancer via a prospective trial. This trial assessed anxiety and distress via questionnaire at the time of diagnosis and 9 months after diagnosis. The good news is that there did not appear to be a significant increase in either anxiety or distress for these patients during their first 9 months of active surveillance. Just how applicable this would be for men in the United States is not known and should be evaluated prospectively. In addition, it would be of interest to assess the level of distress and anxiety at an additional later time point to help reinforce these results and this option for low-risk prostate cancer patients.

C. A. Lawton, MD

Effect of Dutasteride on the Risk of Prostate Cancer

Andriole GL, for the REDUCE Study Group (Washington Univ School of Medicine in St Louis, MO; et al)

N Engl J Med 362:1192-1202, 2010

Background.—We conducted a study to determine whether dutasteride reduces the risk of incident prostate cancer, as detected on biopsy, among men who are at increased risk for the disease.

Methods.—In this 4-year, multicenter, randomized, double-blind, placebo-controlled, parallel-group study, we compared dutasteride, at a dose of 0.5 mg daily, with placebo. Men were eligible for inclusion in the study if they were 50 to 75 years of age, had a prostate-specific antigen (PSA) level of 2.5 to 10.0 ng per milliliter, and had one negative prostate biopsy (6 to 12 cores) within 6 months before enrollment. Subjects underwent a 10-core transrectal ultrasound-guided biopsy at 2 and 4 years.

Results.—Among 6729 men who underwent a biopsy or prostate surgery, cancer was detected in 659 of the 3305 men in the dutasteride group, as compared with 858 of the 3424 men in the placebo group, representing a relative risk reduction with dutasteride of 22.8% (95% confidence interval, 15.2 to 29.8) over the 4-year study period ($P<0.001$). Overall, in years 1 through 4, among the 6706 men who underwent a needle biopsy, there were 220 tumors with a Gleason score of 7 to 10 among 3299 men in the dutasteride group and 233 among 3407 men in the placebo group ($P=0.81$). During years 3 and 4, there were 12 tumors with a Gleason score of 8 to 10 in the dutasteride group, as compared with only 1 in the placebo group (P = 0.003). Dutasteride therapy, as compared with placebo, resulted in a reduction in the rate of acute urinary retention (1.6% vs. 6.7%, a 77.3% relative reduction). The incidence of adverse events was similar to that in studies of dutasteride therapy for benign prostatic hyperplasia, except that in our study, as compared with previous studies, the relative incidence of the composite category of cardiac failure was higher in the dutasteride group than in the placebo group (0.7% [30 men] vs. 0.4% [16 men], P = 0.03).

Conclusions.—Over the course of the 4-year study period, dutasteride reduced the risk of incident prostate cancer detected on biopsy and improved the outcomes related to benign prostatic hyperplasia. (ClinicalTrials.gov number, NCT00056407.)

▶ Adenocarcinoma of the prostate is the second leading cause of cancer deaths in American men. It deserves our attention in terms of ways to decrease its incidence, especially in high-risk populations. One potential to decrease the incidence is the use of 5α-reductase inhibitors, which are used to treat benign prostate hypertrophy. These drugs block the conversion of testosterone to dihydrotestosterone, and this may decrease the risk of prostate cancer. The first study of these drugs used finasteride (the Prostate Cancer Prevention Trial). It did show a decrease in the incidence of prostate cancer, but of the tumors that were detected, there was an increase in the Gleason score of 7 to 10 tumors. So caution was the operative mode for consideration of finasteride to prevent prostate cancer.

This trial evaluated dutasteride, a drug that inhibits both forms of 5α reductase in a double-blinded placebo-controlled parallel group study. Once again a decrease in prostate cancer incidence was found. In the first 4 years of the study, there was no difference in the detection of Gleason score of 7 to 10 tumors between the placebo versus the dutasteride groups. Yet during years 3 and 4, there was a large difference in the Gleason score of 8 to 10 tumors with 12 found in the dutasteride group and only 1 in the placebo group. The cause of these high-grade tumors in patients treated with these drugs is not known. Until it is better understood, caution should be used when considering 5α-reductase inhibitors to prevent prostate cancer.

C. A. Lawton, MD

Long-term toxicity following 3D conformal radiation therapy for prostate cancer from the RTOG 9406 phase I/II dose escalation study

Michalski JM, Bae K, Roach M, et al (Washington Univ Med School, St Louis, MO; Radiation Therapy Oncology Group, Philadelphia, PA; Univ of California-San Francisco; et al)

Int J Radiat Oncol Biol Phys 76:14-22, 2010

Purpose.—To update the incidence of late toxicity of RTOG 9406, a three-dimensional conformal radiation therapy (3DCRT) dose escalation trial for prostate cancer.

Methods and Materials.—A total of 1,084 men were registered to this Phase I/II trial of 3DCRT (eligible patients, 1,055). The dose for level I was 68.4 Gy; 73.8 Gy for level II; 79.2 Gy for level III; 74 Gy for level IV; and 78 Gy for level V. Patients in levels I to III received 1.8 Gy/fraction, and those in levels IV to V received 2.0 Gy/fraction. Disease group I patients were treated at the prostate only, group 2 patients were treated at the prostate and at the seminal vesicles with a prostate boost, and group 3 patients were treated at the prostate and seminal vesicles. The median follow-up period for surviving patients was 6.1 y (level V) to 12.1 y (level I).

Results.—The incidence rates of RTOG grade 3 or less gastrointestinal or genitourinary toxicity were 3%, 4%, 6%, 7%, and 9% in group 1 and 6%, 2%, 6%, 9%, and 12% in group 2 at dose levels of I, II, III, IV, and V, respectively. In group 1, level V patients had a higher probability of grade 2 late or greater gastrointestinal or genitourinary toxicity than those in levels I, II, and III (hazard ratio [HR] = 1.93, $p = 0.0101$; HR = 2.29, $p = 0.0007$; HR = 2.52, $p = 0.0002$, respectively). In group 2, dose level V patients had a higher probability of grade 2 or greater late gastrointestinal or genitourinary toxicity than those in dose levels II, III, and IV (HR = 2.61, $p = 0.0002$; HR = 2.22, $p = 0.0051$; HR = 1.60, $p = 0.0276$, respectively).

Conclusions.—Tolerance to high-dose 3DCRT remains excellent. There is significantly more grade 2 or greater toxicity with a dose of 78 Gy at 2 Gy/fraction than with 68.4 Gy to 79.2 Gy at 1.8 Gy/fraction and with 74 Gy at 2 Gy/fraction.

▶ Late toxicity with regard to radiation in prostate cancer is an important topic for 2 reasons. First, we need to compare the toxicity to other treatments for localized disease, such as surgery or brachytherapy. Second, as we push the doses higher and higher so as to cure more patients, we need to understand the potential consequences of this dose escalation.

This review by the Radiation Therapy Oncology Group (RTOG) of the late toxicities following dose escalated 3-dimensional (3D) conformal radiation therapy is just the type of data from which we can learn. RTOG institutions had to pass certain standards to accrue patients to this trial. So these results are not certain to be equal to the nationwide radiation therapy community as a whole. Yet they are some of the best data that we can look to for results from multiple institutions, and they don't suffer from single-institution biases.

Given the dose level of 68.4 to 79.2 Gy and the relatively low level of grade > 2 toxicity, both gastrointestinal and genitourinary, 3D dose escalated radiation therapy for localized prostate cancer is likely very safe treatment. The question of dose per fraction 1.8 versus 2.0 Gy needs to be investigated further.

C. A. Lawton, MD

Natural History of Clinically Staged Low- and Intermediate-Risk Prostate Cancer Treated With Monotherapeutic Permanent Interstitial Brachytherapy

Taira AV, Merrick GS, Galbreath RW, et al (Univ of Washington, Seattle; Schiffler Cancer Ctr and Wheeling Jesuit Univ, WV)

Int J Radiat Oncol Biol Phys 76:349-354, 2010

Purpose.—To evaluate the natural history of clinically staged low- and intermediate-risk prostate cancer treated with permanent interstitial seed implants as monotherapy.

Methods and Materials.—Between April 1995 and May 2005, 463 patients with clinically localized prostate cancer underwent brachytherapy as the sole definitive treatment. Men who received supplemental external beam radiotherapy or androgen deprivation therapy were excluded. Dosimetric implant quality was determined based on the minimum dose that covered 90% of the target volume and the volume of the prostate gland receiving 100% of the prescribed dose. Multiple parameters were evaluated as predictors of treatment outcomes.

Results.—The 12-year biochemical progression-free survival (bPFS), cause-specific survival, and overall survival rates for the entire cohort were 97.1%, 99.7%, and 75.4%, respectively. Only pretreatment prostate-specific antigen level, percent positive biopsy cores, and minimum dose that covered 90% of the target volume were significant predictors of biochemical recurrence. The bPFS, cause-specific survival, and overall survival rates were 97.4%, 99.6%, and 76.2%, respectively, for low-risk patients and 96.4%, 100%, and 74.0%, respectively, for intermediate-risk patients. The bPFS rate was 98.8% for low-risk patients with high-quality implants versus 92.1% for those with less adequate implants ($p < 0.01$), and it was 98.3% for intermediate-risk patients with high-quality implants versus 86.4% for those with less adequate implants ($p < 0.01$).

Conclusions.—High-quality brachytherapy implants as monotherapy can provide excellent outcomes for men with clinically staged low- and intermediate-risk prostate cancer. For these men, a high-quality implant can achieve results comparable to high-quality surgery in the most favorable pathologically staged patient subgroups.

► Prostate seed implants have become a standard-of-care option for low-risk prostate cancer patients. Long-term outcomes of >10 years have shown equivalence to surgery and high-dose external beam irradiation. Yet we also know that many of these low-risk patients have been overtreated by all of these modalities. Watchful waiting or active surveillance is likely an equivalent option for many of these low-risk patients.

The bigger question to answer is whether prostate cancer patients with more aggressive disease (ie, those with intermediate-risk disease) who are more likely to need some form of treatment are well served with seed implants as monotherapy. These authors have looked at both low- and intermediate-risk patients treated with interstitial brachytherapy alone and found it to be an excellent treatment option for both groups in terms of biochemical progression-free survival, cause-specific survival, and overall survival. The data have long-term follow-up and are an important contribution to the question of seed implants as monotherapy for intermediate-risk disease patients. It is very important to note, however, that the intermediate-risk patients in this cohort are at the more favorable end of the intermediate-risk spectrum with a median pretreatment prostate-specific antigen of 5.9 and a Gleason score <7 and 89% of the patients with clinical T2a or less disease. Whether prostate brachytherapy alone is appropriate for higher risk intermediate-risk patients is not known.

C. A. Lawton, MD

Overall survival analysis of a phase II randomized controlled trial of a Poxviral-based PSA-targeted immunotherapy in metastatic castration-resistant prostate cancer

Kantoff PW, Schuetz TJ, Blumenstein BA, et al (BN ImmunoTherapeutics, Mountain View, CA)

J Clin Oncol 28:1099-1105, 2010

Purpose.—Therapeutic prostate-specific antigen (PSA) -targeted poxviral vaccines for prostate cancer have been well tolerated. PROSTVAC-VF treatment was evaluated for safety and for prolongation of progression-free survival (PFS) and overall survival (OS) in a randomized, controlled, and blinded phase II study.

Patients and Methods.—In total, 125 patients were randomly assigned in a multicenter trial of vaccination series. Eligible patients had minimally symptomatic castration-resistant metastatic prostate cancer (mCRPC). PROSTVAC-VF comprises two recombinant viral vectors, each encoding transgenes for PSA, and three immune costimulatory molecules (B7.1, ICAM-1, and LFA-3). Vaccinia-based vector was used for priming followed by six planned fowlpox-based vector boosts. Patients were allocated (2:1) to PROSTVAC-VF plus granulocyte-macrophage colony-stimulating factor or to control empty vectors plus saline injections.

Results.—Eighty-two patients received PROSTVAC-VF and 40 received control vectors. Patient characteristics were similar in both groups. The primary end point was PFS, which was similar in the two groups (P = .6). However, at 3 years post study, PROSTVAC-VF patients had a better OS with 25 (30%) of 82 alive versus 7 (17%) of 40 controls, longer median survival by 8.5 months (25.1 v 16.6 months for controls), an estimated hazard ratio of 0.56 (95% CI, 0.37 to 0.85), and stratified log-rank P = .0061.

Conclusion.—PROSTVAC-VF immunotherapy was well tolerated and associated with a 44% reduction in the death rate and an 8.5-month improvement in median OS in men with mCRPC. These provocative data provide preliminary evidence of clinically meaningful benefit but need to be confirmed in a larger phase III study.

► Prostate cancer continues to claim the lives of over 25 000 American men every year. While most prostate cancers are diagnosed via an elevation in prostate-specific antigen and many of these cancers don't require any immediate therapy, there remains a subset of prostatic adenocarcinoma that is aggressive and can be lethal.

Treatment for these aggressive tumors often includes the use of antiandrogen hormone therapy to address systemic or possible systemic disease. Once the cancer becomes hormone refractory (castrate resistance), the options narrow significantly. Second-line hormone therapy and/or Taxol-based chemotherapy are the usual choices. Response rates to these options support their use but are less than ideal. Thus research to develop new options for these cancer patients is well justified.

These authors have reported on a phase II randomized trial of a vaccine to address castrate-resistant prostate cancer. The results support further research of PROSTVAC-VF with an improvement in overall survival. While this vaccine is not the answer for all castrate-resistant prostate cancer patients, it certainly is work headed in the right direction.

C. A. Lawton, MD

Patient-reported long-term outcomes after conventional and high-dose combined proton and photon radiation for early prostate cancer

Talcott JA, Rossi C, Shipley WU, et al (Massachusetts General Hosp, Boston)

JAMA 303:1046-1053, 2010

Context.—Increased radiation doses improve prostate cancer control but also increase toxicity to adjacent normal tissue. Proton radiation may attenuate adverse effects.

Objective.—To determine long-term, patient-reported, dose-related toxicity.

Design, Setting, and Patients.—We performed a post hoc cross-sectional survey of surviving participants in the Proton Radiation Oncology Group (PROG) 9509—a randomized trial comparing 70.2 Gy vs 79.2 Gy of combined photon and proton radiation for 393 men with clinically localized prostate cancer (stage T1b-T2b, prostate-specific antigen <15 ng/mL, and no radiographic evidence of metastasis). The estimated 10-year biochemical progression rate for patients receiving standard dose was 32% (95% confidence interval, 26%-39%) compared with 17% (95% confidence interval, 11%-23%) for patients receiving high dose ($P < .001$). We surveyed 280 of the surviving 337 patients (83%) from April 2007 to September 2008.

Main Outcome Measures.—Prostate Cancer Symptom Indices, a validated measure of urinary incontinence, urinary obstruction and irritation, bowel problems, and sexual dysfunction, and related quality-of-life instruments.

Results.—At a median of 9.4 years after treatment (range, 7.4-12.1 years), participants' demographic and clinical characteristics were similar. Patient-reported outcomes were reported as mean (SD) scale score for standard dose vs high dose: urinary obstruction/irritation (23.3 [13.7] vs 24.6 [14.0]; $P = .36$), urinary incontinence (10.6 [17.7] vs 9.7

[15.8]; P = .99), bowel problems (7.7 [7.8] vs 7.9 [9.1]; P = .70), sexual dysfunction (68.2 [34.6] vs 65.9 [34.7]; P = .65), and most other outcomes were also similar, although patients receiving standard dose whose cancers had more often progressed expressed less confidence that their cancers were under control (mean [SD] scale score for standard dose, 76.0 [25.4] vs high dose, 86.2 [17.9]; P < .001). Many patients characterized their urinary and bowel function as normal despite reporting symptoms that, for other prostate cancer patients before and early after cancer treatment, caused substantial distress.

Conclusion.—Among men with clinically localized prostate cancer, treatment with higher-dose radiation compared with standard dose was not associated with an increase in patient-reported prostate cancer symptoms after a median of 9.4 years.

▶ External beam radiation therapy is and has been considered a standard-of-care treatment option for localized adenocarcinoma of the prostate for decades. Recent randomized trials have shown a biochemical progression-free survival benefit to dose escalation, especially in intermediate-risk patients and potentially for low-risk patients. Dose escalation may be fraught with increased complications to surrounding rectum and bladder, as these organs at risk will likely see some increase in dose as well.

It is well understood that patient-reported outcomes are much closer to the true quality of life outcomes compared with physician-reported patient outcomes. Thus, this article is of significance as the data are patient-reported and addressed both bowel and bladder measures via validated instruments.

The results showing no significant difference between the standard doses of 70.2 Gy versus the escalated dose of 79.2 Gy in terms of urinary, sexual, or bowel problems are comforting in terms of pursuing dose escalation for appropriate patients. Yet it does not say that patients are having a perfect quality of life following these radiation fractionation schemes. Two-thirds of the patients developed sexual dysfunction, 10% had urinary incontinence, and 8% had bowel problems. We need to continue to evaluate our radiation therapy techniques to decrease these toxicities as much as possible.

C. A. Lawton, MD

Prostate cancer-specific mortality and the extent of therapy in healthy elderly men with high-risk prostate cancer

Hoffman KE, Chen M-H, Moran BJ, et al (Brigham and Women's Hosp and Dana-Farber Cancer Inst, Boston)

Cancer 116:2590-2595, 2010

Background.—The risk of prostate cancer-specific mortality (PCSM) in healthy elderly men may depend on extent of treatment. The authors of this report compared the use of brachytherapy alone with combined brachytherapy, external-beam radiation to the prostate and seminal vesicles, and androgen-suppression therapy (CMT) in this population.

Methods.—The study cohort comprised 764 men aged ≥65 years with high-risk prostate cancer (T3 or T4N0M0, prostate-specific antigen >20 ng/mL, and/or Gleason score 8-10) who received either brachytherapy alone (n = 206) or CMT (n = 558) at the Chicago Prostate Cancer Center or at a 21st Century Oncology facility. Men either had no history of myocardial infarction (MI) or had a history of MI treated with a stent or surgical intervention. Fine and Gray regression analysis was used to identify the factors associated with PCSM.

Results.—The median patient age was 73 years (interquartile range, 70-77 years). After a median follow-up of 4.9 years, 25 men died of prostate cancer. After adjusting for age and prostate cancer prognostic factors, the risk of PCSM was significantly less (adjusted hazard ratio, 0.29; 95% confidence interval, 0.12-0.68; *P* =.004) for men who received CMT than for men who received brachytherapy alone. Other factors that were associated significantly with an increased risk of PCSM included a Gleason score of 8 to 10 (*P* =.017).

Conclusions.—Elderly men who had high-risk prostate cancer without cardiovascular disease or with surgically corrected cardiovascular disease had a lower risk of PCSM when they received CMT than when they received brachytherapy alone. These results support aggressive locoregional treatment in healthy elderly men with high-risk prostate cancer.

▶ Prostate cancer claims the lives of over 25 000 American men annually and is one of the top 3 causes of death in patients older than 60 years of age. Yet many men—especially if diagnosed with the disease in their 70s—are not offered definitive and aggressive therapy.

With clear predictors of aggressive prostate cancers well understood to be prostate-specific antigen level > 20 ng/mL, Gleason score > 8, or T-stage > 3, one would assume that these cancers would routinely be treated aggressively. Yet if they occur in current patients in their 70s and 80s, noncurative hormone therapy alone or less-than-ideal local radiation alone is often pursued.

These data help the treating physician to understand that for elderly patients in reasonable health who are diagnosed with these aggressive tumors, standard aggressive therapy which includes radiation and androgen suppression, is absolutely appropriate so as to avoid unnecessary prostate cancer-related deaths.

C. A. Lawton, MD

Randomized Trial Comparing Conventional-Dose With High-Dose Conformal Radiation Therapy in Early-Stage Adenocarcinoma of the Prostate: Long-Term Results From Proton Radiation Oncology Group/American College of Radiology 95-09

Zietman AL, Bae K, Slater JD, et al (Loma Linda Univ Med Ctr, CA; Massachusetts General Hosp, Boston; American College of Radiology, Philadelphia, PA)

J Clin Oncol 28:1106-1111, 2010

Purpose.—To test the hypothesis that increasing radiation dose delivered to men with early-stage prostate cancer improves clinical outcomes.

Patients and Methods.—Men with T1b-T2b prostate cancer and prostate-specific antigen ≤ 15 ng/mL were randomly assigned to a total dose of either 70.2 Gray equivalents (GyE; conventional) or 79.2 GyE (high). No patient received androgen suppression therapy with radiation. Local failure (LF), biochemical failure (BF), and overall survival (OS) were outcomes.

Results.—A total of 393 men were randomly assigned, and median follow-up was 8.9 years. Men receiving high-dose radiation therapy were significantly less likely to have LF, with a hazard ratio of 0.57. The 10-year American Society for Therapeutic Radiology and Oncology BF rates were 32.4% for conventional-dose and 16.7% for high-dose radiation therapy ($P < .0001$). This difference held when only those with low-risk disease (n = 227; 58% of total) were examined: 28.2% for conventional and 7.1% for high dose ($P < .0001$). There was a strong trend in the same direction for the intermediate-risk patients (n = 144; 37% of total; 42.1% *v* 30.4%, $P = .06$). Eleven percent of patients subsequently required androgen deprivation for recurrence after conventional dose compared with 6% after high dose ($P = .047$). There remains no difference in OS rates between the treatment arms (78.4% *v* 83.4%; $P = .41$). Two percent of patients in both arms experienced late grade ≥ 3 genitourinary toxicity, and 1% of patients in the high-dose arm experienced late grade ≥ 3 GI toxicity.

Conclusion.—This randomized controlled trial shows superior long-term cancer control for men with localized prostate cancer receiving high-dose versus conventional-dose radiation. This was achieved without an increase in grade ≥ 3 late urinary or rectal morbidity.

▶ The role of proton therapy in prostate cancer continues to be debated. Proponents of proton treatment cite ultra conformal radiation therapy dosimetry as a benefit with resulting decrease in acute and late radiation toxicity. Yet there are no randomized trials with other conformal radiation therapy techniques to prove this. In addition, both 3-dimensional and intensity-modulated radiation therapy as conformal radiation therapy options in localized prostate cancer have safe, acute, and late toxicity profiles. So the debate rages on.

This trial fortunately is not an effort to prove the benefit of protons over photons (as it used both) but to look at the dose question for localized disease patients. In this update with a median follow-up of 8.9 years, once again a benefit was found for the 79.2 Gy equivalent arm over the 70.2 Gy equivalent arm. This benefit was seen for both low- and intermediate-risk subsets. Interestingly, when first published, this analysis had a problem with the low-risk results, which was corrected (see reference 7 of this article). Yet even in this updated analysis the 70.2 Gy arm for the low-risk patients had biochemical failure approaching 30% at 10 years, which seems high compared with other known data. The statistical difference for the low-risk group was $P < .0001$ and $P = .0581$ for the intermediate-risk group, which is the opposite of the other US randomized trial from MD Anderson. The MD Anderson trial showed the intermediate-risk group as benefiting most from dose escalation. Interesting results to ponder.

C. A. Lawton, MD

Reimbursement Policy and Androgen-Deprivation Therapy for Prostate Cancer

Shahinian VB, Kuo Y-F, Gilbert SM (Univ of Michigan, Ann Arbor; Univ of Texas Med Branch, Galveston; Univ of Florida College of Medicine, Gainesville)

N Engl J Med 363:1822-1832, 2010

Background.—The Medicare Modernization Act led to moderate reductions in reimbursement for androgen-deprivation therapy (ADT) for prostate cancer, starting in 2004 and followed by substantial changes in 2005. We hypothesized that these reductions would lead to decreases in the use of ADT for indications that were not evidence based.

Methods.—Using the Surveillance, Epidemiology, and End Results (SEER) Medicare database, we identified 54,925 men who received a diagnosis of incident prostate cancer from 2003 through 2005. We divided these men into groups according to the strength of the indication for ADT use. The use of ADT was deemed to be inappropriate as primary therapy for men with localized cancers of a low-to-moderate grade (for whom a survival benefit of such therapy was improbable), appropriate as adjuvant therapy with radiation therapy for men with locally advanced cancers (for whom a survival benefit was established), and discretionary for men receiving either primary or adjuvant therapy for localized but high-grade tumors. The proportion of men receiving ADT was calculated according to the year of diagnosis for each group. We used modified Poisson regression models to calculate the effect of the year of diagnosis on the use of ADT.

Results.—The rate of inappropriate use of ADT declined substantially during the study period, from 38.7% in 2003 to 30.6% in 2004 to 25.7% in 2005 (odds ratio for ADT use in 2005 vs. 2003, 0.72; 95% confidence interval [CI], 0.65 to 0.79). There was no decrease in the appropriate use of adjuvant ADT (odds ratio, 1.01; 95% CI, 0.86 to 1.19). In cases involving discretionary use, there was a significant decline in use in 2005 but not in 2004.

Conclusions.—Changes in the Medicare reimbursement policy in 2004 and 2005 were associated with reductions in ADT use, particularly among men for whom the benefits of such therapy were unclear. (Funded by the American Cancer Society.)

▶ Prostate cancer remains the most common non–skin cancer diagnosed in American men. More than 25 000 US men die of this disease annually. The appropriate use of surgery, radiation, and hormone therapy is pivotal in attaining the best outcomes for prostate cancer patients. Overuse of any of these modalities results in unnecessary toxicity.

Reimbursement for hormone therapy in the form of gonadotropin-releasing hormone (GnRH) agonist injections was inappropriately high during the 1990s, resulting in urologic practices whose revenues were heavily based on GnRH use. The federal government, through Medicare Part B, paid out almost $1 billion in 2003 for these drugs. At the same time, the surgical alternative to this (ie, orchiectomy) decreased substantially. The federal government, realizing the probable inappropriate use of much of the GnRH agonists, changed the reimbursement in both 2004 and 2005.

This study of more than 54 000 men from the SEER (Surveillance, Epidemiology, and End Results) registry of prostate cancer patients looking at the use of these drugs shows that the Medicare changes decrease the incidence of inappropriate use of these drugs. Fortunately, these data also show that these Medicare changes did not decrease the appropriate use of these drugs.

C. A. Lawton, MD

Salvage radiotherapy for rising prostate-specific antigen levels after radical prostatectomy for prostate cancer: dose–response analysis

Bernard JR Jr, Buskirk SJ, Heckman MG, et al (Mayo Clinic, Jacksonville, FL; et al)

Int J Radiat Oncol Biol Phys 76:735-740, 2010

Purpose.—To investigate the association between external beam radiotherapy (EBRT) dose and biochemical failure (BcF) of prostate cancer in patients who received salvage prostate bed EBRT for a rising prostate-specific antigen (PSA) level after radical prostatectomy.

Methods and Materials.—We evaluated patients with a rising PSA level after prostatectomy who received salvage EBRT between July 1987 and October 2007. Patients receiving pre-EBRT androgen suppression were excluded. Cox proportional hazards models were used to investigate the association between EBRT dose and BcF. Dose was considered as a numeric variable and as a categoric variable (low, <64.8 Gy; moderate, 64.8–66.6 Gy; high, >66.6 Gy).

Results.—A total of 364 men met study selection criteria and were followed up for a median of 6.0 years (range, 0.1–19.3 years). Median pre-EBRT PSA level was 0.6 ng/mL. The estimated cumulative rate of BcF at 5 years after EBRT was 50% overall and 57%, 46%, and 39% for the low-, moderate-, and high-dose groups, respectively. In multivariable analysis adjusting for potentially confounding variables, there was evidence of a linear trend between dose and BcF, with risk of BcF decreasing as dose increased (relative risk [RR], 0.77 [5.0-Gy increase]; $p = 0.05$). Compared with the low-dose group, there was evidence of a decreased risk of BcF for the high-dose group (RR, 0.60; $p = 0.04$), but no difference for the moderate-dose group (RR, 0.85; $p = 0.41$).

Conclusions.—Our results suggest a dose response for salvage EBRT. Doses higher than 66.6 Gy result in decreased risk of BcF.

► Data from multiple randomized trials of adjuvant postoperative irradiation for patients with prostate cancer with pathologic T3 disease and/or positive margins show an obvious benefit to the postoperative radiation. Benefit has been measured in terms of clinical progression-free survival, biochemical progression-free survival, cause-specific survival, and overall survival. The doses of 60 to 64 Gy conventionally fractionated and the volumes treated are well accepted. Yet the majority of patients referred for postoperative radiation to date are not this group of patients, but those with rising prostate-specific antigen (PSA) after surgery. Many of these patients have pathologic T3 disease and/or positive surgical margins. The disease burden in these cases is likely greater and thus one would assume that the dose of radiation needed to eradicate the disease would also be greater.

These authors have looked at this question in terms of doses of a < 64.8 Gy, 64.8 to 66.6 Gy, and > 66.6 Gy (isocenter-defined doses). Their results show a trend toward an improvement in biochemical progression-free survival with the higher doses, although a direct comparison of 64.8 to 66.66 Gy versus > 66 Gy was not statistically different.

These data do not tell us the exact dose to use in these salvage cases. It certainly should make the treating radiation oncologist consider doses > 60 to 64 Gy as used in the adjuvant phase III trials when treating patients with rising PSA after surgery for adenocarcinoma of the prostate.

C. A. Lawton, MD

Statin Use and Risk of Prostate Cancer Recurrence in Men Treated With Radiation Therapy

Gutt R, Tonlaar N, Kunnavakkam R, et al (Univ of Chicago, IL)

J Clin Oncol 28:2653-2659, 2010

Purpose.—There has been growing interest in the potential anticancer activity of statins based on preclinical evidence of their antiproliferative, proapoptotic, and radiosensitizing properties. The primary objective of this study was to determine whether statin use is associated with improved clinical outcomes in patients treated with radiotherapy (RT) for prostate cancer.

Patients and Methods.—In total, 691 men with prostate adenocarcinoma treated with curative-intent RT between 1988 and 2006 were retrospectively analyzed. Of those, 189 patients (27%) were using statins, either during initial consultation or during follow-up. Lipid panels were collected (n = 298) a median of 5 months before RT start. Median follow-up was 50 months after RT.

Results.—Statin use was associated with improved freedom from biochemical failure (FFBF; $P < .001$), freedom from salvage androgen deprivation therapy (FFADT; $P = .0011$), and relapse-free survival (RFS; $P < .001$). Improved FFBF for statin users was seen in low-, intermediate-, and high-risk groups ($P = .0401$, $P = .0331$, and $P = .0034$, respectively). The improvement in FFBF with statin use was independent of ADT use or radiation dose. On multivariable analysis, statin use was associated with improved FFBF ($P < .001$) along with pretreatment prostate-specific antigen ≤ 8.4 ($P < .001$), stage less than T2b ($P = .0111$), and Gleason score < 7 ($P = .0098$). On univariate analysis, pretreatment total cholesterol < 187 (89% *v* 80%; $P = .0494$) and low-density lipoprotein (LDL) < 110 (96% *v* 85%; $P = .0462$) were associated with improved 4-year FFBF.

Conclusion.—Statin use was associated with a significant improvement in FFBF, FFADT, and RFS in this cohort of men treated with RT for prostate cancer. The favorable effect of statins may be mediated by direct effect or via the LDL-lowering effect of these medications.

▶ Given that obesity is an epidemic in the United States and that this disease also leads to increased cholesterol levels (especially low-density lipoprotein [LDL]), it is not surprising that many cancer patients are taking cholesterol-lowering medications, especially statin drugs. Statin drugs have been shown to be associated with a decrease in the risk of advanced prostate cancer, and this may be related to their antiproliferative and proapoptotic properties.

These authors have shown an improvement in biochemical disease-free survival (bNED) in their retrospective analysis for patients with radiation therapy—treated prostate cancers who use statin drugs. The exact cause of the improvement in bNED may be related to the statin drug itself or to the decrease in LDL or both.

Regardless of the cause of the improvement of bNED with statin drug use, these data provide additional support for trials evaluating the benefit of statin drugs. With the widespread use of these medications, a large prospective clinical trial should be run to further quantitate the potential benefit seen to date in these retrospective data.

C. A. Lawton, MD

The rate of secondary malignancies after radical prostatectomy versus external beam radiation therapy for localized prostate cancer: a population-based study on 17,845 patients

Bhojani N, Capitanio U, Suardi N, et al (Univ of Montreal Health Ctr, Quebec, Canada; Vita-Salute San Raffaele, Milan, Italy; et al)

Int J Radiat Oncol Biol Phys 76:342-348, 2010

Purpose.—External-beam radiation therapy (EBRT) may predispose to secondary malignancies that include bladder cancer (BCa), rectal cancer (RCa), and lung cancer (LCa). We tested this hypothesis in a large French Canadian population-based cohort of prostate cancer patients.

Methods and Materials.—Overall, 8,455 radical prostatectomy (RP) and 9,390 EBRT patients treated between 1983 and 2003 were assessed with Kaplan-Meier and Cox regression analyses. Three endpoints were examined: (*1*) diagnosis of secondary BCa, (*2*) LCa, or (*3*) RCa. Covariates included age, Charlson comorbidity index, and year of treatment.

Results.—In multivariable analyses that relied on incident cases diagnosed 60 months or later after RP or EBRT, the rates of BCa (hazard ratio [HR], 1.4; $p = 0.02$), LCa (HR, 2.0; $p = 0.004$), and RCa (HR 2.1; $p < 0.001$) were significantly higher in the EBRT group. When incident cases diagnosed 120 months or later after RP or EBRT were considered, only the rates of RCa (hazard ratio 2.2; $p = 0.003$) were significantly higher in the EBRT group. In both analyses, the absolute differences in incident rates ranged from 0.7 to 5.2% and the number needed to harm (where harm equaled secondary malignancies) ranged from 111 to 19, if EBRT was used instead of RP.

Conclusions.—EBRT may predispose to clinically meaningfully higher rates of secondary BCa, LCa and RCa. These rates should be included in informed consent consideration.

► Secondary malignancies following radiation therapy for prostate cancer continue to be a concern for patients and radiation oncologists alike. While patients who develop 1 cancer such as prostate cancer certainly can develop other malignancies, concern for an increase in this problem via the addition of radiation therapy is important. Data exist that both support and refute the secondary malignancy concern. Thus, we as oncologists must continue to evaluate new research on the topic so as to best understand the risk, if present.

The data from this trial performed through the Quebec Health Plan represent a large population of prostate cancer patients treated with radiation therapy 9390 or surgery 8455 with reasonable follow-up. Interestingly, if one assumes that it takes at least 10 years for radiation therapy to cause a secondary malignancy than these data suggest, then lung cancer may be an important problem. If one uses the 5-year cutoff, then bladder, rectum, and lung cancers are concerns for secondary malignancies.

Certainly, 1 huge question for this data set is the question of smoking. Since smoking is so correlated with lung and bladder cancer, one would need to know whether patients were smokers or not to really understand the potential correlation or lack thereof with radiation therapy. Not knowing the smoking status and finding fewer secondary malignancy correlates at 10 years than 5 years are of concern for adopting these results. Yet we continue to need more studies to get a real handle on the potential for secondary malignancies after radiation therapy for prostate cancer.

C. A. Lawton, MD

Time of decline in sexual function after external beam radiotherapy for prostate cancer

Siglin J, Kubicek GJ, Leiby B, et al (Jefferson Med College of Thomas Jefferson Univ, Philadelphia, PA; Thomas Jefferson Univ Hosp, Philadelphia, PA; et al)

Int J Radiat Oncol Biol Phys 76:31-35, 2010

Purpose.—Erectile dysfunction is one of the most concerning toxicities for patients in the treatment of prostate cancer. The inconsistent evaluation of sexual function (SF) and limited follow-up data have necessitated additional study to clarify the rate and timing of erectile dysfunction after external beam radiotherapy (EBRT) for prostate cancer.

Methods and Materials.—A total of 143 men completed baseline data on SF before treatment and at the subsequent follow-up visits. A total of 1187 validated SF inventories were analyzed from the study participants. Multiple domains of SF (sex drive, erectile function, ejaculatory function, and overall satisfaction) were analyzed for ≤8 years of follow-up.

Results.—The median follow-up was 4.03 years. The strongest predictor of SF after EBRT was SF before treatment. For all domains of SF, the only statistically significant decrease in function occurred in the first 24 months after EBRT. SF stabilized 2 years after treatment completion, with no statistically significant change in any area of SF >2 years after the end of EBRT.

Conclusion.—These data suggest that SF does not have a continuous decline after EBRT. Instead, SF decreases maximally within the first 24 months after EBRT, with no significant changes thereafter.

▶ Discussion of side effects of radiation therapy for patients with prostate cancer usually centers on bowel and bladder issues. Yet sexual function remains a very important aspect of the patient's overall health and in some cases, patients place it as a number one concern for potential toxicity. In addition, it is well known that patient-reported toxicities versus physician-reported ones are different with patient-reported outcomes being much more reliable, (ie, real). These authors have done an excellent job of assessing the effects of radiation therapy on sexual function by evaluating over 1000 patient-reported and validated sexual function inventories on 143 men treated with radiation therapy for localized prostate cancer.

With a median follow-up of just over 4 years, these authors have shown that contrary to the traditional belief that sexual function declines continuously after radiation therapy, their data show a maximal decrease in sexual function within the first 24 months after radiation and no significant changes after that. These data do confirm previous reports that the strongest predictor of sexual function after radiation therapy is sexual functioning prior to radiation therapy.

C. A. Lawton, MD

Kidney

Evaluation of late adverse events in long-term Wilms' tumor survivors

van Dijk IWEM, Oldenburger F, Cardous-Ubbink MC, et al (Academic Med Ctr (AMC), Amsterdam, the Netherlands; Outpatient Clinic for Late Effects (Polikliniek Late Effecten Kindertumoren; PLEK)/AMC, Amsterdam, the Netherlands; et al)

Int J Radiat Oncol Biol Phys 78:370-378, 2010

Purpose.—To evaluate the prevalence and severity of adverse events (AEs) and treatment-related risk factors in long-term Wilms' tumor (WT) survivors, with special attention to radiotherapy.

Methods and Materials.—The single-center study cohort consisted of 185 WT survivors treated between 1966 and 1996, who survived at least 5 years after diagnosis. All survivors were invited to a late-effects clinic for medical assessment of AEs. AEs were graded for severity in a standardized manner. Detailed radiotherapy data enabled us to calculate the equivalent dose in 2 Gy fractions (EQD_2) to compare radiation doses in a uniform way. Risk factors were evaluated with multivariate logistic regression analysis.

Results.—Medical follow-up was complete for 98% of survivors (median follow-up, 18.9 years; median attained age, 22.9 years); 123 survivors had 462 AEs, of which 392 had Grade 1 or 2 events. Radiotherapy to flank/abdomen increased the risk of any AE (OR, 1.08 Gy^{-1} [CI, 1.04–1.13]). Furthermore, radiotherapy to flank/abdomen was associated with orthopedic events (OR, 1.09 Gy^{-1} [CI, 1.05–1.13]) and second tumors (OR, 1.11 Gy^{-1} [CI, 1.03–1.19]). Chest irradiation increased the risk of pulmonary events (OR, 1.14 Gy^{-1} [CI, 1.06–1.21]). Both flank/abdominal and chest irradiation were associated with cardiovascular events (OR, 1.05 Gy^{-1} [CI, 1.00–1.10], OR, 1.06 Gy^{-1} [CI, 1.01–1.12]) and tissue hypoplasia (OR, 1.17 Gy^{-1} [CI, 1.10–1.24], OR 1.10 Gy^{-1} [CI, 1.03–1.18]).

Conclusion.—The majority of AEs, overall as well as in irradiated survivors, were mild to moderate. Nevertheless, the large amount of AEs emphasizes the importance of follow-up programs for WT survivors.

▶ Wilms' tumors or neuroblastomas treated with surgery and postoperative radiation therapy were likely lethal diseases for patients prior to the chemotherapy era. Once effective chemotherapeutic agents were added to the surgery and radiation, the overall survival for these patients increased dramatically. The subsequent challenge for these survivors is to document the potential late sequelae from these treatments so as to diagnosis and treat them early in an effort to mitigate their effects.

These authors have evaluated 185 Wilms' tumor survivors. The minimum follow-up is 5 years, but the median is 18.9 years. They have tried to document any and all adverse events and correlate the events with the type of treatment delivered. Fortunately, they found that the majority of the adverse events were mild to moderate, yet 68% of patients had at least 1 adverse event. In the patients who had radiation as part of their treatment regimen, 30% had at least one > grade 3 adverse event. The adverse events associated with radiation in the treatment regimen were hypoplasia, fertility issues, pulmonary issues, and cardiovascular and orthopedic events. These data stress the absolute requirement for patients treated in their youth with radiation for a malignancy to be followed vigilantly for such adverse events so that they can be diminished. Both the patients and their parents need to be made aware of the need for this meticulous follow-up.

C. A. Lawton, MD

Bladder

Racial Differences in Treatment and Outcomes Among Patients With Early Stage Bladder Cancer

Hollenbeck BK, Dunn RL, Ye Z, et al (Univ of Michigan, Ann Arbor)

Cancer 116:50-56, 2010

Background.—Black patients are at greater of risk of death from bladder cancer than white patients. Potential explanations for this disparity include a more aggressive phenotype and delays in diagnosis resulting in higher stage disease. Alternatively, black patients may receive a lower quality of care, which may explain this difference.

Methods.—Using Surveillance, Epidemiology, and End Results (SEER)-Medicare data for the years from 1992 through 2002, the authors identified patients with early stage bladder cancer. Multivariate models were fitted to measure relations between race and mortality, adjusting for differences in patients and treatment intensity. Next, shared-frailty proportional hazards models were fitted to evaluate whether the disparity was explained by differences in the quality of care provided.

Results.—Compared with white patients (n = 14,271), black patients (n = 342) were more likely to undergo restaging resection (12% vs 6.5%; $P < .01$) and urine cytologic evaluation (36.8% vs 29.7%; $P < .01$), yet they received fewer endoscopic evaluations (4 vs 5; $P < .01$). The use of aggressive therapies (cystectomy, systemic chemotherapy, radiation) was found to be similar among black patients and white patients (12% vs 10.2%, respectively; $P = .31$). Although black patients had a greater risk of death compared with white patients (hazards ratio [HR], 1.23; 95% confidence interval [95% CI], 1.07-1.42), this risk was attenuated only modestly after adjusting for differences in treatment intensity and provider effects (HR, 1.22; 95% CI, 1.06-1.42).

Conclusions.—Although differences in initial treatment were evident, they did not appear to be systematic and had unclear clinical significance.

Whereas black patients are at greater risk of death, this disparity did not appear to be caused by differences in the intensity or quality of care provided.

▶ When disparities in outcomes for any cancer occur between white and black Americans, there is a concern on many levels. The largest concern has to do with quality of health care and the question of decreased access for the black population and/or potential decrease in state of the art treatment for this population. This article is an excellent example of research on this topic for early-stage bladder cancer.

Data show that black patients in the United States have a significantly worse 10-year disease-specific survival for localized bladder cancer compared with white patients. This article looks at Surveillance, Epidemiology, and End Results-Medicare data from 1992-2002 to evaluate possible causes for this decrease in outcome. The good news is that these authors did not find any access to care or quality of care issue as the source of the poor results for the black patients diagnosed with localized bladder cancer. Although comforting, these data do suggest that other factors such as smoking may play a role here. Future research is needed to get at the source of the disparity in bladder cancer outcomes so as to improve on the outcomes for black patients.

C. A. Lawton, MD

Radiation dose–volume effects of the urinary bladder

Viswanathan AN, Yorke ED, Marks LB, et al (Brigham and Women's Hosp/ Dana-Farber Cancer Inst and Harvard Med School, Boston, MA; Memorial Sloan-Kettering Cancer Ctr, NY; Univ of North Carolina, Chapel Hill; et al)

Int J Radiat Oncol Biol Phys 76:S116-S122, 2010

An in-depth overview of the normal-tissue radiation tolerance of the urinary bladder is presented. The most informative studies consider whole-organ irradiation. The data on partial-organ/nonuniform irradiation are suspect because the bladder motion is not accounted for, and many studies lack long enough follow-up data. Future studies are needed.

▶ QUANTEC is an effort on the part of radiation oncology as a specialty to confirm or redefine as appropriate dose volume effects on all normal organs of the body based on the available data. In some cases, specific dose and volume data have been arrived at with associated recommendations for safe radiation delivery. This article is a specific look at the data for radiation dose and volume toxicities for the bladder. The mainstay of the data comes from 3 pelvic malignancies: prostate, bladder, and cervix.

These authors report a relative lack of evidence to make strong dose volume recommendations. They point to a need for more careful assessment (both patient and physician-reported assessments) of bladder toxicity with associated dose and volume data. The authors do, however, give some guidelines based on the disease treated, bladder versus prostate versus gynecologic malignancies. Given the extensive literature evaluation done by this group, the recommendations they suggest should be followed until new data suggest changes.

C. A. Lawton, MD

5 Hematologic Malignancies

Leukemia and Myelodysplastic Syndrome

A phase 2 study of high-dose lenalidomide as initial therapy for older patients with acute myeloid leukemia

Fehniger TA, Uy GL, Trinkaus K, et al (Washington Univ School of Medicine, St Louis, MO)

Blood 117:1828-1833, 2011

Older patients with acute myeloid leukemia (AML) have limited treatment options and a poor prognosis, thereby warranting novel therapeutic strategies. We evaluated the efficacy of lenalidomide as frontline therapy for older AML patients. In this phase 2 study, patients 60 years of age or older with untreated AML received high-dose (HD) lenalidomide at 50 mg daily for up to 2 28-day cycles. If patients achieved a complete remission (CR)/CR with incomplete blood count recovery (CRi) or did not progress after 2 cycles of HD lenalidomide, they received low-dose lenalidomide (10 mg daily) until disease progression, an unacceptable adverse event, or completion of 12 cycles. Thirty-three AML patients (median age, 71 years) were enrolled with intermediate (55%), unfavorable (39%), or unknown (6%) cytogenetic risk. Overall CR/CRi rate was 30%, and 53% in patients completing HD lenalidomide. The CR/CRi rate was significantly higher in patients presenting with a low (<1000/μL) circulating blast count (50%, $P=.01$). The median time to CR/CRi was 30 days, and duration of CR/CRi was 10 months (range, 1- ≥17 months). The most common grades ≥3 toxicities were thrombocytopenia, anemia, infection, and neutropenia. HD lenalidomide has evidence of clinical activity as initial therapy for older AML patients, and further study of lenalidomide in AML and MDS is warranted. This study is registered at www.clinicaltrials.gov as #NCT00546897.

► The outcome for patients aged over 60 with acute myeloid leukemia (AML) has not seen the dramatic improvements observed for children and younger adults. In this older population, median survival is less than 1 year. Furthermore, the incidence of AML continues to rise with age, and AML in this group of patients represents nearly two-thirds of all AML. Intensification of treatment in particular has not been as successful in this group of patients as it has in younger patients in part because of comorbidities and likely more chemotherapy-resistant disease. Thus, alternative strategies, for example, with lower doses of chemotherapy or novel agents such as chromatin remodeling drugs, have become more desirable for testing in this group. The report by Fehniger et al represents one such phase II study in which lenalidomide, whose mechanism of action is unclear, is tested at somewhat higher doses than has been used in the previous studies. At doses that result in some myelosuppression, they report a complete remission (CR)/CR with incomplete platelet recovery (CRi) of 53% in patients who were able to complete the high-dose lenalidomide, although 30% CR/CRi in the overall group. The median duration of these responses was 10 months. Ironically, as with chemotherapy, the most common grade 3 or greater toxicities included thrombocytopenia, anemia, infection, and neutropenia—importantly, major toxicities involving mucositis and other nonhematologic toxicities. The responses and their duration observed with lenalidomide appear to be in the same range as with conventional chemotherapy or other treatment approaches in this high-risk group of patients. With the somewhat improved toxicity profile compared with conventional chemotherapy, lenalidomide would potentially be an important agent to test in combination with other nonconventional chemotherapy agents that display non—cross-resistant drug profiles and nonoverlapping toxicities.

R. J. Arceci, MD, PhD

Aberrant DNA hypermethylation signature in acute myeloid leukemia directed by EVI1

Lugthart S, Figueroa ME, Bindels E, et al (Erasmus Univ Med Ctr, Rotterdam, The Netherlands; Weill Cornell Med College, NY; et al)

Blood 117:234-241, 2011

DNA methylation patterns are frequently dysregulated in cancer, although little is known of the mechanisms through which specific gene sets become aberrantly methylated. The *ecotropic viral integration site 1* (*EVI1*) locus encodes a DNA binding zinc-finger transcription factor that is aberrantly expressed in a subset of acute myeloid leukemia (AML) patients with poor outcome. We find that the promoter DNA methylation signature of *EVI1* AML blast cells differs from those of normal CD34$^+$ bone marrow cells and other AMLs. This signature contained 294 differentially methylated genes, of which 238 (81%) were coordinately hypermethylated. An unbiased motif analysis revealed an overrepresentation of EVI1 binding sites among these aberrantly hypermethylated loci. EVI1 was capable of binding to these promoters in 2 different *EVI1*-expressing cell lines, whereas no binding was observed in an *EVI1*-negative cell line. Furthermore, EVI1 was observed to interact with DNA methyl transferases 3A and 3B. Among the *EVI1* AML cases, 2 subgroups were recognized, of which 1 contained AMLs with many more methylated genes, which was associated with significantly higher levels of *EVI1* than in the cases of the other subgroup. Our data point to a role for EVI1 in directing aberrant promoter DNA methylation patterning in *EVI1* AMLs.

▶ Our understanding of the role of epigenetics in acute myeloid leukemia (AML) is beginning to emerge. An important issue is whether it is a driver or mediator of the malignant phenotype. Some data certainly point to key methylation events involving, for instance, the transcriptional repression of selective tumor suppressor genes. Other reports have stressed the association of methylation patterns with specific genetic abnormalities. In this regard, the report by Lugthart et al shows that a distinctive pattern of hypermethylation occurs in AML characterized by aberrant expression of the oncogene *EVI1*. These leukemias are usually associated with a poor outcome, so the description of such alterations may help to shed light on the reasons underlying such outcome results. Of particular note is that Lugthart et al not only demonstrate altered promoter hypermethylation but also show an overrepresentation of *EVI1* binding sites in those promoters, actual binding of *EVI1* to those sites, and an interaction of *EVI1* with DNMT3A and 3B. These results help to close the linkage between the methylation patterns and altered *EVI1* in this subtype of AML, hopefully then leading to a more focused approach to epigenetic-directed therapy.

R. J. Arceci, MD, PhD

A randomized comparison of 4 courses of standard-dose multiagent chemotherapy versus 3 courses of high-dose cytarabine alone in postremission therapy for acute myeloid leukemia in adults: the JALSG AML201 Study

Miyawaki S, Ohtake S, Fujisawa S, et al (Saiseikai Maebashi Hosp, Japan; Kanazawa Univ Graduate School of Med Science, Kanazawa, Japan; Yokohama City Univ Med Ctr, Japan; et al)

Blood 117:2366-2372, 2011

We conducted a prospective randomized study to assess the optimal postremission therapy for adult acute myeloid leukemia in patients younger than 65 years in the first complete remission. A total of 781 patients in complete remission were randomly assigned to receive consolidation chemotherapy of either 3 courses of high-dose cytarabine (HiDAC, 2 g/m^2 twice daily for 5 days) alone or 4 courses of conventional standard-dose multiagent chemotherapy (CT) established in the previous JALSG AML97 study. Five-year disease-free survival was 43% for the HiDAC group and 39% for the multiagent CT group (P =.724), and 5-year overall survival was 58% and 56%, respectively (P =.954). Among the favorable cytogenetic risk group (n = 218), 5-year disease-free survival was 57% for HiDAC and 39% for multiagent CT (P =.050), and 5-year overall survival was 75% and 66%, respectively (P =.174). In the HiDAC group, the nadir of leukocyte counts was lower, and the duration of leukocyte less than

1.0×10^9/L longer, and the frequency of documented infections higher. The present study demonstrated that the multiagent CT regimen is as effective as our HiDAC regimen for consolidation. Our HiDAC regimen resulted in a beneficial effect on disease-free survival only in the favorable cytogenetic leukemia group. This trial was registered at www.umin.ac.jp/ctr/ as #C000000157.

▶ The question of how many courses of postremission treatment are necessary to optimize the cure for younger patients with acute myeloid leukemia (AML) remains an important question. Usually postremission therapy includes 3 to 5 courses of intensive chemotherapy with non-cross-resistant agents. Unfortunately, many studies, although not all, provide comparisons of disparate postremission regimens rather than a carefully controlled comparison. The study by Miyawaki et al is one such study that randomizes 2 different induction regimens and then either 3 courses of high-dose cytarabine (HiDAC) or 4 courses of less intense combination chemotherapy. There was no difference in induction complete remissions between the 2 arms, and the analysis of the postremission outcome was balanced by the induction regimen received. The only difference in outcome between the 2 postremission regimens was a statistically significant disease-free survival (but not overall survival) in the group of patients with AML characterized by favorable cytogenetics. The HiDAC regimen was, however, more toxic. This study puts into question previous studies that have concluded that HiDAC is beneficial in overall outcome for patients with AML and favorable cytogenetics. It is also still astonishing that 3 consecutive courses of a single agent would be a sensible approach to optimizing cancer care, when such an approach is used to efficiently generate drug resistance. Nevertheless, this study does show that there are several ways to cure patients with AML, and until more effective regimens are developed, achieving less toxicity for the same survival may make sense.

R. J. Arceci, MD, PhD

BEACOPP chemotherapy is a highly effective regimen in children and adolescents with high-risk Hodgkin lymphoma: a report from the Children's Oncology Group

Kelly KM, Sposto R, Hutchinson R, et al (Columbia Univ Med Ctr, NY; Univ of Southern California, Los Angeles, CA; Univ of Michigan Med School, Ann Arbor; et al)

Blood 117:2596-2603, 2011

Dose-intensified treatment strategies for Hodgkin lymphoma (HL) have demonstrated improvements in cure but may increase risk for acute and long-term toxicities, particularly in children. The Children's Oncology Group assessed the feasibility of a dose-intensive regimen, BEACOPP (bleomycin, etoposide, doxorubicin, cyclophosphamide, vincristine, procarbazine, prednisone) in children with high-risk HL (stage IIB or IIIB with bulk disease, stage IV). Rapidity of response was assessed after 4 cycles of BEACOPP. Rapid responders received consolidation therapy with guidelines to reduce the risk of sex-specific long-term toxicities of therapy. Females received 4 cycles of COPP/ABV (cyclophosphamide, vincristine, procarbazine, prednisone, doxorubicin, bleomycin, vinblastine) without involved field radiation therapy (IFRT). Males received 2 cycles of ABVD (doxorubicin, bleomycin, vinblastine, and dacarbazine) with IFRT. Slow responders received 4 cycles of BEACOPP and IFRT. Ninety-nine patients were enrolled. Myelosuppression was frequent. Rapid response was achieved by 74% of patients. Five-year event-free-survival is 94%, IFRT with median follow-up of 6.3 years. There were no disease progressions on study therapy. Secondary leukemias occurred in 2 patients. Overall survival is 97%. Early intensification followed by less intense response-based therapy for rapidly responding patients is an effective strategy for achieving high event-free survival in children with high-risk HL. This trial is registered at http://www.clinicaltrials.gov as #NCT00004010.

▶ Cure rates for patients with Hodgkin lymphoma are relatively high for all stages. The improvement in outcomes for these patients has, however, raised the important question as to whether decreased intensity regimens or regimens limiting certain treatment modalities could maintain the high cure rate while reducing early and late toxicities. To this end, the article by Kelly et al describes the Children's Oncology Group results using BEACOPP (bleomycin, etoposide, doxorubicin, cyclophosphamide, vincristine, procarbazine, prednisone) and response-adjusted therapy in high-risk Hodgkin lymphoma. The rapidity of response was determined after 4 cycles of therapy. Female rapid early responders were then given COPP/ABV (cyclophosphamide, vincristine, procarbazine, prednisone, doxorubicin, bleomycin, vinblastine) treatment without involved field radiation (IFRT), whereas male rapid early responders received 2 more courses of BEACOPP followed by IFRT. Slow early responders, regardless of gender, received 4 more courses of BEACOPP followed by IFRT. Most (74%) patients were classified as having an early rapid response with an overall 5-year event-free survival of 94%. Of interest, 2 patients developed secondary leukemias (2%). However, a large percentage of females were spared IFRT and higher-intensity therapy. In addition, a significant number of males were spared 2 additional courses of BEACOPP. These results are encouraging and should help set a standard of response-adapted therapy for patients with Hodgkin lymphoma; however, the follow-up is still relatively short for these patients in terms of long-term adverse sequelae. Time will be the final arbiter as to the success of this approach, which attempts to be a better cure with less toxicity.

R. J. Arceci, MD, PhD

Cytarabine Dose of 36 g/m² Compared With 12 g/m² Within First Consolidation in Acute Myeloid Leukemia: Results of Patients Enrolled Onto the Prospective Randomized AML96 Study

Schaich M, Röllig C, Soucek S, et al (Universitätsklinikum C.G. Carus, Dresden, Germany; und Stammzell-transplantation, Hamburg, Germany; Klinikum Nord, Nürnberg, Germany; et al)

J Clin Oncol 29:2696-2702, 2011

Purpose.—To assess the optimal cumulative dose of cytarabine for treatment of young adults with acute myeloid leukemia (AML) within a prospective multicenter treatment trial.

Patients and Methods.—Between 1996 and 2003, 933 patients (median age, 47 years; range 15 to 60 years) with untreated AML were randomly assigned at diagnosis to receive cytarabine within the first consolidation therapy at either a intermediate-dose of 12 g/m² (I-MAC) or a high-dose of 36 g/m² (H-MAC) combined with mitoxantrone. Autologous hematopoietic stem-cell transplantation or intermediatedose cytarabine (10 g/m²) were offered as second consolidation. Patients with a matched donor could receive an allogeneic transplantation in a risk-adapted manner.

Results.—After double induction therapy including intermediate-dose cytarabine (10 g/m²), mitoxantrone, etoposide, and amsacrine, complete remission was achieved in 66% of patients. In the primary efficacy analysis population, a consolidation with either I-MAC or H-MAC did not result in significant differences in the 5-year overall (30% *v* 33%; $P = .77$) or disease-free survival (37% v 38%; $P = .86$) according to the intention-to-treat analysis. Besides a prolongation of neutropenia and higher transfusion demands in the H-MAC arm, rates of serious adverse events were comparable in the two groups.

Conclusion.—In young adults with AML receiving intermediate-dose cytarabine induction, intensification of the cytarabine dose beyond 12 g/m² within first consolidation did not improve treatment outcome.

▶ The use of cytarabine arabinoside (ARAC) for the treatment of patients with acute myeloid leukemia (AML) has been part of treatment regimens since the 1970s. Nearly 20 years ago, Mayer et al[1] showed that 4 courses of high-dose ARAC resulted in a significantly improved outcome in adults with AML compared with low doses. The high-dose ARAC had a cumulative value of 72 g/m². Since then, other reports have tried to answer the question of whether fewer cycles would be equivalent to the 4 cycles and have shown that 2 cycles appear to be equivalent. The study by Schaich et al randomized young adult patients with AML to receive, after 2 courses of induction therapy, either a first consolidation course of intermediate-dose (12 g/m²) versus a high dose of 36 g/m². They found no significant difference in 5-year overall or disease-free survival. Although this study demonstrates that the higher dose of ARAC does not confer an improved survival when given as part of a first consolidation, the study does not address the question as to how many courses are optimal. In addition, this study demonstrates that more ARAC may not be better than somewhat less and that it is more toxic. These results strongly suggest that alternative agents need to be added that can synergize with ARAC but not necessarily target the same pathways.

R. J. Arceci, MD, PhD

Reference

1. Mayer RJ, Davis RB, Schiffer CA, et al. Intensive postremission chemotherapy in adults with acute myeloid leukemia. Cancer and Leukemia Group B. *N Engl J Med.* 1994;331:896-903.

ETV6/RUNX1-positive relapses evolve from an ancestral clone and frequently acquire deletions of genes implicated in glucocorticoid signaling

Kuster L, Grausenburger R, Fuka G, et al (St Anna Kinderkrebsforschung, Vienna, Austria; et al)
Blood 117:2658-2667, 2011

Approximately 25% of childhood acute lymphoblastic leukemias carry the *ETV6/RUNX1* fusion gene. Despite their excellent initial treatment response, up to 20% of patients relapse. To gain insight into the relapse mechanisms, we analyzed single nucleotide polymorphism arrays for DNA copy number aberrations (CNAs) in 18 matched diagnosis and relapse leukemias. CNAs were more abundant at relapse than at diagnosis (mean 12.5 vs 7.5 per case; $P = .01$) with 5.3 shared on average. Their patterns revealed a direct clonal relationship with exclusively new aberrations at relapse in only 21.4%, whereas 78.6% shared a common ancestor and subsequently acquired distinct CNA. Moreover, we identified recurrent, mainly nonoverlapping deletions associated with glucocorticoid-mediated apoptosis targeting the Bcl2 modifying factor (*BMF*) (n = 3), glucocorticoid receptor *NR3C1* (n = 4), and components of the mismatch repair pathways (n = 3). Fluorescence in situ hybridization screening of additional 24 relapsed and 72 nonrelapsed ETV6/RUNX1-positive cases demonstrated that *BMF* deletions were significantly more common in relapse cases (16.6% vs 2.8%; $P = .02$). Unlike *BMF* deletions, which were always already present at diagnosis, NR3C1 and mismatch repair aberrations prevailed at relapse. They were all associated with leukemias, which poorly responded to treatment. These findings implicate glucocorticoid-associated drug resistance in ETV6/RUNX1-positive relapse pathogenesis and therefore might help to guide future therapies.

▶ The elucidation of the molecular mechanisms underlying relapse of leukemia is an important goal from the point of view of basic science but also has enormous potential repercussions for patients. Identification of such mechanisms could direct treatment by avoiding certain drugs to which the relapsed leukemia would likely be resistant as well as developing alternative strategies to circumvent resistance. Kuster et al advance this field of inquiry by examining the molecular changes that occur in relapsed ETV6/RUNX1-characterized acute lymphoblastic leukemia (ALL) compared with findings at the time of diagnosis. Using single nucleotide polymorphism arrays for DNA copy number variations, they report that about 21% of relapsed samples develop distinct and new copy number abnormalities (CNAs), whereas about 79% of relapse samples clearly share a common ancestor and later develop unique CNAs. Of particular interest is that nonoverlapping deletions of the Bcl2 modifying factor (BMF) were detectable at diagnosis and relapse but that such abnormalities in the glucocorticoid receptor, NR3C1, and members of the mismatch repair pathway were mostly present in relapse samples. ALL characterized by the ETV6/RUNX1 translocation occurs in approximately 25% of children with ALL and usually portends a superb prognosis, although late relapses occur in 20% of patients. The identification of the clonal evolution and mechanisms characterizing relapse will hopefully provide the foundation upon which more effective treatments can be developed both to prevent the emergence of specific mechanisms of resistance and to direct treatment to circumvent those resistance mechanisms when they do arise.

R. J. Arceci, MD, PhD

Evolution of human *BCR–ABL1* lymphoblastic leukaemia-initiating cells

Notta F, Mulligan CG, Wang JCY, et al (Campbell Family Inst for Cancer Res/Ontario Cancer Inst, Toronto, Canada; St Jude Children's Res Hosp, Memphis, TN; et al)

Nature 469:362-367, 2011

Many tumours are composed of genetically diverse cells; however, little is known about how diversity evolves or the impact that diversity has on functional properties. Here, using xenografting and DNA copy number alteration (CNA) profiling of human *BCR–ABL1* lymphoblastic leukaemia, we demonstrate that genetic diversity occurs in functionally defined leukaemia-initiating cells and that many diagnostic patient samples contain multiple genetically distinct leukaemia-initiating cell subclones. Reconstructing the subclonal genetic ancestry of several samples by CNA profiling demonstrated a branching multi-clonal evolution model of leukaemogenesis, rather than linear succession. For some patient samples, the predominant diagnostic clone repopulated xenografts, whereas in others it was outcompeted by minor subclones. Reconstitution with the predominant diagnosis clone was associated with more aggressive growth properties in xenografts, deletion of *CDKN2A* and *CDKN2B*, and a trend towards poorer patient outcome. Our findings link clonal diversity with leukaemia-initiating-cell function and underscore the importance of developing therapies that eradicate all intratumoral subclones.

▶ The underlying mechanisms for the development and subsequent changes in leukemia cell phenotypes, including such characteristics as drug resistance, remain an important avenue for research and therapeutic target discovery.

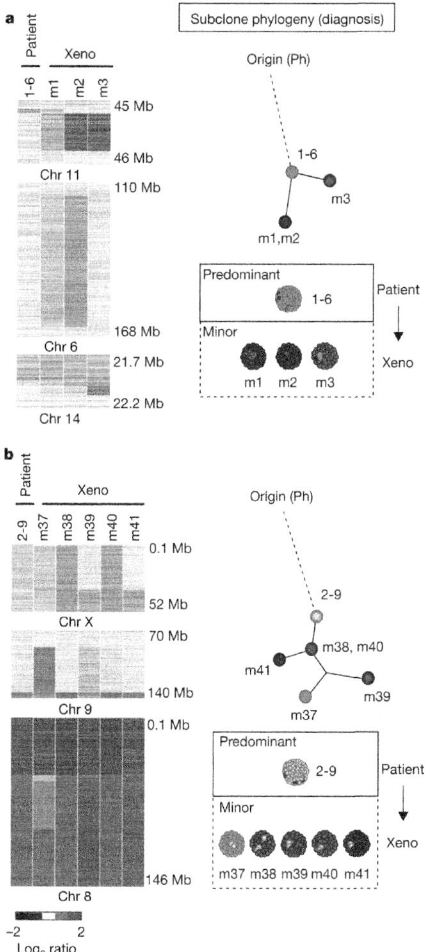

FIGURE 3.—Detection of genetically diverse leukaemia-initiating cells in Ph+ ALL. a, CNA profiling shows that three engrafted recipients from sample 1-6 share a common CNA on Chr 11 (top) that is not detected in the diagnostic sample, but each is distinct for CNA on Chr 6 (middle) and Chr 14 (bottom). b, In sample 2-9, all five engrafted recipients shared a deletion (at varying degrees) in a region of Chr Xp (top), two recipients displayed a common CNA region of Chr 9q (middle; m37, m39), and three recipients had deletions (m37) and duplications (m39, 41) on regions of Chr 8p (bottom). A phylogenetic tree depicting the relationship between major and minor genetic subclones present in the diagnostic sample and a summary of the distinct xenograft subclones are shown to the right of each sample. The dashed line represents clonal evolution from disease origin (Ph, Philadelphia chromosome). (Reprinted by permission from Macmillan Publishers Ltd: Nature, Notta F, Mullighan CG, Wang JCY, et al. Evolution of human *BCR–ABL1* lymphoblastic leukaemia-initiating cells. *Nature.* 2011;469:362-367, copyright 2011.)

Many studies have shown that during the course of treatment, leukemias change the expression and/or mutate different types of genes regulating drug resistance. However, the molecular evolution of these changes has not always been easy to track. Notta et al now show molecular changes in diagnostic samples of *BCR-ABL1* lymphoblastic leukemia–initiating cells, proving that while a dominant clone may be responsible for most diseases at diagnosis, multiple clones of leukemia-initiating cells exist. Further, different clones may come and go during the course of therapy (Fig 3). The predominant diagnostic clone was also shown to correlate with more aggressive growth properties in xenografts and be associated with deletions of *CDKN2A* and *CDKN2B*, both regulators of cell cycle. Thus, Darwin's approach to evolution may, in the end, prove to be prescient in terms of the evolution of leukemia and possibly cancer in general.

R. J. Arceci, MD, PhD

Exome sequencing identifies somatic mutations of DNA methyltransferase gene *DNMT3A* in acute monocytic leukemia

Yan X-J, Xu J, Gu Z-H, et al (Shanghai Jiao Tong Univ School of Medicine, China; Shanghai Jiao Tong Univ, China)

Nat Genet 43:309-315, 2011

Abnormal epigenetic regulation has been implicated in oncogenesis. We report here the identification of somatic mutations by exome sequencing in acute monocytic leukemia, the M5 subtype of acute myeloid leukemia (AML-M5). We discovered mutations in *DNMT3A* (encoding DNA methyltransferase 3A) in 23 of 112 (20.5%) cases. The DNMT3A mutants showed reduced enzymatic activity or aberrant affinity to histone H3 *in vitro*. Notably, there were alterations of DNA methylation patterns and/or gene expression profiles (such as *HOXB* genes) in samples with *DNMT3A* mutations as compared with those without such changes. Leukemias with *DNMT3A* mutations constituted a group of poor prognosis with elderly disease onset and of promonocytic as well as monocytic predominance among AML-M5 individuals. Screening other leukemia subtypes showed Arg882 alterations in 13.6% of acute myelomonocytic leukemia (AML-M4) cases. Our work suggests a contribution of aberrant DNA methyltransferase activity to the pathogenesis of acute monocytic leukemia and provides a useful new biomarker for relevant cases.

► The initial report of *DNMT3A* mutations by Ley et al[1] reported a 22.1% incidence of *DNMT3A* (DNA methyltransferase 3A) in a cohort of adult patients with acute myeloid leukemia (AML); in addition, this was associated with a poor prognosis. Of interest, *DNMT3A* mutations were not observed in a population of pediatric patients with AML.[2] However, there were no significant associated molecular changes associated with the *DNMT3A* changes noted in the Ley et al report. Yan et al now report on another cohort and observe a similar (20.5%) percentage of adult patients with *DNMT3A* mutations and AML. Of particular importance is that they observe decreased enzymatic activity and affinity to histone H3 as well as altered methylation and expression profiles of a subset of genes such as *HOXB*. They also demonstrate that such *DNMT3A* mutations appear preferentially associated with the monocytic subtype of AML, poor prognosis, and elderly disease onset. These results are important as they now link these *DNMT3A* mutations with AML cell molecular and physiologic characteristics. While much remains to be learned about these mutations affecting epigenetic machinery, this article represents an important step forward.

R. J. Arceci, MD, PhD

References

1. Ley TJ, Ding L, Walter MJ, et al. DNMT3A mutations in acute myeloid leukemia. *N Engl J Med.* 2010;363:2424-2433.
2. Ho PA, Kutny MA, Alonzo TA, et al. Leukemic mutations in the methylation-associated genes DNMT3A and IDH2 are rare events in pediatric AML: a report from the Children's Oncology Group. *Pediatr Blood Cancer.* 2011;57:204-209.

Identification of Patients With Acute Myeloblastic Leukemia Who Benefit From the Addition of Gemtuzumab Ozogamicin: Results of the MRC AML15 Trial

Burnett AK, Hills RK, Milligan D, et al (Cardiff Univ School of Medicine, UK; Cardiff and Vale Univ Health Board, UK; Birmingham Heartlands Hosp, UK; et al)

J Clin Oncol 29:369-377, 2010

Purpose.—Antibody-directed chemotherapy for acute myeloid leukemia (AML) may permit more treatment to be administered without escalating toxicity. Gemtuzumab ozogamicin (GO) is an immunoconjugate between CD33 and calicheamicin that is internalized when binding to the epitope. We previously established that it is feasible to combine GO with conventional chemotherapy. We now report a large randomized trial testing the addition of GO to induction and/or consolidation chemotherapy in untreated younger patients.

Patients and Methods.—In this open-label trial, 1,113 patients, predominantly younger than age 60 years, were randomly assigned to receive a single dose of GO (3 mg/m^2) on day 1 of induction course 1 with one of the following three induction schedules: daunorubicin and cytarabine; cytarabine, daunorubicin, and etoposide; or fludarabine, cytarabine, granulocyte colony-stimulating factor, and idarubicin. In remission, 948 patients were randomly assigned to GO in course 3 in combination with amsacrine, cytarabine, and etoposide or high-dose cytarabine. The primary end points were response rate and survival.

Results.—The addition of GO was well tolerated with no significant increase in toxicity. There was no overall difference in response or survival in either induction or consolidation. However, a predefined analysis by cytogenetics showed highly significant interaction with induction GO (P =.001), with significant survival benefit for patients with favorable cytogenetics, no benefit for patients with poor-risk disease, and a trend for benefit in intermediate-risk patients. An internally validated prognostic index identified approximately 70% of patients with a predicted benefit of 10% in 5-year survival.

Conclusion.—A substantial proportion of younger patients with AML have improved survival with the addition of GO to induction chemotherapy with little additional toxicity.

▶ Although dose intensification of treatment for younger patients with acute myeloid leukemia (AML) has improved overall outcomes, it has come with a significant cost in terms of morbidity and mortality. Thus, the introduction of new agents into the backbone of therapy for AML that do not have significant or overlapping toxicities with conventional chemotherapy represents an area of intense clinical research. One class of such agents includes immunotherapeutic approaches, such as AML-directed monoclonal antibodies. Gemtuzumab ozogamicin (GO or Mylotarg) is a calicheamicin-tagged conjugated murine anti-CD33 monoclonal antibody that was developed to selectively target AML cells while sparing normal hematopoietic stem cells. Phase I and II trials appeared positive. Phase III trials are just starting to be reported. The article by Burnett et al reports the Medical Research Council (MRC) AML15 Trial that randomized GO during induction and course 3 of treatment. Although the results showed no overall difference in response or survival when all patients were considered, a planned subgroup analysis demonstrated a significant survival difference for patients with favorable cytogenetics. There was a similar trend in patients with AML with intermediate-risk cytogenetics. Although somewhat odd that these critical data on subgroups are present in the Supplemental Data, it is a good example of the need to read all of an article and not just what is in the primary printed version. Further studies will be needed to establish the addition of GO to MRC-based chemotherapy to declare this a standard of care.

R. J. Arceci, MD, PhD

Impact of *TET2* mutations on response rate to azacitidine in myelodysplastic syndromes and low blast count acute myeloid leukemias

Itzykson R, on behalf of the Groupe Francophone des Myelodysplasies (GFM) (Université Paris 13, France; et al)

Leukemia 25:1-6, 2011

The impact of ten-eleven-translocation 2 (*TET2*) mutations on response to azacitidine (AZA) in MDS has not been reported. We sequenced the *TET2* gene in 86 MDS and acute myeloid leukemia (AML) with 20–30% blasts treated by AZA, that is disease categories wherein this drug is approved by Food and Drug Administration (FDA). Thirteen patients (15%) carried *TET2* mutations. Patients with mutated and wild-type (WT) *TET2* had mostly comparable pretreatment characteristics, except for lower hemoglobin, better cytogenetic risk and longer MDS duration before AZA in *TET2* mutated patients (P=0.03, P=0.047 and P=0.048, respectively). The response rate (including hematological improvement) was 82% in MUT versus 45% in WT patients (P=0.007). Mutated *TET2* (P=0.04) and favorable cytogenetic risk (intermediate risk: $P=0.04$, poor risk: $P=0.048$ compared with good risk) independently predicted a higher response rate. Response duration and overall survival were, however, comparable in the MUT and WT groups. In higher risk MDS and AML with low blast count, *TET2* status may be a genetic predictor of response to AZA, independently of karyotype.

▶ The discovery of mutations in the ten-eleven-translocation 2 (*TET2*) gene, which encodes a dioxygenase that converts 5-methylcytosine to 5-hydroxymethylcytosine, thus altering specific methylation marks on DNA in acute myeloid leukemia (AML) and myelodysplastic syndromes (MDS), has generated a novel mechanism for altered epigenetic patterns. While interesting in itself, the implications of such mutations are in response to specific therapies and the outcome of patients. Itzykson et al report that patients with MDS and AML characterized by mutations in *TET2* show an improved response to the demethylating agent azacytidine. However, overall survival was not improved. This result is perplexing and may reflect the all too frequent confusion of response with truly effective, curative therapy. In addition, the heterogeneity of the population studied, as well as no evidence on combinations of azacytidine with chemotherapy, may have contributed to that lack of a definitive survival advantage. Regardless of the biological basis, these findings may still serve as another piece of important information in the quest to find molecular lesions that can be therapeutically exploited.

R. J. Arceci, MD, PhD

Incidence and Prognostic Influence of *DNMT3A* Mutations in Acute Myeloid Leukemia

Thol F, Damm F, Lüdeking A, et al (Hannover Med School, Germany; et al)
J Clin Oncol 29:2889-2896, 2011

Purpose.—To study the incidence and prognostic impact of mutations in DNA methyltransferase 3A (*DNMT3A*) in patients with acute myeloid leukemia.

Patients and Methods.—A total of 489 patients with AML were examined for mutations in *DNMT3A* by direct sequencing. The prognostic impact of *DNMT3A* mutations was evaluated in the context of other clinical prognostic markers and genetic risk factors (cytogenetic risk group; mutations in *NPM1, FLT3, CEBPA, IDH1, IDH2, MLL1, NRAS, WT1*, and *WT1* SNPrs16754; expression levels of *BAALC, ERG, EVI1, MLL5, MN1*, and *WT1*).

Results.—*DNMT3A* mutations were found in 87 (17.8%) of 489 patients with AML who were younger than 60 years of age. Patients with *DNMT3A* mutations were older, had higher WBC and platelet counts, more often had a normal karyotype and mutations in *NPM1, FLT3*, and *IDH1* genes, and had higher *MLL5* expression levels as compared with patients with wild-type *DNMT3A*. Mutations in *DNMT3A* independently predicted a shorter overall survival (OS; hazard ratio [HR], 1.59; 95% CI, 1.15 to 2.21; $P = .005$) by multivariate analysis, but were not associated with relapse-free survival (RFS) or complete remission (CR) rate when the entire patient cohort was considered. In cytogenetically normal (CN) AML, 27.2% harbored *DNMT3A* mutations that independently predicted shorter OS (HR = 2.46; 95% CI, 1.58 to 3.83; $P < .001$) and lower CR rate (OR, 0.42; 95% CI, 0.21 to 0.84; $P = .015$), but not RFS ($P = .32$). Within patients with CN-AML, *DNMT3A* mutations had an unfavorable effect on OS, RFS, and CR rate in *NPM1/FLT3*-ITD high-risk but not in low-risk patients.

Conclusion.—DNMT3A mutations are frequent in younger patients with AML and are associated with an unfavorable prognosis.

▶ The first description of mutations of *DNMT3A* was obtained from whole genome sequencing of a single patient's acute myeloid leukemia (AML) and normal germ line genome.[1] Other reports have also established some of the potential molecular consequences and outcomes of patients with AML characterized by *DNMT3A* mutations. One might conclude that the story regarding *DNMT3A* is mostly solved. The article by Thol et al proves this possibility to be incorrect. They examined 489 adult patients with AML for *DNMT3A* mutations and analyzed outcomes in the context of an extensive number of known molecular prognostic factors. The presence of *DNMT3A* mutations predicted an overall poorer survival but not a relapse-free survival in the entire cohort, suggesting a potentially interesting difference in drug resistance mechanisms (Fig 3 in the original article). In cytogenetically normal AML, they observed a 27.2% frequency of *DNMT3A* mutations that independently predicted a lower complete remission rate and a shorter overall survival but not a relapse-free survival. The *DNMT3A* mutations also independently conferred a negative prognosis for patients with *FLT3* mutations. This study was also able to examine the role of *DNMT3A* mutations in the context of hematopoietic stem cell transplantation (HSCT); in this setting, no significant difference was obtained in the presence or absence of a *DNMT3A* mutation, suggesting that HSCT may in part overcome the poorer prognosis associated with mutations of *DNMT3A*. While these results will need validation by others, they represent a comprehensive analysis of *DNMT3A*. The conclusion by the authors that demethylating agents should be tested in patients with *DNMT3A* mutations is not a necessarily logical one in that mutated *DNMT3A* results in decreased methylation in many key genes. Nevertheless, alternative therapeutic approaches are certainly warranted in this group of patients.

R. J. Arceci, MD, PhD

Reference

1. Ley TJ, Ding L, Walter MJ, et al. DNMT3A mutations in acute myeloid leukemia. *N Engl J Med.* 2010;363:2424-2433.

Prognostic Importance of Histone Methyltransferase *MLL5* Expression in Acute Myeloid Leukemia

Damm F, Oberacker T, Thol F, et al (Hannover Med School, Germany; Univ of Freiburg Med Ctr, Germany; Univ of Tübingen, Germany; et al)
J Clin Oncol 29:682-689, 2011

Purpose.—To assess the prognostic importance of mixed lineage leukemia 5 (*MLL5*) expression in acute myeloid leukemia (AML).

Patients and Methods.—*MLL5* transcript levels from 509 patients with AML who were treated in multicenter trials AML SHG 0199 and AML SHG 0295 and 48 healthy volunteers were analyzed by real-time reverse-transcription polymerase chain reaction in the context of other molecular markers (*NPM1, FLT3, CEBPA, IDH1/IDH2, NRAS, KIT, MN1, BAALC, ERG*, and *WT1*).

Results.—Patients with high (n = 127) compared with low (n = 382) *MLL5* expression had a higher complete response rate in multivariate analysis (odds ratio, 1.87; 95% CI, 1.08 to 3.24; *P* = .026). In multivariate analysis, high *MLL5* expression was a favorable prognostic marker for overall survival (OS; hazard ratio [HR], 0.66; 95% CI, 0.49 to 0.89; *P* = .007) and relapse-free survival (RFS; HR, 0.72; 95% CI, 0.52 to 1.01; *P* = .057). Patient characteristics, cytogenetic aberrations, and gene mutations were similarly distributed between patients with high and low *MLL5* expression except for a higher platelet count in those with high *MLL5* expression. *MLL5* expression independently predicted prognosis in cytogenetically normal AML patients (n = 268; OS: HR, 0.53; 95% CI, 0.33 to 086; *P* = .011; RFS: HR, 0.61; 95% CI, 0.38 to 0.99; *P* = .05) and in patients with core-binding factor leukemias (n = 81; OS: HR, 0.12; 95% CI, 0.02 to 0.91; *P* = .04; RFS: HR, 0.18; 95% CI, 0.04 to 0.77; *P* = .02). The prognostic importance of high *MLL5* expression was independently validated in 167 patients treated in the AMLSG 07/04 trial (OS: HR, 0.5; 95% CI, 0.27 to 0.92; *P* = .023; RFS: HR, 0.49; 95% CI, 0.25 to 0.96; *P* = .033).

Conclusion.—High *MLL5* expression levels are associated with a favorable outcome and may improve risk and treatment stratification in AML.

► The role of chromatin remodeling proteins in the etiology of acute myeloid leukemia (AML) and myelodysplastic syndromes (MDS) is becoming increasingly important in terms of risk stratification as well as providing potential therapeutic targets. For instance, the identification of *DNMT3a* mutations in adult AML appears to independently predict a poor outcome. The finding of the polycomb-associated histone modifier EZH2 mutations in MDS appears to mark an early etiologic alteration. The *MLL5* (mixed lineage leukemia 5) gene is an H3 histone methyltransferase located on the long arm of chromosome 7, a known hotspot for deletions of monosomy in high-risk AML. Damm et al report that increased expression levels of *MLL5* transcripts are independently associated with a favorable outcome in a large cohort of adults with AML. For example, patients with a high expression level of *MLL5* RNA had a 55% survival compared with 36% with a lower expression level. The result was confirmed in a separate, albeit smaller, cohort of patients. Unfortunately, this article did not show a continuous variable analysis of the data but instead showed data based only on quartiles. In addition, no analysis of AML subtypes was shown. Finally, no biological correlations with molecular or cellular consequences of different levels of *MLL5* were shown. Nevertheless, the results are intriguing and potentially useful but await mechanistic appraisal.

R. J. Arceci, MD, PhD

6-Thioguanine reactivates epigenetically silenced genes in acute lymphoblastic leukemia cells by facilitating proteasome-mediated degradation of DNMT1

Yuan B, Zhang J, Wang H, et al (Univ of California, Riverside)
Cancer Res 71:1904-1911, 2011

Thiopurines including 6-thioguanine ((S)G), 6-mercaptopurine, and azathioprine are effective anticancer agents with remarkable success in clinical practice, especially in effective treatment of acute lymphoblastic leukemia (ALL). (S)G is understood to act as a DNA hypomethylating agent in ALL cells, however, the underlying mechanism leading to global cytosine demethylation remains unclear. Here we report that (S)G treatment results in reactivation of epigenetically silenced genes in T leukemia cells. Bisulfite genomic sequencing revealed that (S)G treatment universally elicited demethylation in the promoters and/or first exons of the genes that were reactivated. (S)G treatment also attenuated the expression of histone lysine-specific demethylase 1 (LSD1), thereby stimulating lysine methylation of the DNA methylase DNMT1 and triggering its degradation via the ubiquitin-proteasomal pathway. Taken together, our findings reveal a previously uncharacterized but vital mechanistic link between (S)G treatment and DNA hypomethylation.

▶ The molecular mechanisms contributing to the efficacy of low-dose, antimetabolite maintenance therapy in patients with acute lymphoblastic leukemia (ALL) are largely not understood, even though they have been in clinical use for more than 35 years. The article by Yuan et al sheds some light on one possible mechanism. Their article examined the previously established observation that DNA hypomethylation of ALL cells is associated with exposure to 6-thioguane. The results demonstrate that in addition to demethylating and thus activating transcription of a subset of genes, thioguanine specifically also leads to the decreased expression of the histone lysine-specific demethylase I (LSD1) that in turn leads to the increased methylation-mediated degradation of the maintenance DNA methylase DNMT1 via the ubiquitin-proteasomal machinery of the cell. Thus, these results show a molecular linkage of thioguanine and hypomethylation in ALL. Although showing the physiological consequences of the effects of hypomethylation on leukemic cell survival or drug sensitivity would have enhanced this article, the results nevertheless form a new step on which to build a better mechanistic understanding of maintenance therapy in ALL.

R. J. Arceci, MD, PhD

AIDA0493 protocol for newly diagnosed acute promyelocytic leukemia: very long-term results and role of maintenance

Avvisati G, EORTC Cooperative Groups (Università Campus Bio-Medico, Roma, Italy; et al)

Blood 117:4716-4725, 2011

All-*trans*-retinoic acid (ATRA) has greatly modified the prognosis of acute promyelocytic leukemia; however, the role of maintenance in patients in molecular complete remission after consolidation treatment is still debated. From July 1993 to May 2000, 807 genetically proven newly diagnosed acute promyelocytic leukemia patients received ATRA plus idarubicin as induction, followed by 3 intensive consolidation courses. Thereafter, patients reverse-transcribed polymerase chain reaction—negative for the *PML-RARA* fusion gene were randomized into 4 arms: oral 6-mercaptopurine and intramuscular methotrexate (arm 1); ATRA alone (arm 2); 3 months of arm1 alternating to 15 days of arm 2 (arm 3); and no further therapy (arm 4). Starting from February 1997, randomization was limited to ATRA-containing arms only (arms 2 and 3). Complete remission was achieved in 761 of 807 (94.3%) patients, and 681 completed the consolidation program. Of these, 664 (97.5%) were evaluated for the PML-RARA fusion gene, and 586 of 646 (90.7%) who tested reverse-transcribed polymerase chain reaction—negative were randomized to maintenance. The event-free survival estimate at 12 years was 68.9% (95% confidence interval, 66.4%-71.4%), and no differences in disease-free survival at 12 years were observed among the maintenance arms.

▶ The discovery of the effectiveness of all-trans-retinoic acid (ATRA) in the treatment of patients with acute promyelocytic leukemia (APL) transformed this subtype of myeloid leukemia from one of the deadliest to one of the most curable. In addition, the treatment of patients with APL reintroduced the concept of maintenance therapy during the postremission period. The role of maintenance therapy, including the types of drugs and the duration, has been the subject of multiple clinical trials. Avvisati et al now report on the AIDA0493 protocol, which randomly assigned 4 different maintenance arms with 1 including no maintenance therapy and the others including 6-mercaptopurine plus methotrexate, ATRA alone, or a combination of these 2 approaches. The results show an overall event-free survival rate of 68.9% at 12 years and no difference in outcome with the different types of maintenance or no maintenance at all for patients who had a negative reverse transcriptase polymerase chain reaction for the *PML-RARA* fusion transcript. Thus, it seems that if induction chemotherapy with ATRA and 3 relatively intensive consolidation courses result in a *PML-RARA*—negative disease status, maintenance therapy may not be required. These results stand in contrast to those from North America, although several key differences exist between the AIDA and North American trials; for instance, the AIDA trials use idarubicin in induction and in 2 of the three consolidation courses. In the end, it is clear that some patients with good-risk APL who become *PML-RARA* negative after 3 intensive consolidation courses, as per the AIDA0493 study, do not appear to need further continuation therapy.

R. J. Arceci, MD, PhD

Allogeneic hematopoietic cell transplantation for hematologic malignancy: relative risks and benefits of double umbilical cord blood

Brunstein CG, Gutman JA, Weisdorf DJ, et al (Univ of Minnesota Med Ctr, Minneapolis; Fred Hutchison Cancer Res Ctr, Seattle, WA)

Blood 116:4693-4699, 2010

Effectiveness of double umbilical cord blood (dUCB) grafts relative to conventional marrow and mobilized peripheral blood from related and unrelated donors has yet to be established. We studied 536 patients at the Fred Hutchinson Cancer Research Center and University of Minnesota with malignant disease who underwent transplantation with an human leukocyte antigen (HLA)—matched related donor (MRD, n = 204), HLA allele—matched unrelated donor (MUD, n = 152) or 1-antigen—mismatched unrelated adult donor (MMUD, n = 52) or 4-6/6 HLA matched dUCB (n = 128) graft after myeloablative conditioning. Leukemia-free survival at 5 years was similar for each donor type (dUCB 51% [95% confidence interval (CI), 41%-59%]; MRD 33% [95% CI, 26%-41%]; MUD 48% [40%-56%]; MMUD 38% [95% CI, 25%-51%]). The risk of relapse was lower in recipients of dUCB (15%, 95% CI, 9%-22%) compared with MRD (43%, 95% CI, 35%-52%), MUD (37%, 95% CI, 29%-46%) and MMUD (35%, 95% CI, 21%-48%), yet nonrelapse mortality was higher for dUCB (34%, 95% CI, 25%-42%), MRD (24% (95% CI, 17%-39%), and MUD (14%, 95% CI, 9%-20%). We conclude that leukemia-free survival after dUCB transplantation is comparable with that observed after MRD and MUD transplantation. For patients without an available HLA matched donor, the use of 2 partially HLA-matched UCB units is a suitable alternative.

▶ The introduction of cord blood donors for hematopoietic stem cell transplantation generated an entirely new source of transplant donors as well as the hope that this approach would provide donors to patients in need of transplantation but without matched sibling or unrelated bone marrow donors. Cord blood transplantation, however, appeared to suffer from a somewhat increased graft failure rate and possibly more relapse, in part because of the decreased graft-versus-host disease observed in patients with leukemia. In addition, cord blood units often had a limited number of stem cells, thus preventing their use in larger patients. The use of 2 or more cord blood donors was in part an attempt to avoid such limitations. Although the immunological complexity of using 2 disparate donors has not been worked out, the double cord blood approach has become the subject of several single-arm trials. To answer whether double cord blood transplants are comparable with other types of transplantation, Brunstein et al compared double cord blood to matched and partially matched family or unrelated donor outcome of such patients. The non-cord blood transplants were done at the Fred Hutchison Cancer Research Center and the double cord blood transplants at the University of Minnesota. The conclusions are that leukemia-free survival is comparable across the different types of donors. Of note, there were significant age differences in the separate groups (younger in the double cord blood group) as well as differences in the leukemia status at the time of transplantation and the nucleated cell dose patients received. Does such a comparison lead to a definitive conclusion that double cord blood transplantation is equivalent to conventional donor transplants? The answer is no, although the suggestion of these results begs for a more definitive test of the question.

R. J. Arceci, MD, PhD

Analysis of the Role of Hematopoietic Stem-Cell Transplantation in Infants With Acute Lymphoblastic Leukemia in First Remission and *MLL* Gene Rearrangements: A Report From the Children's Oncology Group

Dreyer ZE, Dinndorf PA, Camitta B, et al (Texas Children's Hosp, Houston; US Food and Drug Administration, Silver Spring, MD; Midwest Children's Cancer Ctr, Milwaukee, WI; et al)

J Clin Oncol 29:214-222, 2011

Purpose.—Although the majority of children with acute lymphoblastic leukemia (ALL) are cured with current therapy, the event-free survival (EFS) of infants with ALL, particularly those with mixed lineage leukemia (*MLL*) gene rearrangements, is only 30% to 40%. Relapse has been the major source of treatment failure for these patients. The parallel Children's Cancer Group (CCG) 1953 and Pediatric Oncology Group (POG) 9407 studies were designed to test the hypothesis that more intensive therapy, including dose intensification of chemotherapy, and hematopoietic stem-cell transplantation (HSCT) would improve the outcome for this group of patients.

Patients and Methods.—One hundred eighty-nine infants (CCG 1953, n = 115; POG 9407, n = 74) were enrolled between October 1996 and August 2000. For infants with the *MLL* gene rearrangement and an appropriate donor, HSCT was the preferred treatment on CCG 1953 and investigator option on POG 9407 after completion of the second phase of therapy. Fifty-three infants underwent HSCT.

Results.—The 5-year EFS rate was 48.8% (95% CI, 33.9% to 63.7%) in patients who received HSCT and 48.7% (95% CI, 33.8% to 63.6%) in patients treated with chemotherapy alone (P =.60). Transplantation outcomes were not affected by the preparatory regimen or donor source.

Conclusion.—Our data suggest that routine use of HSCT for infants with *MLL*-rearranged ALL is not indicated. However, limited by small numbers, this study should not be considered the definitive answer to this question.

▶ While approximately 85% of acute lymphoblastic leukemia in children can be cured, there are important exceptions, including that subtype in infants characterized by rearrangements of the mixed lineage leukemia (*MLL*) gene. The *MLL* gene encodes a critical histone methyltransferase and has been associated with distinctive changes in epigenetic patterning and gene expression. In order to try to improve on the 30% to 40% event-free survival (EFS) observed in infants with this subtype of leukemia, the Children's Cancer Group and the Pediatric Oncology Group, now combined as the Children's Oncology Group, report on the results of comparing treatment intensification with hematopoietic stem cell transplantation (HSCT) with chemotherapy alone. No significant difference in EFS was observed with 5-year EFS of 48.8% and 48.7% for the HSCT versus chemotherapy-only–treated groups. There was also no significant difference observed in patients who received total body irradiation (TBI) compared with a non–TBI-based transplant preparative regimen. These disappointing results suggest that this unique form of leukemia will require alternative treatment approaches that will need to exploit its distinctive biological characteristics.

R. J. Arceci, MD, PhD

Assessment of dexrazoxane as a cardioprotectant in doxorubicin-treated children with high-risk acute lymphoblastic leukaemia: long-term follow-up of a prospective, randomised, multicentre trial

Lipshultz SE, Scully RE, Lipsitz SR, et al (Univ of Miami Leonard M Miller School of Medicine, FL; Brigham and Women's Hosp, Boston, MA; et al)
Lancet Oncol 11:950-961, 2010

Background.—Doxorubicin chemotherapy is associated with cardiomyopathy. Dexrazoxane reduces cardiac damage during treatment with doxorubicin in children with acute lymphoblastic leukaemia (ALL). We aimed to establish the long-term effect of dexrazoxane on the subclinical state of cardiac health in survivors of childhood high-risk ALL 5 years after completion of doxorubicin treatment.

Methods.—Between January, 1996, and September, 2000, children with high-risk ALL were enrolled from nine centres in the USA, Canada, and Puerto Rico. Patients were assigned by block randomisation to receive ten doses of 30 mg/m^2 doxorubicin alone or the same dose of doxorubicin preceded by 300 mg/m^2 dexrazoxane. Treatment assignment was obtained through a telephone call to a centralised registrar to conceal allocation. Investigators were masked to treatment assignment but treating physicians and patients were not; however, investigators, physicians, and patients were masked to study serum cardiac troponin-T concentrations and echocardiographic measurements. The primary endpoints were late left ventricular structure and function abnormalities as assessed by echocardiography; analyses were done including all patients with data available after treatment completion. This trial has been completed and is registered with ClinicalTrials.gov, number NCT00165087.

Findings.—100 children were assigned to doxorubicin (66 analysed) and 105 to doxorubicin plus dexrazoxane (68 analysed). 5 years after the completion of doxorubicin chemotherapy, mean left ventricular fractional shortening and end-systolic dimension Z scores were significantly worse than normal for children who received doxorubicin alone (left ventricular fractional shortening: −0·82, 95% CI −1·31 to −0·33; end-systolic dimension: 0·57, 0·21–0·93) but not for those who also received dexrazoxane (−0·41, −0·88 to 0·06; 0·15, −0·20 to 0·51). The protective effect of dexrazoxane, relative to doxorubicin alone, on left ventricular wall thickness (difference between groups: 0·47, 0·46–0·48) and thickness-to-dimension ratio (0·66, 0·64–0·68) were the only statistically significant characteristics at 5 years. Subgroup analysis showed dexrazoxane protection (p=0·04) for left ventricular fractional shortening at 5 years in girls (1·17, 0·24–2·11), but not in boys (−0·10, −0·87 to 0·68). Similarly, subgroup analysis showed dexrazoxane protection (p=0·046) for the left ventricular thickness-to-dimension ratio at 5 years in girls (1·15, 0·44–1·85), but not in boys (0·19, −0·42 to 0·81). With a median follow-up for recurrence and death of 8·7 years (range 1·3–12·1), event-free survival was 77% (95% CI 67–84) for children in the doxorubicin-alone group, and 76% (67–84) for children in the doxorubicin plus dexrazoxane group (p=0·99).

Interpretation.—Dexrazoxane provides long-term cardioprotection without compromising oncological efficacy in doxorubicin-treated children with high-risk ALL. Dexrazoxane exerts greater long-term cardioprotective effects in girls than in boys.

► One of most significant adverse late sequelae of anthracycline use in the treatment of patients with cancer is cardiotoxicity. This is especially true in children. While significant efforts have been made to reduce the exposure to anthracyclines in the treatment of patients, this class of drug remains a mainstay in most treatment regimens, especially for leukemia. Dexrazoxane is a free radical scavenger and cardioprotectant that has been used relatively anecdotally or in single-arm clinical trials. Lipshultz et al now report on the longer-term outcome results of a randomized trial of dexrazoxane in children with high-risk acute lymphoblastic leukemia. This group had previously reported that the group of patients who received dexrazoxane had lower troponin levels early after receiving anthracyclines compared with the group that received only anthracycline. In the current report, that difference appears to have been borne out in that the group of patients who received dexrazoxane had improved ventricular fractional shortening and more normal left ventricular thickness-to-dimension ratio. The difference was particularly notable in females. Importantly, leukemia-free survival was the same between the 2 groups, and no increased incidence of secondary malignancies was associated with the use of dexrazoxane. This is an important study and shows what a consortium of institutions can do to move the use of a supportive care agent toward more evidence-based usage.

R. J. Arceci, MD, PhD

Chronic Immune Stimulation Might Act As a Trigger for the Development of Acute Myeloid Leukemia or Myelodysplastic Syndromes

Kristinsson SY, Björkholm M, Hultcrantz M, et al (Karolinska University Hospital Solna and Karolinska Institutet, Stockholm, Sweden; et al)

J Clin Oncol 29:2897-2903, 2011

Purpose.—Patients with acute myeloid leukemia (AML) and myelodysplastic syndrome (MDS) often present with infections, but there are little data to assess whether a personal history of selected infections may act as pathogenic triggers. To additionally expand our knowledge on the role of immune stimulation in the causation of AML and MDS, we have conducted a large, population-based study to evaluate the risk of AML and MDS associated with a prior history of a broad range of infections or autoimmune diseases.

Patients and Methods.—By using population-based central registries in Sweden, we included 9,219 patients with AML, 1,662 patients with MDS, and 42,878 matched controls. We used logistic regression to calculate odds ratios (ORs) and 95% CIs for the association of AML or MDS with infectious and/or autoimmune diseases.

Results.—Overall, a history of any infectious disease was associated with a significantly increased risk of both AML (OR, 1.3; 95% CI, 1.2 to 1.4) and MDS (OR, 1.3; 95% CI, 1.1 to 1.5). These associations were significant even when we limited infections to those occurring 3 or more years before AML/MDS. A previous history of any autoimmune disease was associated with a 1.7-fold (95% CI, 1.5 to 1.9) increased risk for AML and 2.1-fold (95% CI, 1.7 to 2.6) increased risk for MDS. A large range of conditions were each significantly associated with AML and MDS.

Conclusion.—Our novel findings indicate that chronic immune stimulation acts as a trigger for AML/MDS development. The underlying mechanisms may also be due to a common genetic predisposition or an effect of treatment for infections/autoimmune conditions.

▶ The etiologies of myelodysplastic syndromes (MDS) and acute myeloid leukemia (AML) have largely been shown to be the result of chromosomal and gene alternations. However, the causes that underlie these genetic changes are largely not understood, with the exception of some chemical and radiation exposures. This report by Kristinsson et al thus is a novel departure in that it examines and finds significant associations between a history of infections or the presence of an autoimmune disease with the development of MDS and AML. Such a study involves more than 10 000 patients. These results possibly add to the other known causes of MDS and AML that have thus far included certain environmental carcinogenic chemicals and ionizing radiation. While it is difficult to be certain of such results because of the essential absence of clinical data, such as validation of medical records and prior exposures, including treatments that could be leukemogenic, the findings present some tantalizing possibilities that should receive more definitive studies, including mechanistic ones.

R. J. Arceci, MD, PhD

Comparable survival after HLA-well-matched unrelated or matched sibling donor transplantation for acute myeloid leukemia in first remission with unfavorable cytogenetics at diagnosis

Gupta V, Tallman MS, He W, et al (Univ of Toronto, Ontario, Canada; Weill Cornell Med College, NY; Med College of Wisconsin, Milwaukee; et al)
Blood 116:1839-1848, 2010

We compared the outcomes of unrelated donor (URD, n = 358) with human leukocyte antigen (HLA)—matched sibling donor (MSD, n = 226) transplantations in patients with acute myeloid leukemia (AML) in first complete remission (CR1) having unfavorable cytogenetics at diagnosis. Unfavorable cytogenetic abnormalities were: complex (≥ 3 abnormalities), 32%; and noncomplex involving chromosome 7, 25%; chromosome 5, 9%; 11q or MLL rearrangements, 18%; t(6;9), 5%; and other noncomplex, 10%. URDs were HLA-well-matched (n = 254; 71%) or partially-matched (n = 104; 29%). Three-year leukemia-free survival (LFS) for MSD was 42% (95% confidence interval [CI], 35%-48%) compared with 34% (95% CI, 28%-41%) for HLA-well-matched URD and 29%(95% CI, 20%-39%) for partially-matched URD (*P* =.08). In multivariate analysis, HLA-well-matched URD and MSD yielded similar LFS (relative risk [RR] = 1.1, 95% CI, 0.86-1.40, *P* =.44) and overall survival (OS; RR = 1.06, 95% CI, 0.83-1.37, *P* =.63). LFS and OS were significantly inferior for HLA-partially-matched URD recipients, those with prior myelodysplastic syndrome, and those older than 50 years. All cytogenetic cohorts had similar outcomes. Patients with chronic graft-versus-host disease had a significantly lower risk of relapse (RR = 0.68, 95% CI, 0.47-0.99, *P* =.05). Hematopoietic cell transplantation (HCT) using HLA-well-matched URD and MSD resulted in similar LFS and OS in AML patients in CR1 with unfavorable cytogenetics. Outcomes of HCT from HLA-partially-matched URD were inferior.

▶ The optimal approach to treatment for patients with acute myeloid leukemia (AML) characterized by unfavorable high-risk cytogenetics has not been established. Although some studies have supported hematopoietic stem cell transplantation (HSCT) rather than chemotherapy alone for such patients, other studies have reported no significant improvement with HSCT. So the question of what is the best donor for an HSCT in such a group of patients is an interesting twist on this issue and presumes transplantation should be done. Gupta et al report that matched sibling donors and well-matched (ie, no mismatches at the human leukocyte antigen-A, -B, -C, DRB1 loci) unrelated donors (URDs) result in similar outcomes, although there is a trend toward worse outcome in the URD recipients. The donor group that resulted in a significantly worse outcome was the mismatched URDs. These data are potentially important in that they help to set a baseline for donor selection. However, they may be compromised in part by the unequal distribution of several covariates among the 3 donor recipient groups. Details on the type of MLL changes are also not included. In addition, they also are not consistent with other reports demonstrating no outcome differences among donor types in high-risk leukemia, although many of those studies are from registries or single institutions. Gupta et al deserve significant credit for examining the question of donor selection. Whether all patients with AML having unfavorable cytogenetics should undergo transplant remains an important question.

R. J. Arceci, MD, PhD

Demographic, clinical and outcome features of children with acute lymphoblastic leukemia and *CRLF2* deregulation: results from the MRC ALL97 clinical trial

Ensor HM, Schwab C, Russell LJ, et al (Newcastle Univ, Newcastle-upon-Tyne, UK; et al)

Blood 117:2129-2136, 2011

Deregulated expression of *CRLF2* (*CRLF2*-d) arises via its juxtaposition to the *IGH@* enhancer or *P2RY8* promoter. Among 865 BCP-ALL children treated on MRC ALL97, 52 (6%) had *CRLF2*-d but it was more prevalent among Down syndrome patients (54%). *P2RY8-CRLF2* (n=43) was more frequent than *IGH@-CRLF2* (n=9). *CRLF2*-d was not associated with age, sex or white cell count, but *IGH@-CRLF2* patients were older than *P2RY8-CRLF2* patients (median 8 v 4 years, p=0.0017). Patients with *CRLF2*-d were more likely to present with enlarged livers and spleens (38% v 18%, p<0.001). *CRLF2*-d was not seen in conjunction with established chromosomal translocations but 6 (12%) cases had high hyperdiploidy and 5 (10%) iAMP21. Univariate analysis suggested that *CRLF2*-d was associated with an inferior outcome: [EFS HR=2.27 (95% CI 1.48-3.47), p<0.001, OS 3.69 (2.34-5.84), p<0.001]. However, multivariate analysis indicated that its effect was mediated by other risk factors such as cytogenetics and DS status [EFS 1.45 (0.88-2.39), p=0.140, OS 1.90 (1.08-3.36), p=0.027]. Although the outcome of *IGH@-CRLF2* patients appeared inferior compared to *P2RY8-CRLF2* patients the result was not significant [EFS 2.69 (1.15-6.31), p=0.023; OS 2.86 (1.15-6.79), p=0.021]. Therefore, we concluded that patients with *CRLF2*-d should be classified into the intermediate cytogenetic risk group.

▶ Rearrangement through cryptic chromosomal translocations or interstitial deletions of the cytokine receptor gene *CRLF2* has been reported in subsets of children with acute lymphoblastic leukemia (ALL) and has also been reported to be prognostic for a quite poor outcome by both the Children's Oncology Group and BFM Pediatric ALL Study Groups. In contrast, the report from Ensor et al and the United Kingdom's MRC ALL97 trial shows a similar frequency of *CRLF2* alterations of 6% and with a predilection for being more prevalent in patients with Down syndrome with a frequency of 54%. Importantly, in a multivariate analysis, alterations of *CRLF2* were not independently associated with a poor outcome. There was a suggestion that the *IGH@-CRLF2* alteration appeared worse than *P2RY8-CRLF2* alterations, but this did not reach statistical significance. Of note, the *IGH@-CRLF2* alterations are more prevalent among older patients and those of Hispanic ethnicity, both of which represent differences with the North American COG report,[1] although not a likely explanation for differences with the BFM study.[2] However, the BFM study based its analysis on expression rather than genomic abnormalities, thus possibly accounting for some of the observed differences. These results certainly raise the issue about the problems of defining prognostic factors across different populations, studies, and methods of analysis. In such circumstances, a true meta-analysis of multiple studies based on primary data and comparable analyses and end points would seem to be the next best move to make.

R. J. Arceci, MD, PhD

References

1. Harvey RC, Mullighan CG, Chen IM, et al. Rearrangement of CRLF2 is associated with mutation of JAK kinases, alteration of IKZF1, Hispanic/Latino ethnicity, and a poor outcome in pediatric B-progenitor acute lymphoblastic leukemia. *Blood*. 2010;115:5312-5321.
2. Cario G, Zimmermann M, Romey R, et al. Presence of the P2RY8-CRLF2 rearrangement is associated with a poor prognosis in non-high-risk precursor B-cell acute lymphoblastic leukemia in children treated according to the ALL-BFM 2000 protocol. *Blood*. 2010;115:5393-5397.

Effect of mitoxantrone on outcome of children with first relapse of acute lymphoblastic leukaemia (ALL R3): an open-label randomised trial

Parker C, Waters R, Leighton C, et al (Univ of Manchester, UK; Univ of Oxford, UK; et al)

Lancet 376:2009-2017, 2010

Background.—Although survival of children with acute lymphoblastic leukaemia has improved greatly in the past two decades, the outcome of those who relapse has remained static. We investigated the outcome of children with acute lymphoblastic leukaemia who relapsed on present therapeutic regimens.

Methods.—This open-label randomised trial was undertaken in 22 centres in the UK and Ireland and nine in Australia and New Zealand. Patients aged 1–18 years with first relapse of acute lymphoblastic leukaemia were stratified into high-risk, intermediate-risk, and standard-risk groups on the basis of duration of first complete remission, site of relapse, and immunophenotype. All patients were allocated to receive either idarubicin or mitoxantrone in induction by stratified concealed randomisation. Neither patients nor those giving interventions were masked. After three blocks of therapy, all high-risk group patients and those from the intermediate group with postinduction high minimal residual disease ($\geq 10^{-4}$ cells) received an allogenic stem-cell transplant. Standard-risk and intermediate-risk patients with postinduction low minimal residual disease ($<10^{-4}$ cells) continued chemotherapy. The primary outcome was progression-free survival and the method of analysis was intention-to-treat. Randomisation was stopped in December, 2007 because of differences in progression-free and overall survival between the two groups. This trial is registered, reference number ISCRTN45724312.

Findings.—Of 239 registered patients, 216 were randomly assigned to either idarubicin (109 analysed) or mitoxantrone (103 analysed). Estimated 3-year progression-free survival was 35·9% (95% CI 25·9—45·9) in the idarubicin group versus 64·6% (54·2—73·2) in the mitoxantrone group (p=0·0004), and 3-year overall survival was 45·2% (34·5—55·3) versus 69·0% (58·5—77·3; p=0·004). Differences in progression-free survival between groups were mainly related to a decrease in disease events (progression, second relapse, disease-related deaths; HR 0·56, 0·34—0·92, p=0·007) rather than an increase in adverse treatment effects (treatment death, second malignancy; HR 0·52, 0·24—1·11, p=0·11).

Interpretation.—As compared with idarubicin, mitoxantrone conferred a significant benefit in progression-free and overall survival in children with relapsed acute lymphobastic leukaemia, a potentially useful clinical finding that warrants further investigation (Fig 3).

▶ Although many studies have examined the role of various anthracyclines in patients with newly diagnosed leukemia, most studies have concluded that the dose and not the anthracycline itself has been the most critical element. Fewer studies have been performed in patients with relapsed leukemia, and thus the report from Parker et al has potentially even more impact. In this study, they randomized 216 patients with relapsed acute lymphoblastic leukemia (ALL) to receive reinduction therapy with a regimen containing mitoxantrone or idarubicin. Subsequently, patients were directed to further chemotherapy or hematopoietic stem cell transplantation according to risk group stratification. The mitoxantrone and idarubicin were both dosed at 10 mg/m^2 on each of 2 days. The trial was stopped early because of significant differences in progression-free survival of 35.9% for the idarubicin cohort and 64.6% for the mitoxantrone group (Fig 3). Overall survival was also similarly significantly different. These results are important for several reasons, not the least of which is that mitoxantrone is often considered to have a 3:1 ratio of dose-related toxicity compared with doxorubicin, whereas idarubicin has a 5:1 relationship. With such a difference established, it should be important

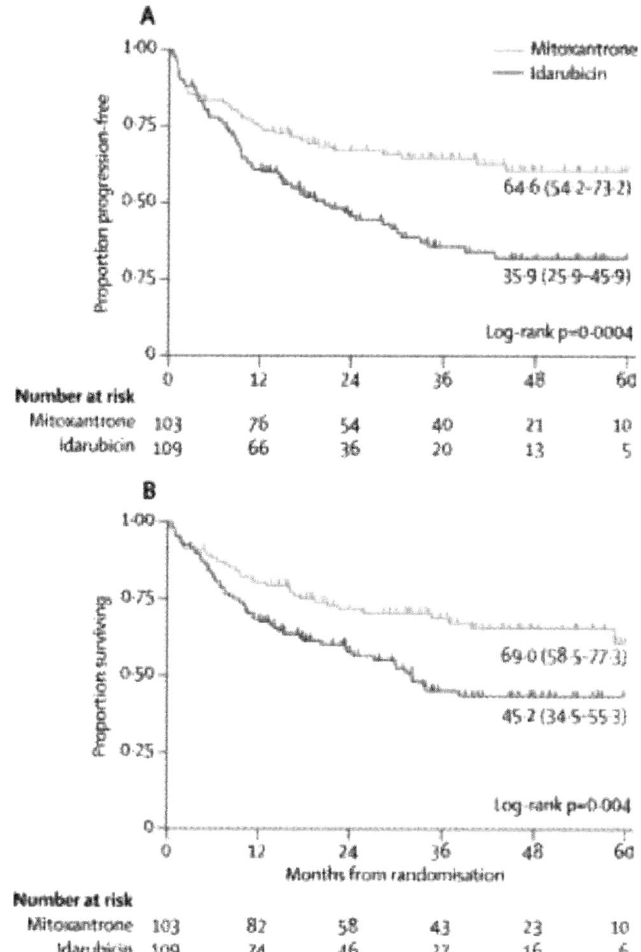

FIGURE 3.—Kaplan Meier estimates of progression-free (A) and overall (B) survival by randomised treatment 3-year estimated survival percentages (95% CI) are presented. (Reprinted from The Lancet, Parker C, Waters R, Leighton C, et al. Effect of mitoxantrone on outcome of children with first relapse of acute lymphoblastic leukaemia (ALL R3): an open-label randomised trial. *Lancet*. 2010;376:2009-2017. Copyright 2010, with permission from Elsevier.)

to determine the potential role of mitoxantrone in the treatment of patients with newly diagnosed ALL.

R. J. Arceci, MD, PhD

Genomic profiling in Down syndrome acute lymphoblastic leukemia identifies histone gene deletions associated with altered methylation profiles

Loudin MG, Wang J, Leung H-CE, et al (Baylor College of Medicine, Houston, TX; New York Univ Cancer Inst; et al)
Leukemia 1-9, 2011

Patients with Down syndrome (DS) and acute lymphoblastic leukemia (ALL) have distinct clinical and biological features. Whereas most DS-ALL cases lack the sentinel cytogenetic lesions that guide risk assignment in childhood ALL, *JAK2* mutations and *CRLF2* overexpression are highly enriched. To further characterize the unique biology of DS-ALL, we performed genome-wide profiling of 58 DS-ALL and 68 non-DS (NDS) ALL cases by DNA copy number, loss of heterozygosity, gene expression and methylation analyses. We report a novel deletion within the 6p22 histone gene cluster as significantly more frequent in DS-ALL, occurring in 11 DS (22%) and only 2 NDS cases (3.1%) (Fisher's exact $P=0.002$). Homozygous deletions yielded significantly lower histone expression levels, and were associated with higher methylation levels, distinct spatial localization of methylated promoters and enrichment of highly methylated genes for specific pathways and transcription factor-binding motifs. Gene expression profiling demonstrated heterogeneity of DS-ALL cases overall, with supervised analysis defining a 45-transcript signature associated with CRLF2 overexpression. Further characterization of pathways associated with histone deletions may identify opportunities for novel targeted interventions.

▶ The fact that children with Down syndrome (DS), or trisomy 21, have a 10- to 20-fold increased risk of the development of acute lymphoblastic leukemia (ALL) has led investigators to pursue how DS ALL might differ from that in other children. Previous studies have demonstrated that children with DS have fewer good prognosis characteristics associated with their leukemia, but there is still a large need to better understand the molecular differences. Loudin et al report genomewide profiling of 58 DS ALL compared with non-DS ALL cases. A particularly interesting finding is the significantly increased association of a 6p22 deletion in DS ALL (22% of cases) compared with only 3.1% in non-DS ALL. This deletion involves a cluster of histone genes, and such cases are shown to lower histone expression levels and altered DNA methylation patterns. They also report a 45-transcript expression signature that is associated with *CRLF2* overexpression, a previously reported abnormality associated with DS ALL. While no functional analyses or independent confirmation of the results are included, studies such as this are beginning to unravel the mystery of DS ALL and possibly open up the door to identifying more effective and less toxic treatments.

R. J. Arceci, MD, PhD

Impact of Pretransplantation Minimal Residual Disease, As Detected by Multiparametric Flow Cytometry, on Outcome of Myeloablative Hematopoietic Cell Transplantation for Acute Myeloid Leukemia

Walter RB, Gooley TA, Wood BL, et al (Fred Hutchinson Cancer Res Ctr, Seattle, WA; Univ of Washington, Seattle)

J Clin Oncol 29:1190-1197, 2011

Purpose.—Allogeneic hematopoietic cell transplantation (HCT) benefits many patients with acute myeloid leukemia (AML) in first remission. Hitherto, little attention has been given to the prognostic impact of pretransplantation minimal residual disease (MRD).

Patients and Methods.—We retrospectively studied 99 consecutive patients receiving myeloablative HCT for AML in first morphologic remission. Ten-color multiparametric flow cytometry (MFC) was performed on bone marrow aspirates before HCT. MRD was identified as a cell population showing deviation from normal antigen expression patterns compared with normal or regenerating marrow. Any level of residual disease was considered MRD positive.

Results.—Before HCT, 88 patients met morphologic criteria for complete remission (CR), whereas 11 had CR with incomplete blood count recovery (CRi). Twenty-four had MRD before HCT as determined by MFC. Two-year estimates of overall survival were 30.2% (range, 13.1% to 49.3%) and 76.6% (range, 64.4% to 85.1%) for MRD-positive and MRD-negative patients; 2-year estimates of relapse were 64.9% (range, 42.0% to 80.6%) and 17.6% (range, 9.5% to 27.9%). After adjustment for all or a subset of cytogenetic risk, secondary disease, incomplete blood count recovery, and abnormal karyotype pre-HCT, MRD-positive HCT was associated with increased overall mortality (hazard ratio [HR], 4.05; 95% CI, 1.90 to 8.62; $P < .001$) and relapse (HR, 8.49; 95% CI, 3.67 to 19.65; $P < .001$) relative to MRD-negative HCT.

Conclusion.—These data suggest that pre-HCT MRD is associated with increased risk of relapse and death after myeloablative HCT for AML in first morphologic CR, even after controlling for other risk factors.

▶ The prognostic impact of having minimal residual disease (MRD) following induction or consolidation therapy has been demonstrated in several studies of patients with newly diagnosed acute myeloid leukemia (AML). While there is some controversy as to the optimal approach to MRD measurements and levels that are optimal, the consensus is that being MRD positive is in most circumstances going to be associated with relapse. Less information has been garnered for MRD status immediately before pre–hematopoietic stem cell transplantation (HSCT). There has been a belief, in fact, that HSCT is able to overcome MRD. Walter et al now help to answer these questions by measuring MRD in 88 patients with AML in morphological remission before HSCT. Approximately 27% of these patients had MRD detected prior to HSCT using a sensitive 10-color flow cytometric assay. They observed a significant

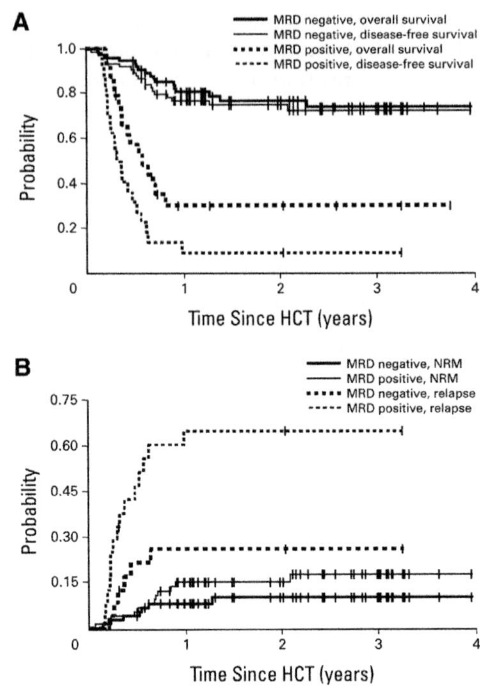

FIGURE 1.—Overall survival (OS), disease-free survival (DFS), relapse, and nonrelapse mortality (NRM). Estimates of the probability of (A) OS and DFS as well as (B) relapse and NRM for patients with acute myeloid leukemia in first morphological remission, with negative versus positive multiparametric flow cytometry results for pre-hematopoietic cell transplantation (HCT) minimal residual disease (MRD). (Reprinted with permission. © 2011 American Society of Clinical Oncology. All rights reserved. Walter RB, Gooley TA, Wood BL, et al. Impact of pretransplantation minimal residual disease, as detected by multiparametric flow cytometry, on outcome of myeloablative hematopoietic cell transplantation for acute myeloid leukemia. *J Clin Oncol.* 2011;29:1190-1197.)

difference in 2-year overall survival (OS), with the MRD-positive and MRD-negative groups having 2-year OSs of 30.2% and 76.6%, respectively (Fig 1). The hazard ratio was 4.07 for increased overall mortality in the MRD-positive group. This study presents important data despite several potential caveats. The retrospective nature of the study could bring up the question of potential bias, and defining a minimal level of MRD that was predictive would have been potentially important. The range of MRD levels went from 0.01% to 3%, with the majority being greater than 0.1%. Nevertheless, this study helps to define a high-risk group of patients who should be considered for additional therapy in conjunction with HSCT, such as immunomodulatory therapy, or alternative approaches to HSCT.

R. J. Arceci, MD, PhD

Outcomes of pediatric bone marrow transplantation for leukemia and myelodysplasia using matched sibling, mismatched related, or matched unrelated donors

Shaw PJ, Kan F, Woo Ahn K, et al (Children's Hosp at Westmead, Sydney, Australia; Natl Marrow Donor Program, Minneapolis, MN; Med College of Wisconsin, Milwaukee; et al)

Blood 116:4007-4015, 2010

Although some trials have allowed matched or single human leukocyte antigen (HLA)–mismatched related donors (mmRDs) along with HLA-matched sibling donors (MSDs) for pediatric bone marrow transplantation in early-stage hematologic malignancies, whether mmRD grafts lead to similar outcomes is not known. We compared patients < 18 years old reported to the Center for International Blood and Marrow Transplant Research with acute myeloid leukemia, acute lymphoblastic leukemia, chronic myeloid leukemia, and myelodysplastic syndrome undergoing allogeneic T-replete, myeloablative bone marrow transplantation between 1993 and 2006. In total, patients receiving bone marrow from 1208 MSDs, 266 8/8 allelic-matched unrelated donors (URDs), and 151 0-1 HLA-antigen mmRDs were studied. Multivariate analysis showed that recipients of MSD transplants had less transplantation-related mortality, acute graft-versus-host disease (GVHD), and chronic GVHD, along with better disease-free and overall survival than the URD and mmRD groups. No differences were observed in transplant-related mortality, acute and chronic GVHD, relapse, disease-free survival, or overall survival between the mmRD and URD groups. These data show that mmRD and 8/8 URD outcomes are similar, whereas MSD outcomes are superior to the other 2 sources. Whether allele level typing could identify mmRD recipients with better outcomes will not be known unless centers alter practice and type mmRD at the allele level.

▶ The optimal selection of a donor for hematopoietic stem cell transplantation in patients with a history of myelodysplastic syndrome or leukemia has not been determined. There are data that would support the concept that some degree of mismatch may augment graft versus leukemia and improve overall survival. However, there is also the chance of increased graft-versus-host disease in such circumstances that can lead to increased treatment-related mortality. This retrospective study by Shaw et al primarily uses data from the Center for International Blood and Marrow Transplant Research (CIBMTR) registry. Data were collected from 1993 to 2006, which certainly raises questions about the conclusions being made, as human leukocyte antigen typing and transplantation have changed significantly since the early 1990s. There are also significant differences in many characteristics of the patients treated with the 3 different donor types being analyzed. Furthermore, survival and other clinical parameters appear to be only carried out to 36 months, even though the last patients included were from 2006. Despite these caveats, the outcome results of 3 different donor types in just over 1200 pediatric patients are potentially important. The results suggest that matched sibling donors provide the best clinical outcomes compared with either matched-unrelated donors or mismatched-related donors. It would certainly have been interesting to see what outcomes might be documented for a large group transplanted with haplo-identical donors.

R. J. Arceci, MD, PhD

Postrelapse survival in childhood acute lymphoblastic leukemia is independent of initial treatment intensity: a report from the Children's Oncology Group

Freyer DR, Devidas M, La M, et al (Univ of Southern California, Los Angeles, CA; Univ of Florida, Gainesville; Children's Oncology Group, Arcadia, CA; et al)

Blood 117:3010-3015, 2011

While intensification of therapy has improved event-free survival (EFS) and survival in newly diagnosed children with acute lymphoblastic leukemia (ALL), postrelapse outcomes remain poor. It might be expected that patients relapsing after inferior initial therapy would have a higher retrieval rate than after superior therapy. In the Children's Oncology Group Study CCG-1961, significantly superior EFS and survival were achieved with an augmented (stronger) versus standard intensity regimen of postinduction intensification (PII) for children with newly diagnosed high-risk ALL and rapid day 7 marrow response (EFS/survival 81.2%/88.7% vs 71.7%/83.4%, respectively). This provided an opportunity to evaluate postrelapse survival (PRS) in 272 relapsed patients who had received randomly allocated initial treatment with augmented or standard intensity PII. As expected, PRS was worse for early versus late relapse, marrow versus extramedullary site, adolescent versus younger age and T versus B lineage. However, no difference in 3-year PRS was detected for having received augmented versus standard intensity PII (36.4% ± 5.7% vs 39.2% ± 4.1%; log rank $P = .72$). Similar findings were noted within subanalyses by timing and site of relapse, age, and immunophenotype. These findings provide insight into mechanisms of relapse in ALL, and are consistent with emergence of a resistant subclone that has acquired spontaneous mutations largely independent of initial therapy. This study is registered at www.clinicaltrials.gov as NCT00002812.

▶ The outcome for patients with relapsed leukemia is usually considered poor but dependent on a variety of prognostic factors, such as initial risk group of the diagnostic leukemia, age, type of relapse (extramedullary or bone marrow) and, critically, time of relapse. An unanswered question has been what role the type of prior treatment plays in outcome following relapse. Freyer et al examine this question in children with acute lymphoblastic leukemia who were initially treated on the Children's Oncology Group Study-1961, which had randomly assigned patients to receive a more intense (augmented) versus standard intensity postremission treatment. In addition to the usual suspects impacting prognosis, the intensity of treatment prior to relapse was notably absent as a significant prognostic factor with 3-year postrelapse survival rate being 36.4% for the augmented treatment group and 39.2% for the standard intensity treated group (Fig 1 in original article). These results imply that alterations in the leukemia at the time of relapse may be independent of the prior treatment. While these data may apply only to the type of prior treatment, they do help to answer and in fact contradict the bias that intensive up-front treatment will always result in more resistant disease that, in turn, is associated with worse outcome.

R. J. Arceci, MD, PhD

Prognostic significance of additional cytogenetic aberrations in 733 de novo pediatric 11q23/*MLL*-rearranged AML patients: results of an international study

Coenen EA, Raimondi SC, Harbott J, et al (Erasmus MC—Sophia Children's Hosp, Rotterdam, The Netherlands; St Jude Children's Res Hosp, Memphis, TN; Justus-Liebig-Univ, Giessen, Germany; et al)

Blood 117:7102-7111, 2011

We previously showed that outcome of pediatric 11q23/*MLL*-rearranged AML depends on the translocation partner (TP). In this multicenter international study on 733 children with 11q23/*MLL*-rearranged AML, we further analyzed which additional cytogenetic aberrations (ACA) had prognostic significance. ACAs occurred in 344/733 (47%) and were associated with unfavorable outcome (5-year overall survival (OS) 47% vs. 62%, P<0.001). Trisomy 8, the most frequent specific ACA (n=130/344, 38%), independently predicted favorable outcome within the ACAs group (OS 61% vs. 39%, P=0.003; Cox model for OS Hazard Ratio (HR) 0.54, P=0.03), based on reduced relapse rate (26% vs. 49%, P<0.001). Trisomy 19 (n=37/344, 11%) independently predicted poor prognosis in ACAs cases, which was partly caused by refractory disease (remission rate 74% vs. 89%, P=0.04; OS 24% vs. 50%, P<0.001; HR 1.77, P=0.01). Structural ACAs had independent adverse prognostic value for event free survival (EFS) (HR 1.36, P=0.01). Complex karyotype, defined as ≥3 abnormalities, was present in 26% (n=192/733), and showed worse outcome than those without complex karyotype (OS 45% vs. 59%, P=0.003) in univariate analysis only. In conclusion, like TP, specific ACAs have independent prognostic significance in pediatric 11q23/*MLL*-rearranged AML, and the mechanism underlying these prognostic differences should be studied.

▶ Translocations involving the MLL (mixed lineage leukemia) gene located on the long arm of chromosome 11 are common in acute myeloid leukemia (AML), and particularly in infant leukemia and secondary AML. Previous reports have documented that the many different translocation partners portend varied prognoses for children with MLL rearrangements. The study by Coenen et al takes a previous international cohort of children with MLL rearranged leukemia a step further with an analysis of the influence of additional chromosome abnormalities on outcome. They find that a high percentage of cases (47%) have such additional cytogenetic abnormalities (ACAs) and that they independently predict a worse outcome. In particular, trisomy 19 predicted a particularly poor prognosis, whereas the presence of trisomy 8 predicted a more favorable prognosis. These results are important in further defining the impact of heterogeneity on outcome. As noted by the authors, the results also show that ACAs can alter the phenotype of AML driven by the powerful MLL oncogene and may lead the way to future studies of which genes involved the ACAs.

R. J. Arceci, MD, PhD

Prognostic significance of the initial cerebro-spinal fluid (CSF) involvement of children with acute lymphoblastic leukaemia (ALL) treated without cranial irradiation: Results of European Organization for Research and Treatment of Cancer (EORTC) Children Leukemia Group study 58881

Sirvent N, Suciu S, Rialland X, et al (CHU Nice, France; EORTC Headquarters, Brussels, Belgium; CHU Angers, France; et al)

Eur J Cancer 47:239-247, 2011

Aim of the Study.—To evaluate the prognostic significance of the initial cerebro-spinal fluid (CSF) involvement of children with ALL enrolled from 1989 to 1996 in the EORTC 58881 trial.

Patients and Methods.—Patients (2025) were categorised according to initial central nervous system (CNS) status: CNS-1 (CNS negative, $n = 1866$), CNS-2 (<5 leucocytes/mm^3, CSF with blasts, $n = 50$), CNS-3 (CNS positive, $n = 49$), TLP+ (TLP with blasts, $n = 60$). CNS-directed therapy consisted in intravenous (i.v.) methotrexate (5 g/sqm) in 4–10 courses, and intrathecal methotrexate injections (10–20), according to CNS status. Cranial irradiation was omitted in all patients.

Results.—In the CNS1, TLP+, CNS2 and CNS3 group the 8-year EFS rate (SE%) was 69.7% (1.1%), 68.8% (6.2%), 71.3% (6.5%) and 68.3% (6.2%), respectively. The 8-year incidence of isolated CNS relapse (SE%) was 3.4% (0.4%), 1.7% (1.7%), 6.1% (3.5%) and 9.4% (4.5%), respectively, whereas the 8-year isolated or combined CNS relapse incidence was 7.6% (0.6%), 3.5% (2.4%), 10.2% (4.4%) and 11.7% (5.0%), respectively. Patients with CSF blasts had a higher rate of initial bad risk features. Multivariate analysis indicated that presence of blasts in the CSF had no prognostic value: (i) for EFS and OS; (ii) for isolated and isolated or combined CNS relapse; WBC count $< 25 \times 10^9$/L and Medac E-coli asparaginase treatment were each related to a lower CNS relapse risk.

Conclusions.—The presence of initial CNS involvement has no prognostic significance in EORTC 58881. Intensification of CNS-directed chemotherapy, without CNS radiation, is an effective treatment of initial meningeal leukaemic involvement.

▶ One of the major discoveries in the treatment of childhood acute lymphoblastic leukemia (ALL) was the preemptive treatment of the central nervous system (CNS) with radiation therapy along with intrathecal chemotherapy. While this significantly reduced the number of patients with relapsed leukemia, it soon became clear that such treatment could have devastating consequences on the neurocognitive development of such young patients. In addition, these adverse sequelae were particularly severe in young females. There has thus been a gradual but important movement to reduce or even eliminate central nervous system radiation by intensifying both intrathecal and systemic chemotherapy. Several groups have now done studies to this end. The article by Sirvent et al describes the analysis of the EORTC 58881 study, which did not deliver CNS radiation to any patients, regardless of the presenting leukemic status in the cerebral spinal fluid. While the cumulative incidence of isolated CNS relapses appeared to be greater in the EORTC study compared with others of the same vintage, the cumulative incidence of combined bone marrow plus CNS was lower in the EORTC study, suggesting that the intensification of system therapy affects the latter more than the former. Indeed, the EORTC 58881 study gave 9 to 10 courses of systemic high-dose methotrexate compared with 4 courses in the BFM 95 and St Jude XV study. Another important aspect of this article is that patients received prednisolone and not dexamethasone during induction; the latter has been shown to have better CNS penetration but more skeletal and infectious complications during induction. The bottom line is that it now appears that CNS radiation may be avoidable in nearly all children with newly diagnosed ALL without risking a reduction in overall survival. More studies on the neurocognitive consequences of intensified intrathecal and systemic therapy now need to be done.

R. J. Arceci, MD, PhD

RUNX1 Mutations in Acute Myeloid Leukemia: Results From a Comprehensive Genetic and Clinical Analysis From the AML Study Group

Gaidzik VI, Bullinger L, Schlenk RF, et al (Univ Hosp of Ulm, Germany; Hannover Med School, Germany; et al)

J Clin Oncol 29:1364-1372, 2011

Purpose.—To evaluate frequency, biologic features, and clinical relevance of *RUNX1* mutations in acute myeloid leukemia (AML).

Patients and Methods.—Diagnostic samples from 945 patients (age 18 to 60 years) were analyzed for *RUNX1* mutations. In a subset of cases (n = 269), microarray gene expression analysis was performed.

Results.—Fifty-nine *RUNX1* mutations were identified in 53 (5.6%) of 945 cases, predominantly in exons 3 (n = 11), 4 (n = 10), and 8 (n = 23). *RUNX1* mutations clustered in the intermediate-risk cytogenetic group

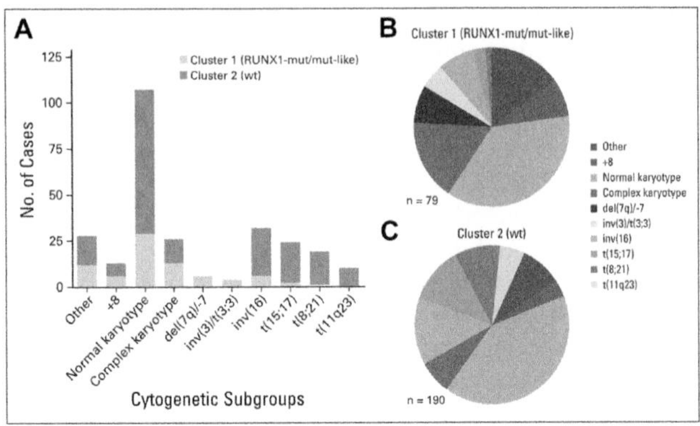

FIGURE 4.—Hierarchical cluster analysis on the basis of the significance analysis of microarrays (SAM)–derived *RUNX1* mutation–associated signature. (A) Comparison of the distribution of cytogenetic subgroups within the hierarchical cluster analysis defined clusters (Data Supplement). Cytogenetic adverse-risk groups with deletion 7q or monosomy 7 [del(7q)/-7] and with inv(3) or t(3;3) were significantly enriched in the *RUNX1* mutation–associated cluster 1 ($P < .0001$, χ^2 test). (B and C) The proportion of AML cases with complex karyotypes (indicated in gray) was significantly higher in (B) the *RUNX1*-mutation–associated cluster 1, whereas almost all inv(16), t(8;21), t(15;17), and t(11q23) cases were present in (C) the *RUNX1*-wild-type–associated cluster 2. mut, mutated; wt, wild-type. (Reprinted from Gaidzik VI, Bullinger L, Schlenk RF, et al. *RUNX1* mutations in acute myeloid leukemia: results from a comprehensive genetic and clinical analysis from the AML study group. *J Clin Oncol.* 2011;29:1364-1372. Reprinted with permission. Copyright 2011 American Society of Clinical Oncology. All rights reserved.)

(46 of 640, 7.2%; cytogenetically normal, 34 of 538, 6.3%), whereas they were less frequent in adverse-risk cytogenetics (five of 109, 4.6%) and absent in core-binding-factor AML (0 of 77) and acute promyelocytic leukemia (0 of 61). *RUNX1* mutations were associated with *MLL*-partial tandem duplications ($P = .0007$) and *IDH1/IDH2* mutations ($P = .03$), inversely correlated with *NPM1* ($P < .0001$), and in trend with *CEBPA* ($P = .10$) mutations. *RUNX1* mutations were characterized by a distinct gene expression pattern; this *RUNX1* mutation-derived signature was not exclusive for the mutation, but also included mostly adverse-risk AML [eg, 7q-, -7, inv(3), or t(3;3)]. *RUNX1* mutations predicted for resistance to chemotherapy (rates of refractory disease 30% and 19%, $P = .047$, for *RUNX1*-mutated and wild-type patients, respectively), as well as inferior event-free survival (EFS; $P < .0001$), relapse-free survival (RFS, $P = .022$), and overall survival ($P = .051$). In multivariable analysis, *RUNX1* mutations were an independent prognostic marker for shorter EFS ($P = .007$). Explorative subgroup analysis revealed that allogeneic hematopoietic stem-cell transplantation had a favorable impact on RFS in *RUNX1*-mutated patients ($P < .0001$).

Conclusion.—AML with *RUNX1* mutations are characterized by distinct genetic properties and are associated with resistance to therapy and inferior outcome (Fig 4).

▶ Identification of prognostic markers in acute myeloid leukemia (AML) that in turn could provide possible therapeutic targets remains a major goal. The runt-related transcription factor *RUNX1* has been known to be involved in the canonical translocation t(8;21) of good-risk AML. A previous study by Tang et al[1] had demonstrated that about 13% of adult patients had *RUNX1* mutations associated with their AML and also had an inferior overall survival. The study by Gaidzik et al now reports on a larger cohort of patients ages 18 to 60 years and finds incidence of *RUNX1* mutations present in 5.6% but more associated with groups of patients with AML having cytogenetically normal karyotype, *MLL*-partial tandem duplications, and *IDH1*/*IDH2* mutations (Fig 4). Of note, most of the mutations were frame shift mutations, and all mutations were heterozygous and clustered between exons 3 and 5. Outcome analysis found significantly inferior event-free survival, disease-free survival, and overall survival in patients with AML having mutations in *RUNX1*. A subgroup analysis suggested that allogeneic transplantation improved the relapse-free survival in patients with *RUNX1*-mutated AML, although the post hoc analysis and small numbers lessen the impact of this potentially important observation. These results extend those from earlier reports and provide potentially important insights into the biology of *RUNX1*-mutated AML and the pathways that could be possibly manipulated for new treatment approaches.

R. J. Arceci, MD, PhD

Reference

1. Tang JL, Hou HA, Chen CY, et al. AML1/RUNX1 mutations in 470 adult patients with de novo acute myeloid leukemia: prognostic implication and interaction with other gene alterations. *Blood*. 2009;114:5352-5361.

Secondary solid cancers after allogeneic hematopoietic-cell transplantation using busulfan-cyclophosphamide conditioning

Majhail NS, Brazauskas R, Rizzo JD, et al (Ctr for International Blood and Marrow Transplant Res, Minneapolis, MN; Ctr for International Blood and Marrow Transplant Res, Milwaukee, WI; et al)
Blood 117:316-322, 2011

Risks of secondary solid cancers among allogeneic hematopoietic-cell transplant (HCT) recipients who receive conditioning without total-body irradiation are not well known. We evaluated the incidence and risk-factors for solid cancers after HCT using high-dose busulfan-cyclophosphamide (Bu-Cy) conditioning in 4,318 recipients of first allogeneic HCT for acute myeloid leukemia (AML) in first complete remission (N=1,742) and chronic myeloid leukemia (CML) in first chronic phase (N=2,576). Our cohort represented 22,041 person-years at risk. Sixty-six solid cancers were reported at a median of 6-years after HCT. The cumulative-incidence of solid cancers at 5- and 10-years after HCT was 0.6% and 1.2% among AML and 0.9% and 2.4% among CML patients. In comparison to general population incidence rates, HCT recipients had 1.4 times higher than expected rate of invasive solid cancers (95% CI, 1.08-1.79, P=0.01). Significantly elevated risks were observed for tumors of the oral cavity, esophagus, lung, soft tissue and brain. Chronic graft-versus-host disease was an independent risk-factor for all solid cancers, and especially cancers of the oral cavity. Recipients of allogeneic HCT using Bu-Cy conditioning are at risk for developing solid cancers. Their incidence continues to increase with time since HCT and life-long cancer surveillance is warranted in this population.

▶ Adverse late effects in survivors of cancer has received increasingly more attention as the numbers of survivors has increased and been carefully monitored. Other than recurrence, one of the most dreaded late effects of having had cancer is the development of a secondary cancer. Such secondary cancers, and particularly solid tumors, have not been extensively explored following hematopoietic stem cell transplantation (HSCT). The article by Majhail et al examines these secondary malignancies in 4318 recipients of busulphan-based preparative regimens for HSCT in patients with myeloid malignancies. Approximately 22 000 person-years of risk are examined. Importantly, they include young children as well as young and older adults. They report a solid tumor incidence of 0.6% to 0.9% at 5 years and 1.2% to 2.4% at 10 years in patients who underwent HSCT for acute myeloid leukemia or chronic myeloid leukemia, respectively. These figures represent an approximately 1.4 times higher incidence than expected population rates. A major risk factor was the presence of chronic graft-versus-host disease, which ironically has also been associated with a lower risk of leukemia relapse. This report gives real numbers and risk for the development of secondary malignancies in this group of patients, along with the types of tumors for preemptive screening in the needed lifelong surveillance.

R. J. Arceci, MD, PhD

6 Lymphoproliferative Disorders and Lymphoma

Autoimmune Lymphoproliferative Syndrome Like Disease With Somatic *KRAS* Mutation

Takagi M, Shinoda K, Piao J, et al (Tokyo Med and Dental Univ, Bunkyo-ku, Japan; Gifu Municipal Hosp, Gifu-shi, Japan; et al)

Blood 117:2887-2890, 2011

Autoimmune lymphoproliferative syndrome (ALPS) is classically defined as a disease with defective FAS-mediated apoptosis (Type I–III). Germline *NRAS* mutation was recently identified in Type IV ALPS. We report two cases with ALPS like disease with somatic *KRAS* mutation. Both of the cases were characterized by prominent autoimmune cytopenia and lymphoadenopathy/splenomegaly. These patients did not satisfy the diagnostic criteria for ALPS or juvenile myelomonocytic leukemia (JMML), and are likely to be defined as a new disease entity of RAS associated ALPS like disease (RALD).

▶ Autoimmune lymphoproliferative syndrome (ALPS) results from defects in *FAS*-mediated apoptosis. The disease is characterized by diffuse adenopathy, autoimmune phenomenon, and a propensity for lymphoma development. Mutations in *FAS* or *FASL* are critical for the regulation of lymphocyte expansion. Quite surprisingly, germline mutations in *NRAS* were subsequently identified in a subtype of ALPS. That *NRAS* could be involved in such a syndrome was noteworthy, as it associated an alternative pathway of T lymphocyte proliferation to inherited disease. In their report, Takagi et al show that somatic mutation of *NRAS* is associated with a variant of ALPS. Of note, the disease in the patients they describe does not fit the classical forms of ALPS or of juvenile myelomonocytic leukemia, which is closely linked to *RAS* and *RAS* pathway mutations. These results point to *RAS* in a variety of cancers as well as autoimmune syndromes. Ironically, despite its central importance, it, like *p53*, has not been able to be effectively exploited therapeutically.

R. J. Arceci, MD, PhD

Disruption of MyD88 signaling suppresses hemophagocytic lymphohistiocytosis in mice

Krebs P, Crozat K, Popkin D, et al (The Scripps Res Inst, La Jolla, CA)
Blood 117:6582-6588, 2011

Hemophagocytic lymphohistiocytosis (HLH) is a rare inflammatory disorder with a poor prognosis for affected individuals. To find a means of suppressing the clinical phenotype, we investigated the cellular and molecular mechanisms leading to HLH in *Unc13d*$^{jinx/jinx}$ mice, in which cytolytic function of NK and CD8$^+$ T cells is impaired. *Unc13d*$^{jinx/jinx}$ mutants infected with lymphochoriomeningitis virus (LCMV) present typical clinical features of HLH, including splenomegaly, elevated serum IFNγ, and anemia. Proteins mediating cell-cell contact, cytokine signaling or Toll-like receptor (TLR) signaling were analyzed. We show that neither the integrin CD18, which is involved in adhesion between antigen-presenting cells and effector T cells, nor tumor necrosis factor (TNF) made nonredundant contributions to the disease phenotype. Disruption of IFNγ signaling reduced immune cell activation in *Unc13d*$^{jinx/jinx}$ mice, but also resulted in uncontrolled viral proliferation and exaggerated release of inflammatory cytokines. Abrogating the function of myeloid differentiation primary response gene 88 (MyD88) in *Unc13d*$^{jinx/jinx}$ mice suppressed immune cell activation and controlled cytokine production in an IL-1 receptor 1 (IL-1R1)–independent way. Our findings implicate MyD88 as the key initiator of myeloid and lymphoid proliferation in HLH, and suggest that blockade of this signaling molecule may reduce immunopathology in patients.

▶ Hemophagocytic lymphohistiocytosis (HLH) was an enigmatic disorder of immune dysregulation with decreased or absent natural killer (NK) and cytolytic T-lymphocyte (CTL) function until the first causative gene mutation was discovered. That gene encoded the cytolytic granule perforin, thus explaining in part the inability of NK cells and CTLs to control their target cells, and unleashing a self-perpetuating wheel of hypercytokinemia. Subsequent mutated genes have been discovered and they have essentially all been shown to function in some aspect of cytolytic granule formation and transport. Although such elegant studies of the molecular aspects of HLH were ongoing, treatment of patients also improved but, like many areas of medicine, through relatively empiric approaches directed at immunosuppression and hematopoietic stem cell transplantation. The article by Krebs et al forces thinking about HLH in a possible new direction. Using a murine knockout model of the Unc13d gene, they were able to identify the myeloid differentiation primary response gene 88 (MyD88) as being necessary for essential characteristics of HLH. By abrogating the function of MyD88, these mice did not superactivate the immune system or increase cytokine production. Importantly, this effect was observed to be interleukin (IL)-1 independent. This is important, as IL1-receptor antagonists have been used in anecdotal cases to treat patients with HLH. Also important is that blocking interferon gamma reduced immune activation but also resulted in uncontrolled viral proliferation and exaggerated production of inflammatory cytokines. These results thus point to a potentially novel therapeutic target for these devastating syndromes. The study represents an excellent example of how mouse models can potentially inform us with regard to new treatment approaches.

R. J. Arceci, MD, PhD

Morbidity and mortality in long-term survivors of Hodgkin lymphoma: a report from the Childhood Cancer Survivor Study

Castellino SM, Geiger AM, Mertens AC, et al (Wake Forest Univ Health Sciences, Winston-Salem, NC; Emory Univ School of Medicine, Atlanta GA; et al)

Blood 117:1806-1816, 2011

The contribution of specific cancer therapies, comorbid medical conditions, and host factors to mortality risk after pediatric Hodgkin lymphoma (HL) is unclear. We assessed leading morbidities, overall and cause-specific mortality, and mortality risks among 2742 survivors of HL in the Childhood Cancer Survivor Study, a multi-institutional retrospective cohort study of survivors diagnosed from 1970 to 1986. Excess absolute risk for leading causes of death and cumulative incidence and standardized incidence ratios of key medical morbidities were calculated. Cox regression models were used to estimate hazard ratios (HRs) and 95% confidence intervals (CIs) of risks for overall and cause-specific mortality. Substantial excess absolute risk of mortality per 10 000 person-years was identified: overall 95.5; death due to HL 38.3, second malignant neoplasms 23.9, and cardiovascular disease 13.1. Risks for overall mortality included radiation dose ≥3000 rad (≥30 Gy; supra-diaphragm: HR, 3.8; 95% CI, 1.1-12.6; infradiaphragm + supradiaphragm: HR, 7.8; 95% CI, 2.4-25.1), exposure to anthracycline (HR, 2.6; 95% CI, 1.6-4.3) or alkylating agents (HR, 1.7; 95% CI, 1.2-2.5), non–breast second malignant neoplasm (HR, 2.6; 95% CI 1.4-5.1), or a serious cardiovascular condition (HR, 4.4; 95% CI 2.7-7.3). Excess mortality from second neoplasms and cardiovascular disease vary by sex and persist > 20 years of follow-up in childhood HL survivors.

▶ Hodgkin lymphoma was one of the first cancers to be cured, initially with radiation therapy, followed by multiagent chemotherapy. The dark side of these cures was unfortunately the adverse late effects that have become apparent over subsequent years. The Childhood Cancer Survivor Study has been one of the key programs to report detailed, quantitative information on late effects of therapy in survivors of Hodgkin lymphoma. The study by Castellino et al documents adverse late effects in 2742 survivors of Hodgkin lymphoma diagnosed and treated from 1970 to 1986. The results are sobering, with 70% of survivors having at least 1 chronic condition and 27% having a serious (ie, grade 3 to 4) chronic condition. Some of the most frequent adverse sequelae include secondary malignancies, particularly thyroid cancers (Fig 3) and cardiovascular disease, which occurred more frequently in men than in women. While it could be argued that treatments have considerably improved since the 1970s, many of the same

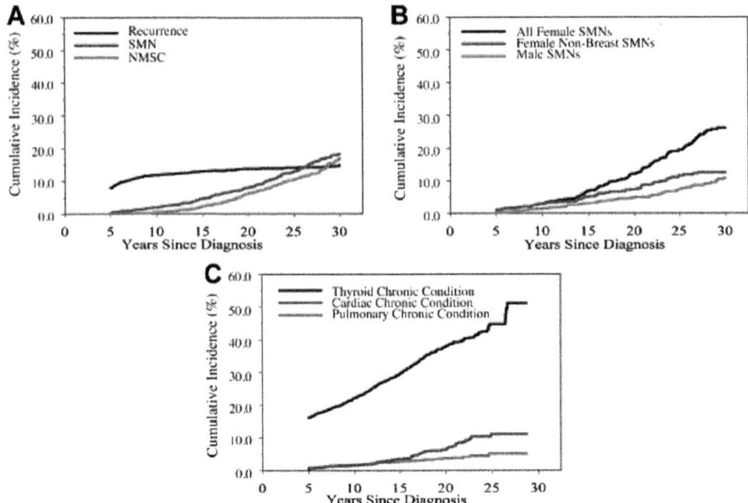

FIGURE 3.—Cumulative incidence of leading chronic medical conditions in 5-year survivors of childhood Hodgkin lymphoma. (A) all neoplasms; (B) invasive second malignant neoplasms (SMNs) by sex (log-rank for women with no breast SMN vs male SMN, $P = .05$); (C) other nonneoplastic conditions. (Reprinted from Castellino SM, Geiger AM, Mertens AC, et al. Morbidity and mortality in long-term survivors of Hodgkin lymphoma: a report from the Childhood Cancer Survivor Study. *Blood.* 2011;117:1806-1816. © The American Society of Hematology.)

therapies are still used, albeit in reduced doses or with alternative agents. Only time will answer the important question as to the incidence of adverse sequelae in more recently treated patients, while even the next generation of treatments, hopefully less toxic, are being introduced.

R. J. Arceci, MD, PhD

Reduced Treatment Intensity in Patients with Early-Stage Hodgkin's Lymphoma

Engert A, Plütschow A, Eich HT, et al (Univ of Cologne, Germany; et al)
N Engl J Med 363:640-652, 2010

Background.—Whether it is possible to reduce the intensity of treatment in early (stage I or II) Hodgkin's lymphoma with a favorable prognosis remains unclear. We therefore conducted a multicenter, randomized trial comparing four treatment groups consisting of a combination chemotherapy regimen of two different intensities followed by involved-field radiation therapy at two different dose levels.

Methods.—We randomly assigned 1370 patients with newly diagnosed early-stage Hodgkin's lymphoma with a favorable prognosis to one of four treatment groups: four cycles of doxorubicin, bleomycin, vinblastine, and dacarbazine (ABVD) followed by 30 Gy of radiation therapy (group 1), four cycles of ABVD followed by 20 Gy of radiation therapy (group 2), two cycles of ABVD followed by 30 Gy of radiation therapy (group 3), or two cycles of ABVD followed by 20 Gy of radiation therapy (group 4). The primary end point was freedom from treatment failure; secondary end points included efficacy and toxicity of treatment.

Results.—The two chemotherapy regimens did not differ significantly with respect to freedom from treatment failure (P=0.39) or overall survival (P=0.61). At 5 years, the rates of freedom from treatment failure were 93.0% (95% confidence interval [CI], 90.5 to 94.8) with the four-cycle ABVD regimen and 91.1% (95% CI, 88.3 to 93.2) with the two-cycle regimen. When the effects of 20-Gy and 30-Gy doses of radiation therapy were compared, there were also no significant differences in freedom from treatment failure (P=1.00) or overall survival (P=0.61). Adverse events and acute toxic effects of treatment were most common in the patients who received four cycles of ABVD and 30 Gy of radiation therapy (group 1).

Conclusions.—In patients with early-stage Hodgkin's lymphoma and a favorable prognosis, treatment with two cycles of ABVD followed by 20 Gy of involved-field radiation therapy is as effective as, and less toxic than, four cycles of ABVD followed by 30 Gy of involved-field radiation therapy. Long-term effects of these treatments have not yet been fully assessed. (Funded by the Deutsche Krebshilfe and the Swiss Federal Government; ClinicalTrials.gov number, NCT00265018.)

▶ Prior to the development of effective chemotherapeutic agents to treat Hodgkin disease, radiation therapy was the mainstay of effective treatment for these patients. Radiation therapy was especially effective for patients with early stage disease, yet there certainly were recurrences after radiation therapy. In addition, when radiation therapy was given as extended field treatment or total lymphoid irradiation, the risk of secondary tumors was significant and concerning. With the development of effective chemotherapy and combining it with radiation therapy, the doses and volumes of radiation therapy can be decreased. However, exactly which combination of chemotherapy and radiation (dose and volume) was the most effective and with the least toxicity remained a serious question.

These authors have looked at both the chemotherapy and radiation therapy question in patients with favorable stage I and II Hodgkin disease and randomly assigned them into this 4-arm study. It is encouraging that 2 cycles of doxorubicin, bleomycin, vinblastine, and dacarbazine (ABVD) chemotherapy were found to be as effective as 4 cycles of ABVD at 5 years. It is also encouraging to note that 20 Gy of involved field radiation therapy was found to be as effective as 30 Gy at 5 years. Clearly, longer follow-up is needed to assess the late effects of the different treatments. Yet one has to assume that the late effects of both less chemotherapy and less radiation will likely result in fewer long-term toxicities. We await that follow-up. In the interim, a new standard has been developed for patients with favorable-prognosis stage I and II Hodgkin disease based on this work.

C. A. Lawton, MD

7 Thoracic Cancer

Biology

Pleural fluid analysis of lung cancer *vs* benign inflammatory disease patients

Kremer R, Best LA, Savulescu D, et al (Rambam Health Care Campus, Haifa, Israel; Technion – Israel Inst of Technology Haifa)
Br J Cancer 102:1180-1184, 2010

Background.—Correct diagnosis of pleural effusion (PE) as either benign or malignant is crucial, although conventional cytological evaluation is of limited diagnostic accuracy, with relatively low sensitivity rates.

Methods.—We identified biological markers accurately detected in a simple PE examination. We analysed data from 19 patients diagnosed with lung cancer (nine adeno-Ca, five non-small-cell Ca (not specified), four squamous-cell Ca, one large-cell Ca) and 22 patients with benign inflammatory pathologies: secondary to trauma, pneumonia or TB.

Results.—Pleural effusion concentrations of seven analysed biological markers were significantly lower in lung cancer patients than in benign inflammatory patients, especially in matrix metalloproteinase (MMP)-9, MMP-3 and CycD1 (lower by 65% ($P < 0.000003$), 40% ($P < 0.0007$) and 34% ($P < 0.0001$), respectively), and in Ki67, ImAnOx, carbonyls and p27. High rates of sensitivity and specificity values were found for MMP-9, MMP-3 and CycD1: 80 and 100%; 87 and 73%; and 87 and 82%, respectively.

Conclusion.—Although our results are of significant merit in both the clinical and pathogenetic aspects of lung cancer, further research aimed at defining the best combination for marker analysis is warranted. The relative simplicity in analysing these markers in any routine hospital laboratory may result in its acceptance as a new diagnostic tool.

► Conventional cytologic pleural fluid evaluation has a low sensitivity (43%-71%), which leads to a high incidence of false-negatives. The authors of this study evaluated how testing pleural fluid for 10 biologic markers (matrix metalloproteinase-9 [MMP-9], MMP-3, MMP-2, p27, Skp-2, Cox-2, CyclinD1 [CycD1], Ki67, IMANOX assay, and carbonyls) would affect the sensitivity and specificity for patients with non-small-cell carcinoma (NSCCA). They compared 2 groups, 1 of 19 patients with lung cancer (9-adenoCA, 5-NSSCA,

4-SCCA, and 1-large-cell CA) with 1 of 22 patients with benign inflammatory pathologies. Of the 19 patients with lung CA, 6 were found to have no malignant cells on cytology. When the pleural fluid was evaluated for these markers, 7 of them were lower in the cancer patients. Specifically, MMP-9, MMP-3, and CycD1 were profoundly lower and highly significant (65%, $P = .000003$; 40%, $P = .0007$; 34% $P = .0001$). The sensitivity and specificity increased from 80% to 87% and 73% to 100%, respectively. The authors addressed the need to repeat this study with a larger patient population and noted that a focused combination of markers may yield better results.

D. D'Angelo-Donovan, DO
T. L. Bauer II, MD

Non-Small-Cell: Early Stage and Adjuvant Therapy

ACR Appropriateness Criteria® on Induction and Adjuvant Therapy for Stage N2 Non–Small-Cell Lung Cancer: Expert Panel on Radiation Oncology–Lung

Gopal RS, Dubey S, Rosenzweig KE, et al (Univ of Texas M. D. Anderson Cancer Ctr, Houston; Univ of California, San Francisco; Memorial Sloan-Kettering Cancer Ctr, NY; et al)
Int J Radiat Oncol Biol Phys 78:969-974, 2010

"The American College of Radiology seeks and encourages collaboration with other organizations on the development of the ACR Appropriateness Criteria through society representation on expert panels. Participation by representatives from collaborating societies on the expert panel does not necessarily imply society endorsement of the final document."

▶ American College of Radiology (ACR) appropriateness criteria regarding the state-of-the-art treatment for multiple malignancies have been developed and updated over many years. The process requires development of an expert panel whose job it is to review all of the important literature related to the question at hand and then through an iterative process develop recommendations for treatment of patients with different clinical scenarios. The final result of this process for patients with N2 non-small-cell lung cancer is presented in this article.

The expert panel reviewed the literature regarding induction and adjuvant treatment for N2 patients and has developed recommendations for 2 clinical scenarios. In each scenario, treatment options from radiation alone to combination therapy with chemotherapy plus or minus surgery were evaluated. The rating scale of 1 through 9 (1 being the least appropriate to 9 being the most appropriate) shows the relative agreement of the experts on each facet of treatment and treatment delivery. These appropriateness criteria are exceedingly helpful to practicing radiation oncologists who are challenged to stay abreast of all the data for all the cancers that we treat. They are guidelines only and not requirements but should be followed unless there are obvious reasons in a given patient to depart from the recommendations.

C. A. Lawton, MD

Early Palliative Care for Patients with Metastatic Non–Small-Cell Lung Cancer

Temel JS, Greer JA, Muzikansky A, et al (Massachusetts General Hosp, Boston; et al)

N Engl J Med 363:733-742, 2010

Background.—Patients with metastatic non–small-cell lung cancer have a substantial symptom burden and may receive aggressive care at the end of life. We examined the effect of introducing palliative care early after diagnosis on patient-reported outcomes and end-of-life care among ambulatory patients with newly diagnosed disease.

Methods.—We randomly assigned patients with newly diagnosed metastatic non–small-cell lung cancer to receive either early palliative care integrated with standard oncologic care or standard oncologic care alone. Quality of life and mood were assessed at baseline and at 12 weeks with the use of the Functional Assessment of Cancer Therapy–Lung (FACT-L) scale and the Hospital Anxiety and Depression Scale, respectively. The primary outcome was the change in the quality of life at 12 weeks. Data on end-of-life care were collected from electronic medical records.

Results.—Of the 151 patients who underwent randomization, 27 died by 12 weeks and 107 (86% of the remaining patients) completed assessments. Patients assigned to early palliative care had a better quality of life than did patients assigned to standard care (mean score on the FACT-L scale [in which scores range from 0 to 136, with higher scores indicating better quality of life], 98.0 vs. 91.5; $P = 0.03$). In addition, fewer patients in the palliative care group than in the standard care group had depressive symptoms (16% vs. 38%, $P = 0.01$). Despite the fact that fewer patients in the early palliative care group than in the standard care group received aggressive end-of-life care (33% vs. 54%, $P = 0.05$), median survival was longer among patients receiving early palliative care (11.6 months vs. 8.9 months, $P = 0.02$).

Conclusions.—Among patients with metastatic non-small-cell lung cancer, early palliative care led to significant improvements in both quality of life and mood. As compared with patients receiving standard care, patients receiving early palliative care had less aggressive care at the end of life but longer survival. (Funded by an American Society of Clinical Oncology Career Development Award and philanthropic gifts; ClinicalTrials.gov number, NCT01038271.)

▶ Patients with metastatic non-small-cell lung cancer can suffer from multiple symptoms related to their disease process. These patients often have painful bony metastasis and symptomatic brain metastasis, in addition to lung symptomatology related to their disease, not to mention psychological issues. Palliative care, which focuses on management of symptoms related to the disease process as well as psychosocial support and decision-making support, has all too often been tapped into too late in a patient's disease course. Thus the ability of palliative care providers to make significant contributions in the patient's end-of-life quality of life becomes limited.

These authors have performed an excellent and much needed trial looking for early palliative care for patients with metastatic non-small-cell lung cancer. These patients not only received early palliative care but in addition received standard oncologic care. The end point of change in quality of life at 12 weeks is the perfect assessment for this group of patients. Given the patient-reported outcomes, which are so important in assessing quality of life, this trial has incorporated essentially all that is needed to point to the pivotal role of early palliative care in these patients. It is fascinating to know that not only did the early palliative care patients have increased quality of life at 12 weeks but also that there was even a survival advantage to early palliative care. This suggests a quantity-of-life improvement with quality-of-life improvement. One hopes that this type of trial is considered for other metastatic cancer patients who would likely benefit from early palliative care intervention.

C. A. Lawton, MD

First-Line Metastatic Non-Small-Cell Lung Cancer

A phase I/II radiation dose escalation study with concurrent chemotherapy for patients with inoperable stages I to III non-small-cell lung cancer: phase I results of RTOG 0117

Bradley JD, Moughan J, Graham MV, et al (Washington Univ School of Medicine, St Louis, MO; RTOG Statistical Headquarters, Philadelphia, PA; Phelps County Med Ctr, Rolla, MO; et al)

Int J Radiat Oncol Biol Phys 77:367-372, 2010

Purpose.—In preparation for a Phase III comparison of high-dose versus standard-dose radiation therapy, this Phase I/II study was initiated to establish the maximum tolerated dose of radiation therapy in the setting of concurrent chemotherapy, using three-dimensional conformal radiation therapy for non-small-cell lung cancer.

Methods and Materials.—Eligibility included patients with histologically proven, unresectable Stages I to III non-small-cell lung cancer. Concurrent chemotherapy consisted of paclitaxel, 50 mg/m^2, and carboplatin, AUC of 2, given weekly. The radiation dose was to be sequentially intensified by increasing the daily fraction size, starting from 75.25 Gy/35 fractions.

Results.—The Phase I portion of this study accrued 17 patients from 10 institutions and was closed in January 2004. After the initial 8 patients were accrued to cohort 1, the trial closed temporarily on September 26, 2002, due to reported toxicity. Two acute treatment-related dose-limiting toxicities (DLTs) were reported at the time: a case of grade 5 and grade 3 radiation pneumonitis. The protocol, therefore, was revised to de-escalate the radiation therapy dose (74 Gy/37 fractions). Patients in cohort 1 continued to develop toxicity, with 6/8 (75%) patients eventually developing grade ≥3 events. Cohort 2 accrued 9 patients. There was one DLT, a grade 3 esophagitis, in cohort 2 in the first 5 patients (1/5 patients) and no DLTs for the next 2 patients (0/2 patients).

Conclusions.—The maximum tolerated dose was determined to be 74 Gy/37 fractions (2.0 Gy per fraction) using three-dimensional conformal radiation therapy with concurrent paclitaxel and carboplatin therapy. This dose level in the Phase II portion has been well tolerated, with low rates of acute and late lung toxicities.

► Radiation therapy has been the mainstay of treatment for inoperable non–small cell lung cancer for decades. The radiation dose limits were established with the results of Radiation Therapy Oncology Group protocol 9311 in 2005. Yet with the understanding of the survival benefit of concurrent chemotherapy with radiation, the question of radiation dose limits has resurfaced. The results of this trial have helped to answer the question of maximally tolerated radiation doses (with concurrent chemotherapy), at least for standard 3D techniques.

The authors found an unacceptable risk of severe toxicity grade 3 or greater with patients receiving 75.25 Gy in 35 fractions (with concurrent paclitaxel and carboplatin). They decreased the dose to 74 Gy in 37 fractions and have found this dose to be the maximum tolerated dose to be used with concurrent paclitaxel and carboplatin. Phase III data are still needed (and currently being done) to evaluate the potential benefit of this dose level versus more conventional 60 Gy doses. In addition, the use of intensity-modulated radiation therapy may offer some further benefit in delivering these doses with decreased toxicity. We await such data.

C. A. Lawton, MD

Clinical Course of Advanced Non–Small-Cell Lung Cancer Patients Experiencing Hypertension During Treatment With Bevacizumab in Combination With Carboplatin and Paclitaxel on ECOG 4599

Dahlberg SE, Sandler AB, Brahmer JR, et al (Dana-Farber Cancer Inst, Boston, MA; Vanderbilt-Ingram Cancer Ctr, Nashville, TN; The Sidney Kimmel Comprehensive Cancer Ctr, Baltimore, MD; et al)

J Clin Oncol 28:949-954, 2010

Purpose.—Bevacizumab is a monoclonal antibody that targets vascular endothelial growth factor (VEGF) with demonstrated efficacy in combination with carboplatin and paclitaxel (PCB) for the treatment of advanced non–small-cell lung cancer (NSCLC). Administration of bevacizumab is postulated to decrease nitric oxide synthesis and lead to hypertension, which may be a physiological sign that the VEGF pathway is more actively being blocked and could result in improved outcomes.

Patients and Methods.—Eastern Cooperative Oncology Group (ECOG) 4599 randomly assigned patients with nonsquamous NSCLC to carboplatin and paclitaxel (PC) versus PCB. Hypertensive patients were compared with nonhypertensive patients with respect to overall survival (OS) and progression-free survival (PFS) using blood pressure data and adverse event data separately. High blood pressure (HBP) by the end of cycle 1 was defined as blood pressure >150/100 at any previous time or at least a 20-mmHg increase in diastolic blood pressure from baseline.

Results.—In a multivariable Cox model adjusting for HBP as a time-varying covariate, comparing those on PCB with HBP with those on PC gave an OS hazard ratio (HR) of 0.60 (95% CI, 0.43 to 0.81; $P = .001$); comparing those on PCB without HBP with those on PC alone, the OS HR was 0.86 (95% CI, 0.74 to 1.00; $P = .05$). Comparing the PCB HBP group with PC gave an adjusted PFS HR of 0.54 (95% CI, 0.41 to 0.73; $P < .0001$) and comparing those on PCB without HBP to those on PC, the HR was 0.72 (95% CI, 0.62 to 0.84; $P < .0001$). The 6-month cumulative incidence of hypertension was 6.2% (95% CI, 3.9% to 8.6%).

Conclusion.—Data from ECOG 4599 suggest that onset of HBP during treatment with PCB may be associated with improved outcomes, and additional studies of the downstream effects of VEGF suppression and hypertension are needed.

▶ Great concern has been expressed recently about the toxicities associated with bevacizumab. The only adverse effect consistently associated with a significant increase in frequency with bevacizumab across all reported phase III trials, however, is hypertension. This study looks specifically at patients with non-small-cell lung cancer treated as a part of Eastern Cooperative Oncology Group 4599 (randomized to paclitaxel/carboplatin/bevacizumab) and evaluates a possible relationship between the appearance of hypertension and subsequent survival. Both progression-free survival (PFS) and overall survival (OS) appear to be enhanced substantially in those patients who incur hypertension as a toxicity. The incidence of hypertension, however, was small (6.2%) and thus identifies a small subset of patients. This observation should be confirmed in other cancers where bevacizumab is commonly used and has been shown to have a positive impact on either PFS or OS (breast cancer, colon cancer, and ovarian cancer). The practical impact of the observation is simply that physicians can now inform the patient who is experiencing hypertension and somewhat frustrated by it that this may actually be a positive sign for a favorable outcome, at least in lung cancer.

J. T. Thigpen, MD

Second-Line Metastatic Non-Small-Cell Lung Cancer

Phase III Trial of Vandetanib Compared With Erlotinib in Patients With Previously Treated Advanced Non–Small-Cell Lung Cancer

Natale RB, Thongprasert S, Greco FA, et al (Cedars-Sinai Outpatient Cancer Ctr, Los Angeles, CA; Sarah Cannon Res Inst, Nashville, TN; Florida Cancer Specialists, Bradenton; et al)

J Clin Oncol 29:1059-1066, 2011

Purpose.—Vandetanib is a once-daily oral inhibitor of vascular endothelial growth factor receptor and epidermal growth factor receptor signaling. This phase III study assessed the efficacy of vandetanib versus erlotinib in unselected patients with advanced non–small-cell lung cancer (NSCLC) after treatment failure with one to two prior cytotoxic chemotherapy regimens.

Patients and Methods.—One thousand two hundred forty patients were randomly assigned to receive vandetanib 300 mg/d (n = 623) or erlotinib 150 mg/d (n = 617). The primary objective was to show superiority in progression-free survival (PFS) for vandetanib versus erlotinib. If the difference did not reach statistical significance for superiority, a noninferiority analysis was conducted.

Results.—There was no significant improvement in PFS for patients treated with vandetanib versus erlotinib (hazard ratio [HR], 0.98; 95.22% CI, 0.87 to 1.10; $P = .721$); median PFS was 2.6 months for vandetanib and 2.0 months for erlotinib. There was also no significant difference for the secondary end points of overall survival (HR, 1.01; $P = .830$), objective response rate (both 12%), and time to deterioration of symptoms for pain (HR, 0.92; $P = .289$), dyspnea (HR, 1.07; $P = .407$), and cough (HR, 0.94; $P = .455$). Both agents showed equivalent PFS and overall survival in a preplanned noninferiority analysis. Adverse events (AEs; any grade) more frequent with vandetanib than erlotinib included diarrhea (50% *v* 38%, respectively) and hypertension (16% *v* 2%, respectively); rash was more frequent with erlotinib than vandetanib (38% *v* 28%, respectively). The overall incidence of grade ≥ 3 AEs was also higher with vandetanib than erlotinib (50% *v* 40%, respectively).

Conclusion.—In patients with previously treated advanced NSCLC, vandetanib showed antitumor activity but did not demonstrate an efficacy advantage compared with erlotinib. There was a higher incidence of some AEs with vandetanib.

▶ The choice of systemic therapy for the first-line treatment of recurrent or advanced non-small-cell lung cancer has been studied extensively in phase III trials. Second- and subsequent-line therapy, on the other hand, has generally been studied in phase II trials. Three approaches for second-line therapy, however, have been evaluated in phase III trials and have been shown to be of benefit: docetaxel, pemetrexed, and erlotinib. This study seeks to evaluate a fourth single agent compared with erlotinib. That approach is single-agent vandetanib, an inhibitor of vascular endothelial growth factor and endothelial growth factor receptor. The study was designed as a superiority study with a preplanned noninferiority analysis if superiority was not demonstrated. The trial shows no superiority, but the noninferiority analysis shows no difference between the 2 approaches. One can therefore assume that vandetanib does in fact confer benefit as second-line therapy, but there is no reason to consider its use when there is no advantage and, in fact, greater toxicity, in this trial. The bottom line? Effective second-line therapy for non-small-cell lung cancer is available.

J. T. Thigpen, MD

Small-Cell Lung Cancer

A Phase 2 Study of Irinotecan, Cisplatin, and Simvastatin for Untreated Extensive-disease Small Cell Lung Cancer

Han J-Y, Lim KY, Yu SY, et al (Natl Cancer Ctr, Goyang-si, Gyeonggi-do, Republic of Korea)

Cancer 117:2178-2185, 2011

Background.—The objective of this study was to investigate the efficacy of simvastatin in combination with irinotecan and cisplatin in chemotherapy-naive patients with extensive-disease small-cell lung cancer (ED-SCLC).

Methods.—In this phase 2 study, 61 patients received treatment with irinotecan (65 mg/m^2) and cisplatin (30 mg/m^2) on Days 1 and 8 every 3 weeks until either death or disease progression occurred. Patients also received oral simvastatin (40 mg daily) during the course of chemotherapy. The primary endpoint was 1-year survival. Secondary endpoints included the response rate (RR), progression-free survival (PFS), and toxicity.

Results.—The 1-year survival rate was 39.3%. The median overall survival (OS) was 11 months, and the median PFS was 6.1 months. Overall, the RR was 75%. The most common grade 3/4 toxicity was neutropenia (67%). Efficacy of the treatment was associated significantly with smoking status. Compared with never-smokers, ever-smokers had a better RR (40% vs 78%; $P=.01$), a longer PFS (2.5 months vs 6.4 months; $P=.018$), and had a trend toward an improved OS (9.0 months vs 11.2 months; $P=.095$). The effect of smoking on survival was apparent when ever-smokers were subdivided according to pack-years (PY) of smoking. Ever-smokers who had smoked >65 PY had a significantly longer OS compared with ever-smokers who had smoked ≤65 PY or never-smokers (20.6 months vs 10.6 months vs 9.0 months, respectively; log-rank $P = 0.032$). In multivariate analysis, PY >65 was predictive of longer survival (hazard ratio, 0.280; 95% confidence interval, 0.113-0.694).

Conclusions.—The current results indicated that simvastatin in combination with irinotecan and cisplatin did not improve the survival of patients with ED-SCLC. Although the subgroup analysis by smoking status was exploratory, the addition of simvastatin to irinotecan and cisplatin may improve the outcome of heavy smokers with ED-SCLC.

▶ Based on preclinical models, the authors hypothesized that simvastatin had an antitumor effect against small-cell lung cancer (SCLC) and a potential synergistic effect with chemotherapy in extensive-disease small-cell lung cancer (ED-SCLC). Unfortunately, it is no surprise that simvastatin did not add any clinical benefit to cisplatin-irinotecan in this single-arm phase II trial in ED-SCLC patients. SCLC is a notoriously difficult disease to treat, and the standard of care for front-line chemo-naïve patients has not changed over the last 15 years. For the Western population, cisplatin-etoposide remains the standard of care, whereas in Japan, either cisplatin-etoposide or cisplatin-irinotecan[1] can be used. A prior phase III trial, JCOG 9511, in Japanese SCLC patients demonstrated a survival benefit with the use of cisplatin-irinotecan and may be related to different pharmacogenetics in Japanese patients.[1] In addition, this article commented on an exploratory subgroup analysis demonstrating that heavy smokers (> 65 pack years) had a better overall survival outcome. Caution should be taken here; there were only 5 never-smokers in this analysis and these patients most likely have a unique (worse) biology, as SCLC is very rarely seen in never-smoking patients. The authors propose that simvastatin may decrease smoking-related comorbidities, which therefore leads to the survival benefit in the heavy smokers. I find this theory difficult to accept, as we know the median overall survival for this population of patients still remains only about 1 year, and to accept this theory would require the belief that a cholesterol-lowering agent could provide a major survival impact within a few months.

A. S. Tsao, MD

Reference

1. Noda K, Nishiwaki Y, Kawahara M, et al. Irinotecan plus cisplatin compared with etoposide plus cisplatin for extensive small-cell lung cancer. *N Engl J Med*. 2002; 346:85-91.

Randomized Phase II Study of Bevacizumab in Combination With Chemotherapy in Previously Untreated Extensive-Stage Small-Cell Lung Cancer: Results From the SALUTE Trial

Spigel DR, Townley PM, Waterhouse DM, et al (Sarah Cannon Res Inst, Nashville, TN; Methodist Estabrook Cancer Ctr, Omaha, NE; Oncology/Hematology Care, Cincinnati, OH; et al)

J Clin Oncol 29:2215-2222, 2011

Purpose.—Because of promising efficacy signals in single-arm studies, a placebo-controlled, double-blind, randomized phase II trial was designed to assess the efficacy and safety of adding bevacizumab to first-line standard chemotherapy for treatment of extensive-stage small-cell lung cancer (SCLC).

Patients and Methods.—Patients with SCLC were randomly assigned to receive bevacizumab or placebo, with cisplatin or carboplatin plus etoposide, for four cycles followed by single-agent bevacizumab or placebo until progression or unacceptable toxicity. The primary end point was progression-free survival (PFS).

Results.—Fifty-two patients were randomly assigned to the bevacizumab group and 50 to the placebo group; 69% versus 66%, respectively, completed four cycles of therapy. Median PFS was higher in the bevacizumab group (5.5 months) than in the placebo group (4.4 months; hazard ratio [HR], 0.53; 95% CI, 0.32 to 0.86). Median overall survival (OS) was similar for both groups (9.4 v 10.9 months for bevacizumab and placebo groups, respectively), with an HR of 1.16 (95% CI, 0.66 to 2.04). Overall response rates were 58% (95% CI, 43% to 71%) for the bevacizumab group and 48% (95% CI, 34% to 62%) for the placebo group. Median duration of response was 4.7 months for the bevacizumab group and 3.2 months for the placebo group. In the bevacizumab and placebo groups, 75% versus 60% of patients, respectively, experienced one or more grade 3 or higher adverse events. No new or unexpected safety signals for bevacizumab were observed.

Conclusion.—The addition of bevacizumab to cisplatin or carboplatin plus etoposide for treatment of extensivestage SCLC improved PFS, with an acceptable toxicity profile. However, no improvement in OS was observed.

▶ The addition of bevacizumab to platinum-etoposide was found to improve response rate, prolong duration of response, and increase progression-free survival (hazard ratio [HR], 0.53) but not overall survival (HR, 1.16) in this randomized placebo-controlled trial in chemo-naïve extensive-stage small-cell lung cancer (SCLC) patients. This clinical benefit from bevacizumab was achieved with only a 15% increase in rate of grade 3 toxicity. The limitations in the Study of Bevacizumab in Previously Untreated Extensive-Stage Small-Cell Lung Cancer (SALUTE) analyses are that data on subsequent lines of therapy were not collected and potential imbalances in salvage therapy usage could affect the negative overall survival results seen in this study. There was also another incongruity: patients who received carboplatin with bevacizumab had a greater magnitude of progression-free survival benefit than those who received cisplatin with bevacizumab. This finding is unexplained and discrepant against the prior CISplatin versus CArboplatin non-small-cell lung cancer meta-analysis, which suggested that cisplatin-based regimens had improved response rates over carboplatin-based regimens. In considering the SALUTE trial results, I would still say that the use of bevacizumab in SCLC still remains investigational; prior studies have attempted to add antiangiogenic agents into the SCLC armaments with mixed results. A subsequent larger randomized phase III trial with bevacizumab and additional ongoing randomized trials using vascular endothelial growth factor receptor inhibitors with chemotherapy will hopefully guide us in determining whether there is a role for antiangiogenics in SCLC therapy.

A. S. Tsao, MD

PET Evaluation of Lung Cancer

Combined use of positron emission tomography and volume doubling time in lung cancer screening with low-dose CT scanning

Ashraf H, Dirksen A, Loft A, et al (Gentofte Univ Hosp, Denmark; Univ of Copenhagen, Denmark)

Thorax 66:315-319, 2011

Background.—In lung cancer screening the ability to distinguish malignant from benign nodules is a key issue. This study evaluates the ability of positron emission tomography (PET) and volume doubling time (VDT) to discriminate between benign and malignant nodules.

Methods.—From the Danish Lung Cancer Screening Trial, participants with indeterminate nodules who were referred for a 3-month rescan were investigated. Resected nodules and indolent nodules (ie, stable for at least 2 years) were included. Between the initial scan and the 3-month rescan, participants were referred for PET. Uptake on PET was categorised as most likely benign to malignant (grades IeIV). VDT was calculated from volume measurements on repeated CT scans using semiautomated pulmonary nodule evaluation software. Receiver operating characteristic (ROC) analyses were used to determine the sensitivity and specificity of PET and VDT.

Results.—A total of 54 nodules were included. The prevalence of lung cancer was 37%. In the multivariate model both PET (OR 2.63, $p<0.01$) and VDT (OR 2.69, $p<0.01$) were associated with lung cancer. The sensitivities and specificities of both PET and VDT were 71% and 91%, respectively. Cut-off points for malignancy were PET >II and VDT <1 year, respectively. Combining PET and VDT resulted in a sensitivity of 90% and a specificity of 82%; ROC cut-off point was either PET or VDT indicating malignancy.

Conclusion.—PET and VDT predict lung cancer independently of each other. The use of both PET and VDT in combination is recommended when screening for lung cancer with low-dose CT.

▶ The management of esophageal cancer requires a multimodality approach. Short of surgical resection, there are a few methods of palliation, including stenting, endoscopic mucosal resection, radiofrequency ablation, cryotherapy, and photodynamic therapy, when radiation therapy is insufficient. The ablative techniques offer the potential for cure if the cancer is sufficiently localized.

The authors of this study looked retrospectively at 79 patients from 10 different institutions, all with esophageal cancer, in whom other therapy had failed or who had refused or were ineligible for surgery or any other therapy. They all received low-pressure liquid nitrogen therapy every 4 to 6 weeks until complete local tumor eradication was observed by appearance and lack of residual disease on endoscopic biopsy. The median number of treatments was 3 (range, 1–25).

Of the 79 subjects who received treatment, no serious adverse events, including perforation and hemorrhage, were reported. Ten percent of patients, all of whom had previous tumor therapy, reported benign stricture. Only 49 of the 79 patients were available for efficacy analysis; the remaining 30 were still undergoing cryotherapy treatments. Of those 49 patients, 61.2% demonstrated a complete response at mean follow-up of 10.6 months.

The authors have shown that endoscopic spray cryotherapy is safe and effective. The authors address the limitations of their study in that it is retrospective and limited in the number of subjects and length of follow-up, but this is the largest reported series on the topic. Further studies with longer follow-up periods will be required before this therapy becomes a mainstay of treatment.

D. D'Angelo-Donovan, DO

T. L. Bauer II, MD

Smoking and Prevention

Lung cancer in 'Never-smokers': a unique entity

Subramanian J, Govindan R (Washington Univ School of Medicine, St Louis, MO)

Oncology 24:29-35, 2010

Lung cancer in "never-smokers" constitutes only a small proportion of patients with lung cancer. Nevertheless, the topic has recently attracted a good deal of attention. Initially this was due to the fact that never-smokers with lung cancer had better outcomes with epidermal growth factor receptor-tyrosine kinase (EGFR-TK) inhibitors, compared to tobacco smokers with lung cancer. More recently the identification of molecular changes unique to lung cancer in never-smokers has generated further interest in this disease. These findings have the potential to enhance our knowledge of lung cancer biology and lead to the development of new, more effective treatments for lung cancer. In this review, we summarize the existing body of knowledge on lung cancer in never-smokers.

▶ While lung cancer used to be virtually always associated with tobacco use, lung cancer in patients who never smoked is a growing facet of all occurrences of lung cancer. The root cause of these cancers is not known, but this article is an excellent review of the potential risk factors. These risk factors range from environmental factors such as tobacco smoke—that is, second-hand smoking—radon, asbestos, and cooking fumes to genetic, viral, and even hormonal factors. The one bit of good news for such patients with lung cancer is that they appear to have better clinical outcomes with epidermal growth factor receptor-tyrosine kinase inhibitors compared with lung cancer in tobacco smokers. This opens up the opportunity to study these patients for a potentially different kind of lung cancer, the treatment of which may be quite different. This article explores some of these different approaches and encourages physicians to think of this entity as a unique form of lung cancer. Research stemming from alternative approaches to this type of lung cancer needs to be explored further.

C. A. Lawton, MD

Advanced Diseases

Phase II Study of Cetuximab in Combination With Chemoradiation in Patients With Stage IIIA/B Non–Small-Cell Lung Cancer: RTOG 0324

Blumenschein GR Jr, Paulus R, Curran WJ, et al (The Univ of Texas MD Anderson Cancer Ctr, Houston; Radiation Therapy Oncology Group Statistical Ctr; Thomas Jefferson Univ Hosp, Philadelphia, PA; et al)

J Clin Oncol 29:2312-2318, 2011

Purpose.—Non–small-cell lung cancer (NSCLC) commonly expresses the epidermal growth factor receptor (EGFR), which is associated with poor clinical outcome. Cetuximab is a chimerized monoclonal antibody that targets the EGFR and, in preclinical models, it demonstrates radiosensitization properties. We report a phase II trial testing the combination of cetuximab with chemoradiotherapy (CRT) in unresectable stage III NSCLC.

Patients and Methods.—Eligibility criteria included unresectable stage III NSCLC, Zubrod performance status ≤ 1, weight loss $\leq 5\%$, forced expiratory volume in 1 second ≥ 1.2 L, and adequate organ function. Patients received an initial dose of cetuximab (400 mg/m^2) on day 1 of week 1 and then weekly doses of cetuximab (250 mg/m^2) until completion of therapy (weeks 2 through 17). During week 2, patients started CRT (63 Gy in 35 fractions) with weekly carboplatin at area under the [concentration-time] curve (AUC) 2 and six doses of paclitaxel at 45 mg/m^2 followed by carboplatin (AUC 6) and two cycles of paclitaxel (200 mg/m^2) during weeks 12 through 17. Primary end points included safety and compliance of concurrent cetuximab and CRT.

Results.—In all, 93 patients were enrolled and 87 were evaluable. Median follow-up was 21.6 months. Response rate was 62% (n = 54), median survival was 22.7 months, and 24-month overall survival was 49.3%. Adverse events related to treatment included 20% grade 4 hematologic toxicities, 8% grade 3 esophagitis, and 7% grade 3 to 4 pneumonitis. There were five grade 5 events.

Conclusion.—The combination of cetuximab with CRT is feasible and shows promising activity. The median and overall survival achieved with this regimen were longer than any previously reported by the Radiation Therapy Oncology Group.

▶ RTOG 0324 was able to demonstrate that cetuximab added to chemoradiation was feasible and could be administered with reasonable compliance across numerous US centers. Although the authors reported that the incidence of grade > 3 nonhematologic adverse events was similar to that in prior studies, there were 6 grade 5 events in the cetuximab arm, and 3 of these patients were found to have had > 20 Gy incorrectly delivered to a significant volume of lung. This suggests that radiation field gating with the addition of chemo-cetuximab must be carefully and stringently delivered to limit risk of death. When compared with prior studies, RTOG 0324 has noteworthy survival results, and the regimen was moved forward and provided the basis for the phase III RTOG 0617 trial, which completed accrual May 12, 2011. Other cooperative groups have also explored the use of cetuximab with other chemotherapy backbones with x-ray therapy; a phase II CALGB 30407 study evaluated radiation plus carboplatin-pemetrexed plus cetuximab and reported similar preliminary overall survival (median overall survival, 22 months) in both arms. The results of all of these trials taken together will help define whether cetuximab will have a role in local regionally advanced non-small-cell lung cancer (NSCLC). Future needs include identifying a biomarker that can predict for improved survival or response to cetuximab-based regimens in NSCLC. Unlike in colorectal cancer, *KRAS* mutations are not negative predictors for cetuximab usage in NSCLC.

A. S. Tsao, MD

Miscellaneous

Bronchopulmonary Carcinoid Tumors: Long-Term Outcomes After Resection

Cao C, Yan TD, Kennedy C, et al (The Univ of Sydney, New South Wales, Australia; Royal Prince Alfred Hosp, Sydney, Australia; The Baird Inst for Applied Heart and Lung Surgical Res, Sydney, New South Wales, Australia)
Ann Thorac Surg 91:339-343, 2011

Background.—Bronchopulmonary carcinoid tumors are considered as a relatively uncommon and less malignant group of lung cancers. However, patients with histologically atypical disease are known to have a worse prognosis. The present study aims to evaluate the long-term outcomes after resection of bronchopulmonary carcinoid tumors according to the new tumor, nodes, metastasis (TNM) staging system.

Methods.—Patients with histologically proven bronchopulmonary carcinoid tumors who underwent surgery in our thoracic unit over the last 25 years were identified from a prospectively collected database.

Results.—One hundred and eighty-six patients were identified from our electronic database. Of these, 164 were known to have typical disease, while 22 had atypical disease. Median overall survival was 20.0 years. The mean follow-up was 8.0 years (median 7.0 years). Univariate analysis found age over 60, atypical disease, TNM staging, N status, and M status to have a statistically significant influence on overall survival. Multivariate analysis found age over 60 and atypical histopathology to have a detrimental impact on overall survival. Patients in the atypical subgroup were found to be significantly older, and presented with higher stage disease.

Conclusions.—It is clear from the current study and previous reports that patients with atypical histopathology have different baseline characteristics, disease behavior, and prognosis compared with patients with typical disease. The proposed TNM staging system appears to be applicable to patients in our surgical experience, and may offer more accurate prognostic information and assist in the management plans for individuals.

▶ In the past, bronchopulmonary carcinoid tumors were classified as low-grade typical, intermediate-grade atypical, high-grade large-cell neuroendocrine carcinomas, and small-cell lung carcinomas. The authors of this study were looking to assess if the newest, seventh edition of the tumor, nodes, metastasis (TMN) staging system would be applicable to patients with bronchopulmonary carcinoid tumors. The authors also evaluated their overall survival results and prognostic factors as they related to overall survival in patients who had undergone surgical resection for their disease.

The authors looked at 186 patients with a mean follow-up of 8 years, with no patients lost to follow-up. They found that their median overall survival was 20.0 years, and their 5-year, 10-year, and 15-year survival rates were 93.7%, 81.7%, and 71.4%, respectively. They found that 4 prognostic factors had a statistically significant effect on overall survival: age >60, atypical histology, presence of metastasis at the time of surgery, and the TMN stage according to the new seventh edition. Most notably, they observed median overall survival of the atypical subtype group to be 5.1 years, whereas the typical subtype group showed median survival of 20.2 years, giving further support to the proposed idea that these 2 subtypes be considered as 2 separate disease entities. They also found the new seventh edition of the TMN staging system could reliably predict overall survival in their patient population. The authors agree that more research needs to be done before the TMN staging system could be routinely applied to bronchopulmonary carcinomas.

D. D'Angelo-Donovan, DO
T. L. Bauer II, MD

8 Gastrointestinal

Esophagus and Stomach

Exposure to Oral Bisphosphonates and Risk of Esophageal Cancer

Cardwell CR, Abnet CC, Cantwell MM, et al (Queen's Univ Belfast, UK; Natl Insts of Health, Rockville, MD)

JAMA 304:657-663, 2010

Context.—Use of oral bisphosphonates has increased dramatically in the United States and elsewhere. Esophagitis is a known adverse effect of bisphosphonate use, and recent reports suggest a link between bisphosphonate use and esophageal cancer, but this has not been robustly investigated.

Objective.—To investigate the association between bisphosphonate use and esophageal cancer.

Design, Setting, and Participants.—Data were extracted from the UK General Practice Research Database to compare the incidence of esophageal and gastric cancer in a cohort of patients treated with oral bisphosphonates between January 1996 and December 2006 with incidence in a control cohort. Cancers were identified from relevant Read/Oxford Medical Information System codes in the patient's clinical files. Cox proportional hazards modeling was used to calculate hazard ratios and 95% confidence intervals for risk of esophageal and gastric cancer in bisphosphonate users compared with nonusers, with adjustment for potential confounders.

Main Outcome Measure.—Hazard ratio for the risk of esophageal and gastric cancer in the bisphosphonate users compared with the bisphosphonate nonusers.

Results.—Mean follow-up time was 4.5 and 4.4 years in the bisphosphonate and control cohorts, respectively. Excluding patients with less than 6 months' follow-up, there were 41 826 members in each cohort (81% women; mean age, 70.0 (SD, 11.4) years). One hundred sixteen esophageal or gastric cancers (79 esophageal) occurred in the bisphosphonate cohort and 115 (72 esophageal) in the control cohort. The incidence of esophageal and gastric cancer combined was 0.7 per 1000 person-years of risk in both the bisphosphonate and control cohorts; the incidence of esophageal cancer alone in the bisphosphonate and control cohorts was 0.48 and 0.44 per 1000 person-years of risk, respectively. There was no difference in risk of esophageal and gastric cancer combined between the cohorts for any bisphosphonate use (adjusted hazard ratio, 0.96 [95% confidence interval,

0.74-1.25]) or risk of esophageal cancer only (adjusted hazard ratio, 1.07 [95% confidence interval, 0.77-1.49]). There also was no difference in risk of esophageal or gastric cancer by duration of bisphosphonate intake.

Conclusion.—Among patients in the UK General Practice Research Database, the use of oral bisphosphonates was not significantly associated with incident esophageal or gastric cancer.

▶ Measuring bone density for both men and women in the United States has become commonplace. The result of this is that osteopenia and osteoporosis have been diagnosed at unprecedented numbers. Given the obesity in this country, these bone problems should not be a surprise to anyone, yet the result of this diagnosis is that thousands of Americans are being placed on bisphosphonate therapy.

Bisphosphonate therapy, like all medical interventions, has side effects. The effect on the jaw with regard to osteonecrosis with dental surgery is a well-documented potential toxicity of this therapy. Esophagitis and gastritis are other well-documented toxicities of bisphosphonate therapy. The concern of esophagitis and gastritis is related to the question of whether inflammation/irritation of a tissue could increase the risk of dysplasia and potentially lead to an increasing carcinoma risk.

These authors have looked at data from the United Kingdom general practice research database to try to assess this question in more than 82 000 patients with a mean follow-up of 4.5 years. They found no difference in the incidence of either esophageal or gastric carcinoma in patients on bisphosphonate therapy versus those not on the therapy, suggesting no association between these drugs and these cancers. Certainly one needs more data and longer follow-up to be certain of the lack of an association between bisphosphonates and esophageal and/or gastric malignancies. But these data are comforting in that if there were a significant risk of developing these cancers on these drugs, it likely would have been seen in this analysis. We await further work on this important topic.

C. A. Lawton, MD

Perioperative Chemotherapy Compared With Surgery Alone for Resectable Gastroesophageal Adenocarcinoma: An FNCLCC and FFCD Multicenter Phase III Trial

Ychou M, Boige V, Pignon J-P, et al (Centre Val d'Aurelle, Montpellier, France; Centre Hospitalier Universitaire Saint-Eloi, Montpellier, France; Institut de Cancérologie Gustave Roussy, Villejuif, France; et al)
J Clin Oncol 29:1715-1721, 2011

Purpose.—After curative resection, the prognosis of gastroesophageal adenocarcinoma is poor. This phase III trial was designed to evaluate the benefit in overall survival (OS) of perioperative fluorouracil plus cisplatin in resectable gastroesophageal adenocarcinoma.

Patients and Methods.—Overall, 224 patients with resectable adenocarcinoma of the lower esophagus, gastroesophageal junction (GEJ), or stomach were randomly assigned to either perioperative chemotherapy and surgery (CS group; n = 113) or surgery alone (S group; n = 111). Chemotherapy consisted of two or three preoperative cycles of intravenous cisplatin (100 mg/m^2) on day 1, and a continuous intravenous infusion of fluorouracil (800 mg/m^2/d) for 5 consecutive days (days 1 to 5) every 28 days and three or four postoperative cycles of the same regimen. The primary end point was OS.

Results.—Compared with the S group, the CS group had a better OS (5-year rate 38% *v* 24%; hazard ratio [HR] for death: 0.69; 95% CI, 0.50 to 0.95; P =.02); and a better disease-free survival (5-year rate: 34% *v* 19%; HR, 0.65; 95% CI, 0.48 to 0.89; P =.003). In the multivariable analysis, the favorable prognostic factors for survival were perioperative chemotherapy (P =.01) and stomach tumor localization (P < .01). Perioperative chemotherapy significantly improved the curative resection rate (84% *v* 73%; P =.04). Grade 3 to 4 toxicity occurred in 38% of CS patients (mainly neutropenia) but postoperative morbidity was similar in the two groups.

Conclusion.—In patients with resectable adenocarcinoma of the lower esophagus, GEJ, or stomach, perioperative chemotherapy using fluorouracil plus cisplatin significantly increased the curative resection rate, disease-free survival, and OS.

► Adenocarcinoma of the esophagus, the gastroesophageal junction (GEJ), and the stomach potentially resectable for cure has a poor prognosis despite complete surgical resection. Intergroup Study 0116 in the United States evaluated postoperative chemoradiation as an adjuvant to surgery and showed an advantage for this approach. As a result, patients with resection of one of these neoplasms generally receive postoperative adjuvant chemoradiation with all of the attendant toxicities. This study evaluates preoperative and postoperative chemotherapy as an adjuvant without radiation. The chemotherapy regimen included cisplatin and continuous infusion 5-fluorouracil given as 2 to 3 preoperative courses and 3 to 4 postoperative courses. The use of the chemotherapy compared with surgery alone improved complete resection rate, disease-free survival, and overall survival. Although the absolutely optimal chemotherapeutic regimen has not been determined, this regimen and the cisplatin/epirubicin/5-fluorouracil regimen used in the MAGIC trial have both been shown to improve disease-free and overall survival significantly. This makes pre- and postoperative chemotherapy a valid option in the treatment of resectable adenocarcinoma of the distal esophagus, the GEJ, and the stomach.

J. T. Thigpen, MD

Pancreas

A national propensity-adjusted analysis of adjuvant radiotherapy in the treatment of resected pancreatic adenocarcinoma

McDade TP, Hill JS, Simons JP, et al (Univ of Massachusetts Med School, Worcester)

Cancer 116:3257-3266, 2010

Background.—The benefit of adjuvant radiotherapy (RT) for resected pancreatic adenocarcinoma remains controversial after randomized clinical trials. In this national-level US study, a propensity score (conditional probability of receiving RT) was used to adjust for potential confounding in nonrandomized designs from treatment group differences.

Methods.—Patients were identified from the Surveillance, Epidemiology, and End Results (SEER) registry (1988-2005 dataset). Multivariate analyses to determine the effect of RT on overall survival were performed using propensity-adjusted Cox proportional hazards and Kaplan-Meier analyses.

Results.—In total, 5676 patients with resected pancreatic adenocarcinoma were identified, and 40.8% of those patients had received adjuvant RT. Univariate predictors of survival included age, race, marital status, disease stage, tumor size, tumor extension, tumor grade, lymph node status, year of diagnosis, type of resection, and receipt of RT (all $P < .002$). In a Cox model, independent predictors of improved survival included white race, married status, earlier stage, smaller tumors, well differentiated tumors, negative lymph node (N0) status, recent diagnosis, and receipt of RT (all $P < .05$). In a propensity-adjusted proportional hazards regression, the benefit of adjuvant treatment that included RT remained significant after adjusting for the likelihood of receiving RT (hazard ratio, 0.773; 95% confidence interval, 0.714-0.836; $P < .0001$). Within all 5 propensity strata, Kaplan-Meier survival differed significantly ($P < .0001$ [lowest and highest probability strata] and $P = .0165$ [middle stratum with a "pseudorandom" probability of RT]).

Conclusions.—Adjuvant RT for resected pancreatic adenocarcinoma was associated with a significant survival advantage in a large national database, even after using propensity score methods to adjust for differences between treatment groups. The authors concluded that adjuvant RT should be considered for all appropriate patients who have resected pancreatic adenocarcinoma.

► Pancreatic adenocarcinoma remains one of the deadliest adenocarcinomas found in humans. The overall survival rates even in completely resected patients are limited. Thus the need for postoperative adjuvant therapy in the form of chemotherapy and radiation has been studied and well documented since the mid 1980s.

Unfortunately, there have been several randomized trials performed which have questioned the benefit of the adjuvant radiation in particular. The authors of this article have used the Surveillance, Epidemiology, and End Results registry to try to address the issue of the need for postoperative radiation therapy in addition to chemotherapy for these patients. Their statistical models of propensity-adjusted Cox proportional hazards and Kaplan-Meier analyses have shown a survival benefit with the addition of adjuvant radiation therapy. Thus, they conclude that adjuvant chemotherapy and radiation therapy remain the standard of care for resected pancreatic adenocarcinoma patients treated within the United States.

While we still need a well-designed, prospective, randomized, phase III trial of surgery plus chemotherapy versus surgery plus chemotherapy and radiation therapy to finally answer this question, these data certainly well support the use of both chemotherapy and radiation therapy adjuvantly in these patients.

C. A. Lawton, MD

A Phase 2 Trial of Gemcitabine, 5-Fluorouracil, and Radiation Therapy in Locally Advanced Nonmetastatic Pancreatic Adenocarcinoma: Cancer and Leukemia Group B (CALGB) 80003

Mamon HJ, for the Cancer and Leukemia Group B (Dana-Farber Cancer Inst, Boston, MA; et al)

Cancer 117:2620-2628, 2011

Background.—The purpose of this study was to assess the efficacy and safety of 5-fluorouracil (5FU) and gemcitabine administered concurrently with radiation in patients with locally advanced, nonmetastatic pancreatic cancer.

Methods.—Eligible patients had histologically confirmed pancreatic adenocarcinoma deemed locally unresectable without evidence of metastatic disease. In addition, all patients underwent laparoscopy or laparotomy before study entry to rule out peritoneal carcinomatosis. Patients received radiation therapy (50.4 Gy) with concurrent infusional 5FU (200 mg/m^2 5 days/week) and weekly gemcitabine (200 mg/m^2). After a 3-week break, patients received weekly gemcitabine at 1000 mg/m^2 for 3 of 4 weeks, for 4 cycles. The primary endpoint of the trial was the proportion of patients surviving 9 months from study entry. Secondary endpoints included objective tumor response, CA19-9 response, overall survival (OS) time to progression (TTP), and toxicity.

Results.—Between November 2001 and October 2004, 81 patients were enrolled, 78 of whom were eligible for analysis. With a median follow-up of 55.2 months, the median OS was 12.2 months (95% confidence interval [CI], 10.9-14.9) and the median TTP was 10 months (95% CI, 6.4-12.0). An objective tumor response was seen in 19 patients (25%), and among 56 patients with an elevated CA19-9 at baseline, 29 (52%) had a sustained CA19-9 response. Overall, 41% of patients had grade 3 or greater treatment-related gastrointestinal adverse events.

Conclusions.—The combination of 5FU, gemcitabine, and radiation is well tolerated. Survival is comparable with the best results of other recent studies of 5FU and radiation or gemcitabine and radiation.

▶ Chemoradiotherapy is an accepted treatment regimen for locally advanced pancreatic cancer. Both 5-fluorouracil (5FU) and gemcitabine have been previously combined with radiotherapy with similar efficacy and median overall survival rates of 10 to 12 months. Mamon et al from Cancer and Leukemia Group B have tested the efficacy of combined gemcitabine and 5FU with radiotherapy followed by gemcitabine in 78 patients with unresectable pancreatic cancer. The primary goal was obtaining a 9-month progression-free survival (PFS) rate of 50% or higher. The trial met its 9-months PFS end point (73%), but the overall survival of 12.2 months was comparable with that obtained with single-agent gemcitabine or 5FU-based chemoradiation. Time to progression was 10 months. The authors noted an improved median overall survival, albeit not statistically significant (13 vs 9 months, $P = .11$), for patients with a sustained CA19-9 decrease of >75%.

Although this combination was reasonably well tolerated, the trial's results do not merit further study in locally advanced pancreatic adenocarcinoma. The authors recommend that future clinical trials in this patient population include an induction chemotherapy regimen followed by chemoradiotherapy, with the potential incorporation of radiosensitizing molecularly targeted agents.

E. G. Chiorean, MD

Colorectal

Comparison of Two Neoadjuvant Chemoradiotherapy Regimens for Locally Advanced Rectal Cancer: Results of the Phase III Trial ACCORD 12/0405-Prodige 2

Gérard J-P, Azria D, Gourgou-Bourgade S, et al (Centre Antoine-Lacassagne, Nice Cedex, France; Université Nice Sofia Antipolis, France; Centre Val d'Aurelle, Montpellier, France; et al)

J Clin Oncol 28:1638-1644, 2010

Purpose.—Neoadjuvant chemoradiotherapy is considered a standard approach for T3-4 M0 rectal cancer. In this situation, we compared neoadjuvant radiotherapy plus capecitabine with dose-intensified radiotherapy plus capecitabine and oxaliplatin.

Patients and Methods.—We randomly assigned patients to receive 5 weeks of treatment with radiotherapy 45 Gy/25 fractions with concurrent capecitabine 800 mg/m^2 twice daily 5 days per week (Cap 45) or radiotherapy 50 Gy/25 fractions with capecitabine 800 mg/m^2 twice daily 5 days per week and oxaliplatin 50 mg/m^2 once weekly (Capox 50). The primary end point was complete sterilization of the operative specimen (ypCR).

Results.—Five hundred ninety-eight patients were randomly assigned to receive Cap 45 ($n = 299$) or Capox 50 ($n = 299$). More preoperative grade 3 to 4 toxicity occurred in the Capox 50 group (25 *v* 1%; $P < .001$).

Surgery was performed in 98% of patients in both groups. There were no differences between groups in the rate of conservative surgery (75%) or postoperative deaths at 60 days (0.3%). The ypCR rate was 13.9% with Cap 45 and 19.2% with Capox 50 (P =.09). When ypCR was combined with yp few residual cells, the rate was respectively 28.9% with Cap 45 and 39.4% with Capox 50 (P =.008). The rate of positive circumferential rectal margins (between 0 and 2 mm) was 19.3% with Cap 45 and 9.9% with Capox 50 (P =.02).

Conclusion.—The benefit of oxaliplatin was not demonstrated and this drug should not be used with concurrent irradiation. Cap 50 merits investigation for T3-4 rectal cancers.

▶ T3 and T4 nonmetastatic rectal cancers are cured more often with the use of preoperative radiation therapy (RT). Furthermore, data from randomized trials support the addition of chemotherapy (5-fluorouracil) to the preoperative radiation regimen to increase pathologic complete response (CR) rates at the time of surgery. Thus, the question today regarding ways to improve the postchemotherapy pathologic CR rates (ypCR rates) centers on RT dose and chemotherapy regimens. These authors have studied both questions in a phase III randomized trial, which has shown some complex results. The dose escalation arm of 50 Gy in 25 fractions was associated with more preoperative grade 3 and 4 toxicity than the 45-Gy arm. Yet the 50-Gy arm was given both capecitabine and oxaliplatin not just capecitabine alone as in the 45-Gy arm. The 50-Gy arm did show a statistical improvement in the rate of positive circumferential radial margins, which is a surrogate for improved local control.

The challenge with these data lies in the treatment design where 2 variables were changed and the results are mixed. The authors do not support the addition of oxaliplatin in future trials but do encourage the use of dose escalation to 50 Gy. Clearly this recommendation warrants further investigation, but the data are encouraging.

C. A. Lawton, MD

Intensity-modulated radiation therapy for anal cancer: toxicity versus outcomes

Zagar TM, Willett CG, Czito BG (Duke Univ School of Medicine, Durham, NC)
Oncology 24:815-823, 2010

The treatment of cancer of the anal canal has changed significantly over the past several decades. Although the abdominoperineal resection (APR) was the historical standard of care, a therapeutic paradigm shift occurred with the seminal work of Nigro, who reported that anal canal cancer could be treated with definitive chemoradiation, with APR reserved for salvage therapy only. This remains an attractive approach for patients and physicians alike and the standard of care in this disease. Now, nearly four decades later, a similar approach continues to be utilized, albeit with higher radiation doses; however, this strategy remains fraught with considerable treatment-related morbidities. With the advent of intensity-modulated radiation therapy (IMRT), many oncologists are beginning to utilize this technology in the treatment of anal cancer in order to decrease these toxicities while maintaining similar treatment efficacy. This article reviews the relevant literature leading up to the modern treatment of anal canal cancer, and discusses IMRT-related toxicity and disease-related outcomes in the context of outcomes of conventionally treated anal cancer.

▶ The use of chemotherapy combined with radiation therapy in anal cancer has replaced mutilating surgery and has resulted in excellent outcomes with this organ-preserving approach. Yet getting patients through the concurrent chemotherapy and radiation therapy with the significant acute morbidity of skin breakdown, infection, and cytopenia is a difficult process at best. One potential improvement for treatment delivery is the use of intensity-modulated radiation therapy (IMRT) as opposed to the standard 3-dimensional (3D) approaches. The obvious benefit of IMRT is decreased acute skin/mucosal toxicity. This potential improvement in acute toxicity must be balanced and analyzed with regard to the possibility of missing disease with this more conformal approach. The dose-volume histograms obtained with an IMRT approach are clearly better than those in the standard 3D approach. But if one spares tumor in an effort to decrease toxicity, the battle is won, but the war is lost. These authors do an excellent job of outlining the strengths and weaknesses of each approach. They appropriately suggest the use of IMRT but with caution, pointing to the importance of clearly understanding the disease process so as to treat all the potential areas of disease while sparing as much normal tissue as possible.

C. A. Lawton, MD

Radiation dose–volume effects in radiation-induced rectal injury

Michalski JM, Gay H, Jackson A, et al (Washington Univ School of Medicine, St Louis, MO; Memorial Sloan-Kettering Cancer Ctr, NY; et al)

Int J Radiat Oncol Biol Phys 76:S123-S129, 2010

The available dose/volume/outcome data for rectal injury were reviewed. The volume of rectum receiving ≥60Gy is consistently associated with the risk of Grade ≥2 rectal toxicity or rectal bleeding. Parameters for the Lyman-Kutcher-Burman normal tissue complication probability model from four clinical series are remarkably consistent, suggesting that high doses are predominant in determining the risk of toxicity. The best overall estimates (95% confidence interval) of the Lyman-Kutcher-Burman model parameters are n = 0.09 (0.04–0.14); m = 0.13 (0.10–0.17); and TD_{50} = 76.9 (73.7–80.1) Gy. Most of the models of late radiation toxicity come from three-dimensional conformal radiotherapy dose-escalation studies of early-stage prostate cancer. It is possible that intensity-modulated radiotherapy or proton beam dose distributions require modification of these models because of the inherent differences in low and intermediate dose distributions.

▶ QUANTEC is an effort on the part of radiation oncology as a specialty to confirm or redefine the radiation dose-volume effects on all normal organs. This article is a specific look at the rectum as an organ at risk. Unlike many normal organs of the body where the data on dose and volume and associated toxicity are sparse, the data for the rectum are fairly voluminous. Also the effects on the rectum, if injured, with issues of stool frequency, bleeding, and potential incontinence, significantly affects quality of life for patients with cancer. Thus, it is very important for the treating radiation oncologist to know these data so as to limit toxicity as much as possible.

These authors have done a nice job of outlining the challenges in defining the rectal volume and reviewing the dose-volume toxicity data. One factor previously not thought to be associated with late rectal injury is severity of acute toxicity. These authors review this topic and report that based on the data available, a high rate of acute radiation rectal toxicity is now recognized as a significant risk factor associated with late radiation rectal injury.

Finally, the rectal dose-volume constraints for conventionally fractionated radiation therapy (up to 78 Gy) using 3-dimensional treatment planning are $V_{50} < 50\%$, $V_{60} < 35\%$, $V_{65} < 25\%$, $V_{70} < 20\%$, and $V_{75} < 15\%$. All radiation oncologists treating pelvic malignancies need to be careful to comply with these constraints.

C. A. Lawton, MD

Colon: Early Stage and Adjuvant

Association Between Time to Initiation of Adjuvant Chemotherapy and Survival in Colorectal Cancer: A Systematic Review and Meta-Analysis

Biagi JJ, Raphael MJ, Mackillop WJ, et al (Queen's Univ, Kingston, Ontario, Canada)

JAMA 305:2335-2342, 2011

Context.—Adjuvant chemotherapy (AC) improves survival among patients with resected colorectal cancer. However, the optimal timing from surgery to initiation of AC is unknown.

Objective.—To determine the relationship between time to AC and survival outcomes via a systematic review and meta-analysis.

Data Sources.—MEDLINE (1975 through January 2011), EMBASE, the Cochrane Database of Systematic Reviews, and the Cochrane Central Register of Controlled Trials were searched to identify studies that described the relationship between time to AC and survival.

Study Selection.—Studies were only included if the relevant prognostic factors were adequately described and either comparative groups were balanced or results adjusted for these prognostic factors.

Data Extraction.—Hazard ratios (HRs) for overall survival and disease-free survival from each study were converted to a regression coefficient (β) and standard error corresponding to a continuous representation per 4 weeks of time to AC. The adjusted β from individual studies were combined using a fixed-effects model. Inverse variance ($1/SE^2$) was used to weight individual studies. Publication bias was investigated using the trim and fill approach.

Results.—We identified 10 eligible studies involving 15 410 patients (7 published articles, 3 abstracts). Nine of the studies were cohort or population based and 1 was a secondary analysis from a randomized trial of chemotherapy. Six studies reported time to AC as a binary variable and 4 as 3 or more categories. Meta-analysis demonstrated that a 4-week increase in time to AC was associated with a significant decrease in both overall survival (HR, 1.14; 95% confidence interval [CI], 1.10-1.17) and disease-free survival (HR, 1.14; 95% CI, 1.10-1.18). There was no significant heterogeneity among included studies. Results remained significant after adjustment for potential publication bias and when the analysis was repeated to exclude studies of largest weight.

Conclusion.—In a meta-analysis of the available literature on time to AC, longer time to AC was associated with worse survival among patients with resected colorectal cancer.

▶ The interval of time between surgery and the initiation of adjuvant chemotherapy is theoretically crucial to the efficacy of the adjuvant treatment. Surgical removal of the bulk of disease can theoretically accelerate the growth and rate at which mutations leading to drug resistance can occur in the residual micrometastases. Delays in the initiation of adjuvant therapy can therefore lead to decreased efficacy by allowing for greater likelihood of the emergence of disease that is resistant for whatever reason. Previous studies have suggested that clinical evidence supports that adjuvant therapy started more than 12 weeks after surgery will have little effect. This meta-analysis evaluated 10 trials that had data on time to start of adjuvant therapy available for study and that included 15 410 patients and found positive evidence that delays in the start of adjuvant therapy to more than 4 weeks after surgery compromised the effectiveness of the therapy. The investigators concluded that a delay to 8 weeks increased the hazard of death by 14% and that a delay to 12 weeks increased the hazard of death by 30%. The one flaw in the study is that no data from the oxaliplatin era are included among the 10 studies evaluated. By the same token, no data from studies including bevacizumab are included either. The bottom line is that adjuvant therapy should be started as soon as possible after surgery and that the start should occur, if possible, no later than 4 weeks after surgery.

J. T. Thigpen, MD

DNA Mismatch Repair Status and Colon Cancer Recurrence and Survival in Clinical Trials of 5-Fluorouracil-Based Adjuvant Therapy

Sinicrope FA, Foster NR, Thibodeau SN, et al (Mayo Clinic, Rochester, MN; et al)

J Natl Cancer Inst 103:863-875, 2011

Background.—Approximately 15% of colorectal cancers develop because of defective function of the DNA mismatch repair (MMR) system. We determined the association of MMR status with colon cancer recurrence and examined the impact of 5-fluorouracil (FU)-based adjuvant therapy on recurrence variables.

Methods.—We included stage II and III colon carcinoma patients (n = 2141) who were treated in randomized trials of 5-FU-based adjuvant therapy. Tumors were analyzed for microsatellite instability by polymerase chain reaction and/or for MMR protein expression by immunohistochemistry to determine deficient MMR (dMMR) or proficient MMR (pMMR) status. Associations of MMR status and/or 5-FU-based treatment with clinicopathologic and recurrence covariates were determined using χ^2 or Fisher Exact or Wilcoxon rank-sum tests. Time to recurrence (TTR), disease-free survival (DFS), and overall survival (OS) were analyzed using univariate and multivariable Cox models, with the latter adjusted for covariates. Tumors showing dMMR were categorized by presumed germline vs sporadic origin and were assessed for their prognostic and predictive impact. All statistical tests were two-sided.

Results.—In this study population, dMMR was detected in 344 of 2141 (16.1%) tumors. Compared with pMMR tumors, dMMR was associated with reduced 5-year recurrence rates (33% vs 22%; $P < .001$), delayed TTR ($P < .001$), and fewer distant recurrences (22% vs 12%; $P < .001$). In multivariable models, dMMR was independently associated with delayed TTR (hazard ratio = 0.72, 95% confidence interval = 0.56 to 0.91, $P = .005$) and improved DFS ($P = .035$) and OS ($P = .031$). In stage III cancers, 5-FU-based treatment vs surgery alone or no 5-FU was associated with reduced distant recurrence for dMMR tumors (11% vs 29%; $P = .011$) and reduced recurrence to all sites for pMMR tumors ($P < .001$). The dMMR tumors with suspected germline mutations were associated with improved DFS after 5-FU-based treatment compared with sporadic tumors where no benefit was observed ($P = .006$).

Conclusions.—Patients with dMMR colon cancers have reduced rates of tumor recurrence, delayed TTR, and improved survival rates, compared with pMMR colon cancers. Distant recurrences were reduced by 5-FU-based adjuvant treatment in dMMR stage III tumors, and a subset analysis suggested that any treatment benefit was restricted to suspected germline vs sporadic tumors.

► Approximately 15% of colorectal cancers (CRC) occur because of a defective DNA mismatch repair (MMR) genetic system, giving rise to deficient MMR (dMMR) colorectal cancers. dMMR tumors are mostly caused by epigenetic alterations in *MLH1* (in sporadic CRC), while few are secondary to germline mutations in *MLH1*, *MSH2*, *MSH6*, and *PMS2* (causing Lynch syndrome). Characteristically, dMMR CRC show high frequency of microsatellite instability (MSI-H), have clinical and pathologic characteristics, mainly located in the proximal colon, and have better clinical outcomes, based on retrospective data. In addition, several studies suggest no benefit from 5-fluorouracil (5-FU) for dMMR colorectal cancers.[1,2] It is unclear whether the lack of survival benefit using 5-FU for stages 2 and 3 CRC varies depending on the epigenetic or mutational inactivation of the DNA mismatch repair genes.

In one of the largest studies reported to date, with a median follow-up of 8 years, Sinicrope et al analyzed the effect of dMMR on patterns of cancer relapse and survival as well as on the effects of 5-FU adjuvant therapy (with no additional oxaliplatin or irinotecan) on clinical outcomes for 2141 patients with stages 2 (n = 778) and 3 (n = 1363) colorectal cancers; participation in international, randomized adjuvant clinical trials with 5-FU; and available tissue specimens for analysis of MSI (by reverse transcriptase polymerase chain reaction) and MMR protein expression by immunohistochemistry (IHC). Several tumors (n = 111) were also tested for the *BRAF* V600E mutation.

Approximately 16% of all patients had dMMR tumors, and the dMMR tumors were more likely to be stage 2, proximal in location, and poorly differentiated. dMMR CRC patients had superior disease-free survival (DFS) (hazard ratio [HR], 0.73; *P* = .004) as well as superior overall survival (HR, 0.73; *P* = .004) compared with proficient MMR tumors, but the significant benefit was limited to patients with stage 3 disease.

In a prior study, Sargent et al[1] reported on the lack of efficacy of 5-FU adjuvant therapy for dMMR colorectal cancer. In the current study, 5-FU therapy was associated with fewer distant recurrences for stage 3 dMMR CRC, but an overall predictive analysis for stage 2 or 3 dMMR CRC was not performed. Nevertheless, the authors intended to analyze the possible predictive effect from 5-FU by categorizing dMMR cancers into sporadic and germline based on dMMR (either loss of *MSH2* and MSI-H and/or loss of *MLH1*) and an age cutoff of 55 years at diagnosis: sporadic if age over 55, and germline (Lynch syndrome) if age 55 or less. All tumors with loss of *MSH2* were presumed germline, and all tumors with BRAF mutation were presumed sporadic. Prognosis was similar for germline and sporadic dMMR CRC. Of note, in patients with presumed germline tumors (n = 66), 5-FU versus no therapy was associated with improved DFS (HR 0.29, *P* = .006), while no benefit was observed for sporadic dMMR CRC (n = 120). This benefit was restricted to stage 3 germline dMMR CRC. No formal analysis in stage 2 dMMR CRC was provided.

These results suggest that the benefit of 5-FU in stage 3 dMMR colorectal cancer depends on the mechanism of epigenetic or mutational inactivation of the MMR genes, and while hypothesis generating, will need validation from larger randomized studies.

The study's limitations reside in its retrospective design, pooling of the patients from multiple randomized trials with incomplete tissue availability, and the categorization of germline versus sporadic on the presumption of MMR analysis in tumor in combination with the age at diagnosis rather than molecular germline DNA testing. Most importantly, the authors have not reported an updated analysis on the predictive value of MMR deficiency on DFS and overall survival based on treatment with 5-FU or observation.

Despite these shortcomings, the implications for clinical practice are important, and while this study did not address the role of 5-FU in stage 2 dMMR CRC, it validated the benefit from 5-FU for stage 3 CRC, including for MSI-H and other dMMR CRC. The predictive value of dMMR on treatment with 5-FU plus oxaliplatin, per standard practice for many stage 3 CRC patients, is currently unknown but will be addressed in future trials.

E. G. Chiorean, MD

References

1. Sargent DJ, Marsoni S, Monges G, et al. Defective mismatch repair as a predictive marker for lack of efficacy of fluorouracil-based adjuvant therapy in colon cancer. *J Clin Oncol.* 2010;28:3219-3226.
2. Jover R, Zapater P, Castells A, et al. The efficacy of adjuvant chemotherapy with 5-fluorouracil in colorectal cancer depends on the mismatch repair status. *Eur J Cancer.* 2009;45:365-373.

Colon: Advanced

Addition of cetuximab to oxaliplatin-based first-line combination chemotherapy for treatment of advanced colorectal cancer: results of the randomised phase 3 MRC COIN trial

Maughan TS, on behalf of the MRC COIN Trial Investigators (Cardiff Univ UK; et al)

Lancet 377:2103-2114, 2011

Background.—In the Medical Research Council (MRC) COIN trial, the epidermal growth factor receptor (EGFR)-targeted antibody cetuximab was added to standard chemotherapy in first-line treatment of advanced colorectal cancer with the aim of assessing effect on overall survival.

Methods.—In this randomised controlled trial, patients who were fit for but had not received previous chemotherapy for advanced colorectal cancer were randomly assigned to oxaliplatin and fluoropyrimidine chemotherapy (arm A), the same combination plus cetuximab (arm B), or intermittent chemotherapy (arm C). The choice of fluoropyrimidine therapy (capecitabine or infused fluouroracil plus leucovorin) was decided before randomisation. Randomisation was done centrally (via telephone) by the MRC Clinical Trials Unit using minimisation. Treatment allocation was not masked. The comparison of arms A and C is described in a companion paper. Here, we present the comparison of arm A and B, for which the primary outcome was overall survival in patients with KRAS wild-type tumours. Analysis was by intention to treat. Further analyses with respect to NRAS, BRAF, and EGFR status were done. The trial is registered, ISRCTN27286448.

Findings.—1630 patients were randomly assigned to treatment groups (815 to standard therapy and 815 to addition of cetuximab). Tumour samples from 1316 (81%) patients were used for somatic molecular analyses; 565 (43%) had KRAS mutations. In patients with KRAS wild-type tumours (arm A, n=367; arm B, n=362), overall survival did not differ between treatment groups (median survival 17·9 months [IQR 10·3–29·2] in the control group vs 17·0 months [9·4–30·1] in the cetuximab group; HR 1·04, 95% CI 0·87–1·23, p=0·67). Similarly, there was no effect on progression-free survival (8·6 months [IQR 5·0–12·5] in the control group vs 8·6 months [5·1–13·8] in the cetuximab group; HR 0·96, 0·82–1·12, p=0·60). Overall response rate increased from 57% (n=209) with chemotherapy alone to 64% (n=232) with addition of cetuximab (p=0·049). Grade 3 and higher skin and gastrointestinal toxic effects were increased with cetuximab (14 vs 114 and 67 vs 97 patients in the control group vs the cetuximab group with KRAS wild-type tumours, respectively). Overall survival differs by somatic mutation status irrespective of treatment received: BRAF mutant, 8·8 months (IQR 4·5–27·4); KRAS mutant, 14·4 months (8·5–24·0); all wild-type, 20·1 months (11·5–31·7).

Interpretation.—This trial has not confirmed a benefit of addition of cetuximab to oxaliplatin-based chemotherapy in first-line treatment of patients with advanced colorectal cancer. Cetuximab increases response rate, with no evidence of benefit in progression-free or overall survival in KRAS wild-type patients or even in patients selected by additional mutational analysis of their tumours. The use of cetuximab in combination with oxaliplatin and capecitabine in first-line chemotherapy in patients with widespread metastases cannot be recommended.

▶ Epidermal growth factor receptor (EGFR)-targeted therapies have a well-defined role in metastatic *KRAS* wild-type colorectal cancer. The monoclonal antibody cetuximab is US Food and Drug Administration approved in combination with irinotecan for metastatic colorectal cancer after progression on irinotecan, and as single agent after failure of any prior chemotherapy. Cetuximab has also demonstrated improved progression-free and overall survival when combined with FOLFIRI (infusional 5-fluorouracil and irinotecan) in the first-line treatment of *KRAS* wild-type metastatic colorectal cancer, with an added 3.5 months' benefit on overall survival (hazard ratio [HR], 0.8) and 1.5 months in progression-free survival (PFS) (HR, 0.7).[1]

The Medical Research Council (MRC) COIN trial investigators have addressed the role of adding cetuximab to an oxaliplatin-based regimen in first-line metastatic colorectal cancer and also analyzed the effect of treatment interruptions on outcomes. Overall, 2445 patients were randomly assigned to have FOLFOX (infusional 5-fluorouracil and oxaliplatin) or XELOX (capecitabine and oxaliplatin) until disease progression (arm A), FOLFOX or XELOX plus cetuximab until disease progression (arm B), or intermittent FOLFOX or XELOX (12 weeks of treatment, and restart at progression; arm C). The primary end point was overall survival in KRAS wild-type tumors, and the secondary end point included overall survival in KRAS mutant, KRAS/NRAS/BRAF wild type, "any" mutant, progression-free survival, response, and quality of life. This article reports on the primary outcome. Approximately 65% versus 35% of patients were treated at the physician's discretion with XELOX versus FOLFOX. Among 367 patients with *KRAS* wild-type disease randomly assigned to FOLFOX/XELOX and 361 patients with *KRAS* wild-type disease randomly assigned to FOLFOX/XELOX plus cetuximab, there was no benefit in overall survival (17.9 vs 17 months) or PFS (8.6 months in both groups) but a modest improvement in response from 57% to 64% ($P = .049$). Patients with wild-type tumors for all genes tested, *KRAS*, *NRAS*, and *BRAF*, similarly did not demonstrate any benefit from the addition of cetuximab. Exploratory analysis for predictive factors on PFS found that 5-fluorouracil, but not capecitabine treatment, was associated with improved PFS when combined with cetuximab (HR 0.72, 95% confidence interval [CI] 0.53–0.98; $P = .037$).

An additional study, NORDIC VII, previously reported at ESMO 2010, had shown similarly disappointing results when bolus 5-fluorouracil and oxaliplatin (FLOX) were combined with cetuximab, indicating no benefit in PFS (7.9 months for FLOX with cetuximab vs 8.7 months with FLOX, HR 1.07).[2]

The possibility of the lack of benefit with cetuximab added to the chemotherapy backbone being caused by capecitabine due to increased toxicity, as suggested by the authors, is unlikely to explain entirely the findings, as the duration of treatment was similar in both groups in the COIN study, especially when corroborated further with the NORDIC study, which used 5-fluorouracil. These results clearly suggest that cetuximab should not be used in combination with oxaliplatin-fluoropyrimidine chemotherapy in metastatic colorectal cancer, and raise the concern of a significant negative drug-drug interaction.

E. G. Chiorean, MD

References

1. Van Cutsem E, Köhne CH, Láng I, et al. Cetuximab plus irinotecan, fluorouracil, and leucovorin as first-line treatment for metastatic colorectal cancer: updated analysis of overall survival according to tumor KRAS and BRAF mutation status. *J Clin Oncol.* 2011;29:2011-2019.
2. Tveit K, Guren T, Glimelius B, et al. Randomized phase III study of 5-fluorouracil/folinate/oxaliplatin given continuously or intermittently with or without cetuximab, as first line treatment of metastatic colorectal cancer: the NORDIC VII study by the Nordic Colorectal Cancer Biomodulation Group. *J Clin Oncol.* 2011;29 [abstract 365].

Addition of cetuximab to oxaliplatin-based first-line combination chemotherapy for treatment of advanced colorectal cancer: results of the randomised phase 3 MRC COIN trial

Maughan TS, on behalf of the MRC COIN Trial Investigators (Cardiff Univ, UK; et al)

Lancet 377:2103-2114, 2011

Background.—In the Medical Research Council (MRC) COIN trial, the epidermal growth factor receptor (EGFR)-targeted antibody cetuximab was added to standard chemotherapy in first-line treatment of advanced colorectal cancer with the aim of assessing effect on overall survival.

Methods.—In this randomised controlled trial, patients who were fit for but had not received previous chemotherapy for advanced colorectal cancer were randomly assigned to oxaliplatin and fluoropyrimidine chemotherapy (arm A), the same combination plus cetuximab (arm B), or intermittent chemotherapy (arm C). The choice of fluoropyrimidine therapy (capecitabine or infused fluouroracil plus leucovorin) was decided before randomisation. Randomisation was done centrally (via telephone) by the MRC Clinical Trials Unit using minimisation. Treatment allocation was not masked. The comparison of arms A and C is described in a companion paper. Here, we present the comparison of arms A and B, for which the primary outcome was overall survival in patients with *KRAS* wild-type tumours. Analysis was by intention to treat. Further analyses with respect to *NRAS, BRAF,* and *EGFR* status were done. The trial is registered, ISRCTN27286448.

Findings.—1630 patients were randomly assigned to treatment groups (815 to standard therapy and 815 to addition of cetuximab). Tumour samples from 1316 (81%) patients were used for somatic molecular analyses; 565 (43%) had *KRAS* mutations. In patients with *KRAS* wild-type tumours (arm A, n=367; arm B, n=362), overall survival did not differ between treatment groups (median survival 17·9 months [IQR 10·3–29·2] in the control group *vs* 17·0 months [9·4–30·1] in the cetuximab group; HR 1·04, 95% CI 0·87–1·23, p=0·67). Similarly, there was no effect on progression-free survival (8·6 months [IQR 5·0–12·5] in the control group *vs* 8·6 months [5·1–13·8] in the cetuximab group; HR 0·96, 0·82–1·12, p=0·60). Overall response rate increased from 57% (n=209) with chemotherapy alone to 64% (n=232) with addition of cetuximab (p=0·049). Grade 3 and higher skin and gastrointestinal toxic effects were increased with cetuximab (14 *vs* 114 and 67 *vs* 97 patients in the control group *vs* the cetuximab group with *KRAS* wild-type tumours, respectively). Overall survival differs by somatic mutation status irrespective of treatment received: BRAF mutant, 8·8 months (IQR 4·5–27·4); *KRAS* mutant, 14·4 months (8·5–24·0); all wild-type, 20·1 months (11·5–31·7).

Interpretation.—This trial has not confirmed a benefit of addition of cetuximab to oxaliplatin-based chemotherapy in first-line treatment of patients with advanced colorectal cancer. Cetuximab increases response rate, with no evidence of benefit in progression-free or overall survival in *KRAS* wild-type patients or even in patients selected by additional mutational analysis of their tumours. The use of cetuximab in combination with oxaliplatin and capecitabine in first-line chemotherapy in patients with widespread metastases cannot be recommended.

► The most commonly used regimens in colorectal cancers use oxaliplatin with a fluoropyrimidine (either fluorouracil or capecitabine). The addition of bevacizumab to this combination has been suggested by some trials to enhance overall survival. The other biological alternative is cetuximab, which has been used primarily with irinotecan-based regimens. This trial seeks to determine whether the addition of cetuximab to an oxaliplatin and fluoropyrimidine regimen is advantageous in those patients with *Kras* wild-type tumors. The data show no advantage and substantial toxicity disadvantages for the addition of cetuximab to an oxaliplatin-based regimen. At least for now, it would appear that the standard of care for the first-line treatment of metastatic colon cancer remains an oxaliplatin and fluoropyrimidine regimen with or without bevacizumab. Cetuximab would appear to be better reserved for use with irinotecan-based regimens in patients with *Kras* wild-type tumors.

J. T. Thigpen, MD

Chemotherapy options in elderly and frail patients with metastatic colorectal cancer (MRC FOCUS2): an open-label, randomised factorial trial

Seymour MT, on behalf of the FOCUS2 Investigators, the National Cancer Research Institute Colorectal Cancer Clinical Studies Group (Univ of Leeds, UK; et al)

Lancet 377:1749-1759, 2011

Background.—Elderly and frail patients with cancer, although often treated with chemotherapy, are under-represented in clinical trials. We designed FOCUS2 to investigate reduced-dose chemotherapy options and to seek objective predictors of outcome in frail patients with advanced colorectal cancer.

Methods.—We undertook an open, 2 × 2 factorial trial in 61 UK centres for patients with previously untreated advanced colorectal cancer who were considered unfit for full-dose chemotherapy. After comprehensive health assessment (CHA), patients were randomly assigned by minimisation to: 48-h intravenous fluorouracil with levofolinate (group A); oxaliplatin and fluorouracil (group B); capecitabine (group C); or oxaliplatin and capecitabine (group D). Treatment allocation was not masked. Starting doses were 80% of standard doses, with discretionary escalation to full dose after 6 weeks. The two primary outcome measures were: addition of oxaliplatin ([A vs B] + [C vs D]), assessed with progression-free survival (PFS); and substitution of fluorouracil with capecitabine ([A vs C] + [B vs D]), assessed by change from baseline to 12 weeks in global quality of life (QoL). Analysis was by intention to treat. Baseline clinical and CHA data were modelled against outcomes with a novel composite measure, overall treatment utility (OTU). This study is registered, number ISRCTN21221452.

Findings.—459 patients were randomly assigned (115 to each of groups A-C, 114 to group D). Factorial comparison of addition of oxaliplatin versus no addition suggested some improvement in PFS, but the finding was not significant (median 5·8 months [IQR 3·3-7·5] vs 4·5 months [2·8-6·4]; hazard ratio 0·84, 95% CI 0·69-1·01, p=0·07). Replacement of fluorouracil with capecitabine did not improve global QoL: 69 of 124 (56%) patients receiving fluorouracil reported improvement in global

QoL compared with 69 of 123 (56%) receiving capecitabine. The risk of having any grade 3 or worse toxic effect was not significantly increased with oxaliplatin (83/219 [38%] vs 70/221 [32%]; p=0·17), but was higher with capecitabine than with fluorouracil (88/222 [40%] vs 65/218 [30%]; p=0·03). In multivariable analysis, fewer baseline symptoms (odds ratio 1·32, 95% CI 1·14-1·52), less widespread disease (1·51, 1·05-2·19), and use of oxaliplatin (0·57, 0·39-0·82) were predictive of better OTU.

Interpretation.—FOCUS2 shows that with an appropriate design, including reduced starting doses of chemotherapy, frail and elderly patients can participate in a randomised controlled trial. On balance, a combination including oxaliplatin was preferable to single-agent fluoropyrimidines, although the primary endpoint of PFS was not met. Capecitabine did not improve QoL compared with fluorouracil. Comprehensive baseline assessment holds promise as an objective predictor of treatment benefit.

▶ There has always been a tendency among oncologists to modify treatment regimens because the patient is, in the opinion of the physician, unable to tolerate full-dose treatment. This flies in the face of the opinion held by many that the intensity of treatment is important, at least up to a certain level. The result has been the development of trials such as this, focusing on the elderly and infirm (those unable to tolerate full-dose therapy in the opinion of the physician). This study basically looks at 3 questions in this patient population with colon cancer. Firstly, the study seeks to determine whether starting therapy at a reduced dose of 80% of full dose resulted in benefit with less toxicity. The population was not randomized for this question, so this issue cannot be answered in this trial. Furthermore, leaving the definition of the patient population in the hands of the individual investigator on a case-by-case basis leaves open the question of exactly what is being studied. Secondly, the addition of oxaliplatin yielded a strong trend in favor of adding the oxaliplatin; hence, the investigators concluded that this was worthwhile. Finally, the substitution of capecitabine for 5-fluorouracil resulted in added toxicity without added benefit. What do we then take from this study for our practice? Firstly, even with reduced doses of drugs, patients benefit from therapy that includes oxaliplatin with 5-fluorouracil. Secondly, the substitution of capecitabine for 5-fluorouracil does not appear to be advantageous. Thirdly, the question as to whether doses can be reduced for older and infirm patients without compromising efficacy remains unanswered.

J. T. Thigpen, MD

Randomized Trial of Two Induction Chemotherapy Regimens in Metastatic Colorectal Cancer: An Updated Analysis

Masi G, Vasile E, Loupakis F, et al (Istituto Toscano Tumori, Pisa, Italy; et al)

J Natl Cancer Inst 103:21-30, 2011

Background.—In a randomized trial with a median follow-up of 18.4 months, 6 months of induction chemotherapy with a three-drug regimen comprising 5-fluorouracil (by continuous infusion)—leucovorin, irinotecan, and oxaliplatin (FOLFOXIRI) demonstrated statistically significant improvements in response rate, radical surgical resection of metastases, progression-free survival, and overall survival compared with 6 months of induction chemotherapy with fluorouracil—leucovorin and irinotecan (FOLFIRI).

Methods.—From November 14, 2001, to April 22, 2005, we enrolled 244 patients with metastatic colorectal cancer. To evaluate if the superiority of FOLFOXIRI is maintained in the long term, we updated the overall and progression-free survival data to include events that occurred up to February 12, 2009, with a median follow-up of 60.6 months. We performed a subgroup and a risk-stratified analysis to examine whether outcomes differed in specific patient subgroups, and we analyzed the results of treatment after progression. Survival curves were estimated by the Kaplan—Meier method. Multivariable Cox regression models were fit to estimate hazard ratios (HRs) and 95% confidence intervals (CIs). All statistical tests were two-sided.

Results.—FOLFOXIRI demonstrated statistically significant improvements in median progression-free survival (9.8 vs 6.8 months, HR for progression = 0.59, 95% CI = 0.45 to 0.76, $P < .001$) and median overall survival (23.4 vs 16.7 months, HR for death = 0.74, 95% CI = 0.56 to 0.96, $P = .026$) with a 5-year survival rate of 15% (95% CI = 9% to 23%) vs 8% (95% CI = 4% to 14%). The improvements in progression-free survival and, to a lesser extent, in overall survival were evident even when the analysis excluded patients who received radical resection of metastases. With regard to the risk-stratified analysis, FOLFOXIRI results in longer progression-free survival and over-all survival than FOLFIRI in all risk subgroups.

Conclusions.—Six months of induction chemotherapy with FOLFOXIRI is associated with a clinically significant improvement in the long-term outcome compared with FOLFIRI with an absolute benefit in survival at 5 years of 7%.

► The outlook for the patient with metastatic colon cancer has improved substantially in the past 15 years as new active agents have been added to 5-fluorouracil. The addition of first irinotecan, then oxaliplatin, and subsequently the monoclonal antibodies cetuximab and bevacizumab has increased the overall median survival from less than a year to more than 2 years. Two chemotherapy doublets have become the standard backbones for treatment: FOLFOX and FOLFIRI. This trial examines a regimen that includes all 3 chemotherapeutic agents as compared with one of the doublets, FOLFIRI. The results suggest an improvement in response rate, progression-free survival, and overall survival with the 3-drug regimen at the expense of a substantial increase in toxicity. In particular, patients receiving the 3-drug regimen had a higher response rate, which led to a greater likelihood that residual disease could be resected after chemotherapy. These data look convincing, but they are contradicted by another phase III trial by the Hellenic Group that found the increased toxicity seen in this trial but no advantage for the 3-drug regimen. These conflicting results have resulted in the continued use of doublets of chemotherapy in combination with bevacizumab as the basis for the therapy of most patients with metastatic disease.

J. T. Thigpen, MD

9 Cancer Biology

Correlation of Somatic Mutation and Expression Identifies Genes Important in Human Glioblastoma Progression and Survival

Masica DL, Karchin R (The Johns Hopkins Univ, Baltimore, MD)

Cancer Res 71:4550-4561, 2011

Cooperative dysregulation of gene sequence and expression may contribute to cancer formation and progression. The Cancer Genome Atlas (TCGA) Network recently cataloged gene sequence and expression data for a collection of glioblastoma multiforme (GBM) tumors. We developed an automated, model-free method to rapidly and exhaustively examine the correlation among somatic mutation and gene expression and interrogated 149 GBM tumor samples from the TCGA. The method identified 41 genes whose mutation status is highly correlated with drastic changes in the expression (z-score ± 2.0), across tumor samples, of other genes. Some of the 41 genes have been previously implicated in GBM pathogenesis (e.g., NF1, TP53, RB1 and IDH1) and others, while implicated in cancer, had not previously been highlighted in studies using TCGA data (e.g., SYNE1, KLF6, FGFR4, and EPHB4). The method also predicted that known oncogenes and tumor suppressors participate in GBM via drastic over- and underexpression, respectively. Additionally, the method identified a known synthetic lethal interaction between TP53 and PLK1, other potential synthetic lethal interactions with TP53, and correlations between IDH1 mutation status and the overexpression of known GBM survival genes.

▶ The generation of DNA sequence and transcriptional patterns in a wide variety of cancers has been a result of the The Cancer Genome Atlas (TCGA). The results of the analysis of such extensive databases have revealed some expected findings, such as the high frequency of p53 mutations, and some unexpected findings, such as mutations in chromatin-modifying proteins. Despite such important findings, the challenge of integrative analysis across such large databases from a variety of tumor types is significant. Masica and Karchin present an elegant, automated, model-free method to determine the correlation among somatic mutations and corresponding gene expression. They use this approach to a set of genes known to be involved in glioblastoma pathogenesis but probably most importantly, identify another set of genes not previously associated with glioblastoma. Even more important is that through pathway analysis they were also able to propose potential synthetic lethal interactions among some of the altered genes. Although biological validation will be essential as a next step for such bioinformatic analyses, such approaches should take on an increasingly important role in helping to make sense out of the sometimes Tower of Babel of sequencing.

R. J. Arceci, MD, PhD

Nuclear ErbB2 Enhances Translation and Cell Growth by Activating Transcription of Ribosomal RNA Genes

Li L-Y, Chen H, Hsieh Y-H, et al (China Med Univ Hosp, Taichung, Taiwan; et al)

Cancer Res 71:4269-4279, 2011

Aberrant regulation of rRNA synthesis and translation control can facilitate tumorigenesis. The ErbB2 growth factor receptor is overexpressed in many human tumors and has been detected in the nucleus, but the role of nuclear ErbB2 is obscure. In this study, we defined a novel function of nuclear ErbB2 in enhancing rRNA gene transcription by RNA polymerase-I (RNA Pol I). Nuclear ErbB2 physically associates with β-actin and RNA Pol I, coinciding with active RNA Pol I transcription sites in nucleoli. RNA interference–mediated knockdown of ErbB2 reduced pre-rRNA and protein synthesis. In contrast, wild-type ErbB2 augmented pre-rRNA level, protein production, and cell size/cell growth, but not by an ErbB2 mutant that is defective in nuclear translocation. Chromatin immunoprecipitation assays revealed that ErbB2 enhances binding of RNA Pol I to rDNA. In addition, ErbB2 associated with rDNA, RNA Pol I, and β-actin, suggesting how it could stimulate rRNA production, protein synthesis, and increased cell size and cell growth. Finally, ErbB2-potentiated RNA Pol I transcription could be stimulated by ligand and was not substantially repressed by inhibition of PI3-K and MEK/ERK (extracellular signal regulated kinase), the main ErbB2 effector signaling pathways. Together, our findings indicate that nuclear ErbB2 functions as a regulator of rRNA synthesis and cellular translation, which may contribute to tumor development and progression.

▶ The control of cell proliferation in all cells, including cancer, is closely coupled with the duplication of cellular components to bequeath sufficient molecular building blocks to progeny. One of the most energy-intensive structures to replace in dividing cells is the ribosome. Despite the importance of ribosome biogenesis and protein synthesis, the regulation of making ribosomes, composed of both ribosomal RNAs and proteins, is not well understood. ErbB2 (also known as HER2 or neu) is a cell surface receptor with tyrosine kinase activity, which, when activated, regulates a variety of key survival and proliferation pathways. ErbB2 is also overexpressed in many tumor types, most notably breast cancer. Li et al now demonstrate that ErbB2 is able to translocate in association with actin from the cytoplasm to the nucleus where it interacts with polymerase type I to enhance the transcription of ribosomal transcripts. In addition, this activation is enhanced by ligand binding to ErbB2. These results are important in that they provide a mechanistic link between an important receptor in cancer and the fundamental and required cell process of ribosomal biogenesis in cancer. Because the effect on ribosomal RNA transcription appears separate from the other effects of ErbB2 on cell signaling pathways, this also suggests that inhibitors of ErbB4 directly may be more effective than targeting only 1 of the affected downstream pathways.

R. J. Arceci, MD, PhD

The Genetic Landscape of the Childhood Cancer Medulloblastoma

Parsons DW, Li M, Zhang X, et al (Johns Hopkins Kimmel Cancer Ctr, Baltimore, MD; et al)

Science 331:435-439, 2011

Medulloblastoma (MB) is the most common malignant brain tumor of children. To identify the genetic alterations in this tumor type, we searched for copy number alterations using high-density microarrays and sequenced all known protein-coding genes and microRNA genes using Sanger sequencing in a set of 22 MBs. We found that, on average, each tumor had 11 gene alterations, fewer by a factor of 5 to 10 than in the adult solid tumors that have been sequenced to date. In addition to alterations in the Hedgehog and Wnt pathways, our analysis led to the discovery of genes not previously known to be altered in MBs. Most notably, inactivating mutations of the histone-lysine N-methyltransferase genes MLL2 or MLL3 were identified in 16% of MB patients. These results demonstrate key differences between the genetic landscapes of adult and childhood cancers, highlight dysregulation of developmental pathways as an important mechanism underlying MBs, and identify a role for a specific type of histone methylation in human tumorigenesis.

► The genetic sequencing of human tumors has received a great deal of financial support and cultural encouragement from the National Institutes of Health–sponsored TCGA (The Cancer Genome Atlas) and TARGET (Therapeutically Applicable Research to Generate Effective Treatments) to separate institutional consortia. The hope is that such studies will identify all the key mutated pathways that exist in various cancer types and then develop effective targeted drug therapies. On the other hand, there has been criticism or at least skepticism that such approaches would produce a lot of sequencing data without a true end point. As Dr Sydney Brenner has said, such approaches are "low input, high throughput, no output." The study by Parsons et al now reports on genomic sequencing of 22 childhood medulloblastomas. Several interesting findings are reported and particularly include the relatively low number of consistently observed mutations (average of 11) compared with most adult tumors, the identification of alterations to genes that are part of the Hedgehog and Wnt pathways, and documentation of mutations in 16% of tumors of the histone-lysine N-methyltransferase genes, *MLL2/MLL3*. While short on biology, the study and those like it are important for establishing the genetic framework upon which cancer is partly built but also in identifying specific pathways that can then be validated functionally and clinically.

R. J. Arceci, MD, PhD

10 Sarcoma

Prognostic Factors After Relapse in Nonmetastatic Rhabdomyosarcoma: A Nomogram to Better Define Patients Who Can Be Salvaged With Further Therapy

Chisholm JC, Marandet J, Rey A, et al (Royal Marsden Hosp, Sutton, UK; Inst of Child Life and Health, Bristol, UK; Institut Gustave Roussy, Villejuif, France; et al)

J Clin Oncol 29:1319-1325, 2011

Purpose.—Previous studies suggest poor outcome in children with relapsed rhabdomyosarcoma (RMS). A better understanding is needed of which patients can be salvaged after first relapse.

Patients and Methods.—The analysis included children with nonmetastatic RMS and embryonal sarcoma enrolled onto the International Society of Paediatric Oncology (SIOP) Malignant Mesenchymal Tumor (MMT) 84, 89, and 95 studies who relapsed after achieving complete local control with primary therapy. All patients included in the analysis had follow-up for ≥ 3.0 years after the last event. The clinical features, initial treatment characteristics, and features of the relapse were correlated with survival in univariate and multivariate analyses.

Results.—In all, 474 eligible patients were identified for the study. At ≥ 3.0 years from the last event, 176 (37%) were alive ("cured"). In a full-model multivariate analysis, the factors identified at first relapse that most strongly associated with poor outcome were metastatic relapse (odds ratio [OR], 4.19; 95% CI, 2.0 to 8.5), prior radiotherapy treatment (OR, 3.64; 95% CI, 2.1 to 6.4), initial tumor size > 5 cm (OR, 2.53; 95% CI, 1.5 to 4.1), and time of relapse < 18 months from diagnosis (OR, 2.20; 95% CI, 1.3 to 3.6). Unfavorable primary disease site, nodal involvement at diagnosis, alveolar histology, and previous three- or six-drug chemotherapy were also independently associated with poor outcome. To estimate chance of cure for individual patients, a nomogram was developed, which allowed for weighting of these significant factors.

Conclusion.—Some children with relapsed RMS remain curable. It is now possible to estimate the chance of salvage for individual children to direct therapy appropriately toward cure, use of experimental therapies, and/or palliation.

▶ While dose intensification has resulted in improved survival for some subgroups of patients with rhabdomyosarcoma (RMS) as characterized by the studies in North America, patients on less-intense European trials have had an inferior event-free survival but an apparently higher survival following relapse. To better understand the factors that might impact survival after relapse, Chisholm et al analyzed a variety of characteristics from 474 patients with initial nonmetastatic RMS who had been treated on 3 International Society of Paediatric Oncology trials from 1984, 1989, and 1995. They identified a wide variety of factors that impacted postrelapse survival, including, most notably, metastatic relapse, initial tumor size > 5 cm, and time of relapse of < 18 months from diagnosis. At 3 or more years from the last event, 37% of patients were alive (Fig 1 in original article). To refine the usefulness of their results, the authors devised a nomogram for integrating and tallying the impact of various factors that can then be used to predict outcome (Fig 2 in original article). While this is an interesting and potentially useful approach to counseling patients and families as well as possibly stratifying patients for future clinical trials after relapse, the results and predictive nomogram (Fig 2 in original article) should be looked upon with caution, as they are based on studies that are 15 to 26 years old. Furthermore, the prognostic nomogram may be relevant only to the treatment paradigms patients received in those studies. The issue of whether to intensify therapy at the time of diagnosis, hoping to cure more patients on the first round of treatment, versus less intense treatment followed by salvage therapy is not answered by this study.

R. J. Arceci, MD, PhD

Prognostic Significance and Tumor Biology of Regional Lymph Node Disease in Patients With Rhabdomyosarcoma: A Report From the Children's Oncology Group

Rodeberg DA, Garcia-Henriquez N, Lyden ER, et al (Univ of Pittsburgh, PA; Nebraska Med Ctr, Omaha, NE; Univ of Oklahoma Health Sciences Ctr, Oklahoma City, OK; et al)

J Clin Oncol 29:1304-1311, 2011

Purpose.—Regional lymph node disease (RLND) is a component of the risk-based treatment stratification in rhabdomyosarcoma (RMS). The purpose of this study was to determine the contribution of RLND to prognosis for patients with RMS.

Patients and Methods.—Patient characteristics and survival outcomes for patients enrolled onto Intergroup Rhabdomyosarcoma Study IV (N = 898, 1991 to 1997) were evaluated among the following three patient groups: nonmetastatic patients with clinical or pathologic negative nodes (N0, 696 patients); patients with clinical or pathologic positive nodes (N1, 125 patients); and patients with a single site of metastatic disease (77 patients).

Results.—Outcomes for patients with nonmetastatic alveolar N0 RMS were significantly better than for patients with N1 RMS (5-year failure-free survival [FFS], 73% v 43%, respectively; 5-year overall survival [OS], 80% v 46%, respectively; $P < .001$). Patients with a single site of alveolar metastasis had even worse FFS and OS (23% FFS and OS, $P = .01$) when compared with patients with N1 RMS; however, the differences were not as large as the differences between patients with N0 RMS and N1 RMS. For embryonal RMS, there was no statistically significant difference in FFS or OS ($P = .41$ and $P = .77$, respectively) for patients with N1 versus N0 RMS. Gene array analysis of primary tumor specimens identified that genes associated with the immune system and antigen presentation were significantly increased in N1 versus N0 alveolar RMS.

Conclusion.—RLND alters prognosis for alveolar but not embryonal RMS. For patients with N1 disease and alveolar histology, outcomes were more similar to distant metastatic disease rather than local disease. Current data suggest that more aggressive therapy for patients with alveolar N1 RMS may be warranted.

▶ The prognosis for metastatic disease in patients with rhabdomyosarcoma (RMS) has been accepted as uniformly poor. However, detailed analysis of patients with nonmetastatic RMS with or without regional lymph node disease involvement has not been accomplished. Rodeberg et al examine this question in about 900 patients treated on the Intergroup Rhabdomyosarcoma Study IV. The results revealed several important findings. First was that 5-year failure-free survival (FFS) was 73% in the node-negative group compared with 43% in the node-positive group; similarly, overall survival (OS) was 80% in the former and 46% in the latter groups. Of note, patients who had single site of alveolar metastasis had FFS and OS of 23%, suggesting that such patients also had a negligible salvage rate. Somewhat surprisingly, patients with embryonal RMS with or without nodal involvement had similar FFS and OS, suggesting a different biology and sensitivity to local and nodal disease. This study also reported that primary tumors associated with more nodal spread had increased RNA expression of a subset of genes preferentially associated with the immune system and antigen presentation. Such data are difficult to interpret without more detailed analysis, and it would have been interesting to compare the alveolar with the embryonal to potentially identify drug or radiation resistance or sensitivity pathways.

R. J. Arceci, MD, PhD

Results of the Intergroup Rhabdomyosarcoma Study Group D9602 Protocol, Using Vincristine and Dactinomycin With or Without Cyclophosphamide and Radiation Therapy, for Newly Diagnosed Patients With Low-Risk Embryonal Rhabdomyosarcoma: A Report From the Soft Tissue Sarcoma Committee of the Children's Oncology Group

Raney RB, Walterhouse DO, Meza JL, et al (The Univ of Texas MD Anderson Cancer Ctr, Houston; Dell Children's Med Ctr of Central Texas, Austin; Children's Memorial Med Ctr, Chicago, IL; et al)

J Clin Oncol 29:1312-1318, 2011

Purpose.—Patients with localized, grossly resected, or gross residual (orbital only) embryonal rhabdomyosarcoma (ERMS) had 5-year failure-free survival (FFS) rates of 83% and overall survival rates of 95% on Intergroup Rhabdomyosarcoma Study Group (IRSG) protocols III/IV. IRSG

D9602 protocol (1997 to 2004) objectives were to decrease toxicity in similar patients by reducing radiotherapy (RT) doses and eliminating cyclophosphamide for the lowest-risk patients.

Patients and Methods.—Subgroup A patients (lowest risk, with ERMS, stage 1 group I/IIA, stage 1 group III orbit, stage 2 group I) received vincristine plus dactinomycin (VA). Subgroup B patients (ERMS, stage 1 group IIB/C, stage I group III nonorbit, stage 2 group II, stage 3 group I/II) received VA plus cyclophosphamide. Patients in group II/III received RT. Compared with IRS-IV, doses were reduced from 41.4 to 36 Gy for stage 1 group IIA patients and from 50 or 59 to 45 Gy for group III orbit patients.

Results.—Estimated 5-year FFS rates were 89% (95% CI, 84% to 92%) for subgroup A patients (n = 264) and 85% (95% CI, 74%, 91%) for subgroup B patients (n = 78); median follow-up: 5.1 years. Estimated 5-year FFS rates were 81% (95% CI, 68% to 90%) for patients with stage 1 group IIA tumors (n = 62) and 86% (95% CI, 76% to 92%) for patients with group III orbit tumors (n = 77).

Conclusion.—Five-year FFS and OS rates were similar to those observed in comparable IRS-III patients, including patients receiving reduced RT doses, but were lower than in comparable IRS-IV patients receiving VA plus cyclophosphamide. Five-year FFS rates were similar among subgroups A and B patients.

▶ The early and late adverse sequelae of chemotherapy and radiation therapy for patients with rhabdomyosarcoma are quite significant. Thus, attempts to systematically reduce these toxicities have become of considerable interest in groups of patients with overall excellent survival outcomes. Raney et al report on the results of the D9602 Intergroup RMS Study Group (IRSG) Protocol, which attempted to reduce toxicity by omitting cyclophosphamide and reducing the dose of radiation therapy in the patients with lowest-risk disease, such as those with stage 1 and 2 orbital disease embryonal histology. Results were compared with those of historical controls from IRSG protocols III and IV. The results suggest that reduced radiation dose gave comparable outcomes, while outcomes appeared lowered in the group not receiving cyclophosphamide, particularly those in subgroup B. While the omission of cyclophospha mide, reducing the level myelosuppression without compromising outcome in subgroup A patients, is a clinically significant finding, it would have been useful to see data on secondary acute myeloid leukemia in patients on this study, as follow-up would have been long enough for the majority of such cases to have been identified. Nevertheless, the results from this trial, while somewhat inconclusive in light of the caveat of using only historical controls, are important and have been used to design the subsequent trial that will examine the question of reducing the dose exposure to cyclophosphamide.

R. J. Arceci, MD, PhD

11 Melanoma

A Randomized Phase 2 Study of Etaracizumab, a Monoclonal Antibody Against Integrin $\alpha_v\beta_3$, ± Dacarbazine in Patients With Stage IV Metastatic Melanoma

Hersey P, for the Etaracizumab Melanoma Study Group (Newcastle Melanoma Unit, Australia; et al)

Cancer 116:1526-1534, 2010

Background.—The alpha $_v$ beta $_3$ ($\alpha_v\beta_3$) integrin is involved in intracellular signaling regulating cell proliferation, migration, and differentiation and is important for tumor-induced angiogenesis.

Methods.—This phase 2, randomized, open-label, 2-arm study was designed to capture safety data and evaluate the antitumor efficacy of etaracizumab (Abegrin), an IgG1 humanized monoclonal antibody against the $\alpha_v\beta_3$ integrin, in patients with previously untreated metastatic melanoma. The objective was to evaluate whether etaracizumab ± dacarbazine had sufficient clinical activity to warrant further study in a phase 3 clinical trial.

Results.—One hundred twelve patients were randomized to receive etaracizumab alone (N = 57) or etaracizumab + dacarbazine (N = 55). Safety of etaracizumab ± dacarbazine was acceptable with infusion-related, gastrointestinal, and metabolic reactions being the most common adverse events (AEs). The majority of AEs were grade 1 or 2 in severity in both study arms; most events were not considered serious, except for cardiovascular (myocardial infarction, atrial fibrillation) and thromboembolic events, which occurred in 3 and 5 patients, respectively. None of the patients in the etaracizumab-alone study arm and 12.7% of patients in the etaracizumab + dacarbazine study arm achieved an objective response. The median duration of objective response in the etaracizumab + dacarbazine study arm was 4.2 months. Stable disease rate, time to progression (TTP), and progression-free survival (PFS) appeared to be similar between the 2 treatment arms. Stable disease occurred in 45.6% of patients in the etaracizumab-alone study arm and 40.0% of patients in the etaracizumab + dacarbazine study arm. Median TTP and median PFS were both 1.8 months in the etaracizumab-alone study arm and 2.5 and 2.6 months in the etaracizumab + dacarbazine study arm, respectively. Median overall survival was 12.6 months in the etaracizumab-alone study arm and 9.4 months in the etaracizumab + dacarbazine study arm.

Conclusions.—The survival results in both treatment arms of this study were considered unlikely to result in clinically meaningful improvement over dacarbazine alone.

▶ In this randomized phase II trial, a monoclonal antibody targeting the alpha $_V$ beta $_3$ ($\alpha_V\beta_3$) integrin was studied alone and in combination with dacarbazine. The overall outcomes including response rate, time to progression, and median survival were not different though the antibody-alone arm did have a slight prolongation of median survival. There is tremendous interest in the use of $\alpha_V\beta_3$ inhibitors in melanoma given the potential application of these agents as antiangiogenic agents. In addition, this target is also of considered value given its presence on the surface of tumor cells including melanoma. The trial highlights the fact that agents thought to be antiangiogenic may play a role as antitumor agents if applied in the correct setting. The inability to select patients whose tumors overexpress $\alpha_V\beta_3$ is a drawback for this trial and suggests that patient selection is critical in these types of trials using targeted agents.

M. S. Gordon, MD

Role of Radiation Therapy in Cutaneous Melanoma

Shuff JH, Siker ML, Daly MD, et al (Med College of Wisconsin, Milwaukee)
Clin Plast Surg 37:147-160, 2010

Background.—In the United States, about 62,000 new cases of cutaneous melanoma were diagnosed in 2008. This disease causes an estimated 8400 deaths each year, with 5-year survival of 92%. Both increased awareness of the disease and screening programs that detect disease at earlier stages have contributed to this high survival. Most patients are treated with surgery, often simple excision of a cutaneous lesion. However, with larger lesions the risk of locoregional recurrence and distant spread increases markedly, with recurrence noted at the primary site, as in-transit lesions, or in nearby lymphatics. Radiotherapy is seldom used in treating cutaneous melanoma because it was considered radioresistant. As modern studies have refuted this status, radiotherapy has been used more often in the definitive, adjuvant, and palliative treatment of melanoma alone or with other modalities. Technologic advances in treatment delivery and targeting make it more useful. The current and future role of radiotherapy in cutaneous melanoma was explored.

Radiobiologic Considerations.—The supposed radioresistance of melanoma was founded on an early clinical review that reported a response rate of 2.5% when radiotherapy was used in about 400 patients with advanced disease. In vitro studies more recently reveal more radioresponsiveness than originally indicated. In addition, the radioresistance may reflect melanoma cells' ability to repair sublethal radiation-induced damage. Hypofractionated delivery of radiotherapy may help overcome the cellular repair processes. However, hypofractionation is not associated with significantly improved outcomes compared to conventional radiotherapy. The perfect schedule for delivering radiotherapy to cutaneous melanoma patients remains to be established.

Adjuvant Therapy.—The recurrence rates after surgical resection are between 15% and 24% for lesions 4 mm or larger and up to 50% for lesions with head or neck desmoplastic melanoma subtype. Although surgical resection is the primary treatment choice, adjuvant radiation therapy should be considered for both the primary site and the regional lymph nodes.

Therapeutic lymph node dissection is the standard of care for patients with lymph node metastases. Sentinel lymph node biopsy is done for patients who have high-risk primary tumors with no lymphatic metastases. Elective nodal irradiation may also be considered. After the surgical approach, nodal irradiation is indicated in patients with high-risk clinicopathologic features, such as node size, number of involved lymph nodes, and presence of extracapsular extension. The risk of distant metastases in these patients is great and the overall prognosis poor. The potential benefits of radiation therapy are weighed against the burden of treatment, often including the possibility of systemic adjuvant therapy when local and distant recurrent disease is highly likely.

Systemic Therapy.—Retrospective reviews show a higher rate of acute and late toxicity when patients receive radiation therapy and interferon, either concomitantly or sequentially. Prospective studies are needed to further assess the toxicity and efficacy of this combination.

Palliative Therapy.—Both locoregional and systemic recurrences are common because of melanoma's aggressive nature and unpredictable behavior. Because of the location of metastatic disease and further progression of disease even while systemic therapy is used, many patients benefit from palliative radiation therapy. The potential benefit of this therapy is shown by retrospective studies. Both as an adjuvant and a palliative treatment, radiotherapy has provoked partial or even complete response in melanomas. In patients with brain metastases, whole brain radiotherapy has been the standard of care for palliation. However, stereotactic radiosurgery, either initially or as salvage, has been effective, so whole brain radiation, resection, or more stereotactic radiosurgery can be reserved for recurrent lesions. Systemic treatment combined with radiotherapy or used alone may also prove effective. Treatment guidelines for patient selection and sequencing of the modalities remain to be determined.

Toxicity.—Toxicity can be acute or long term (late). Acute effects occur during or within 90 days of completing treatment; late toxicity occurs after that time frame. The acute reactions usually seen with cutaneous melanoma treatment are erythema of the skin in the treatment field, dry or moist desquamation of the skin, and potential discomfort, with mucositis and transient parotiditis developing in head and neck locations. The intent of the irradiation—definitive versus adjuvant versus palliative—will influence the toxicity profile, along with location of the radiation treatment field and adjacent normal tissues. Current evidence suggests that the long-term complications in patients with cervical and axillary nodal lesions tend to be mild to moderate but overall are acceptable. Postoperatively for patients with involved inguinal nodes, adverse pathologic factors, risk of systemic involvement, and individual patient characteristics must all be considered, but severe long-term toxicity is usually minimal. Even with acute and potentially long-term complications related to adjuvant radiation therapy after lymph node dissection for melanoma, the benefits of radiation therapy tend to outweigh the morbidity of a regional recurrence in appropriately selected patients.

Future Role.—Advances in the technology of radiation oncology have been significant. This includes highly conformal techniques such as intensity-modulated radiation therapy that avoids normal tissues when delivering radiation to the tumor. This results in a wider therapeutic index and may allow for larger radiation dosing, which could increase the odds of achieving control long term. Image-guided radiation therapy helps clinicians clarify the position of the patient and treatment target before each fraction and may allow adaptive therapy, so treatment delivery can be modified during the course of therapy in concert with changes in tumor size or physiology. By avoiding larger amounts of normal tissues and adjacent organs, making it possible to use larger doses, and safely altering therapy to fit changing conditions, radiotherapy offers a safer way to deliver more aggressive combined treatment.

Conclusions.—Cutaneous melanoma is now understood to demonstrate a broad range of radiosensitivity, so that many fractionation schemes can be used, including standard fractionation and hypofractionation. Persons who have high-risk features benefit from adjuvant treatment but are still at risk for distant failure and often have a poor prognosis. Tolerance for radiation therapy varies with treatment site and the effects of previous, concurrent, and future treatments. Delivered properly, radiation can enhance local and regional control of metastatic disease and provide palliation.

▶ Cutaneous melanoma continues to afflict over 60 000 Americans annually. It was responsible for over 8000 deaths in 2008. While surgery remains the mainstay of treatment for most patients, this review of the role of radiation in this disease is timely and well done.

The authors do an excellent job of outlining the history of radiation as it applies to cutaneous melanoma. In particular, their discussion of the radioresistance fallacy is excellent. Another area of controversy well discussed in the review article is the question of fraction size. While extensive data are explored, suggesting that hypofractionation may be the preferred radiation technique in this disease, the authors correctly point out that the only prospective randomized trial comparing standard fractionation to hypofractionation showed no difference in outcomes.

Finally, the discussions of adjuvant radiation to the primary site and regional lymphatics and the palliative role of radiation in this disease are thorough and a must-read. Cutaneous melanoma is a complex and often fatal disease. The significant role of radiation therapy is important to understand, and these authors are to be commended for an exhaustive review of all the pertinent aspects of radiation in this disease.

C. A. Lawton, MD

12 Cancer Therapies

A Prospective Phase II Evaluation of Esophageal Stenting for Neoadjuvant Therapy for Esophageal Cancer: Optimal Performance and Surgical Safety

Brown RE, Abbas AE, Ellis S, et al (Univ of Louisville, KY; Ochsner Health System, New Orleans, LA)

J Am Coll Surg 212:582-589, 2011

Background.—Many surgeons are reluctant to use esophageal stents during neoadjuvant therapy for esophageal cancer because of concerns about nutritional status, stent-related complications, or added difficulties during esophagogastrectomy. We hypothesized that esophageal stenting during neoadjuvant therapy allows for optimal nutritional intake without adversely affecting perioperative outcomes.

Study Design.—This study is a prospective, dual-institution, single-arm, phase II evaluation of esophageal cancer patients undergoing neoadjuvant therapy before resection. All patients had a self-expanding polymer stent placed before neoadjuvant therapy. We monitored dysphagia symptoms, nutritional status, stent-related complications, and perioperative complications during the course of therapy and 90 days postoperatively.

Results.—We enrolled 32 patients with dysphagia and weight loss who were eligible for neoadjuvant therapy. After stent placement, 2 patients had stent migrations requiring replacement. No erosive complications were observed. During the course of neoadjuvant therapy, we noted improvement in dysphagia, mild weight loss, and maintenance of performance status. At a median of 50 days (range 18 to 92 days) after completion of neoadjuvant therapy, 20 patients underwent margin-negative esophagogastrectomy (16 Ivor Lewis, 4 minimally invasive) without problems with stent removal or difficulty in surgical dissection. Twelve patients did not undergo resection due to development of metastases (n = 8) or rapid decline in functional status (n = 4). Major perioperative complications included pulmonary embolism (n = 2), chyle leak (n = 1), and bronchial injury (n = 1). No surgical complications were attributed to stent placement.

Conclusions.—Use of esophageal stents during neoadjuvant therapy is safe and results in resolution of dysphagia, mild weight loss, and maintenance of performance status without an effect on intraoperative dissection, perioperative complications, or delay in resection after neoadjuvant therapy.

▶ The authors studied the role of esophageal stenting to aid in the administration of induction chemoradiotherapy before esophagectomy. Fifty-six patients were screened, and 32 entered into their nonrandomized phase II study. Two patients had stent migration, 20 went on to surgical resection, and 12 patients did not undergo further surgery (8 secondary to disease progression and 4 because of significant clinical deterioration). The study demonstrates that 20 patients were able to undergo preoperative stenting without adversely impacting the surgical resection. This study provides an additional option for assisting patients in the preoperative phase of induction chemoradiation in the management of esophageal cancer. Mini-laparotomy or laparoscopy allows for preoperative staging at the time of the pretreatment feeding tube placement. However, this approach does delay initiation of treatment slightly and does require an invasive procedure. The authors have demonstrated an apparently safe alternative to feeding tube placement without compromising the surgical resection in patients undergoing induction chemoradiation followed by esophagectomy for esophageal cancer.

T. L. Bauer II, MD

American Society of Clinical Oncology Provisional Clinical Opinion: Epidermal Growth Factor Receptor (*EGFR*) Mutation Testing for Patients With Advanced Non–Small-Cell Lung Cancer Considering First-Line EGFR Tyrosine Kinase Inhibitor Therapy

Keedy VL, Temin S, Somerfield MR, et al (Vanderbilt Univ Med Ctr, Nashville, TN; American Society of Clinical Oncology, Alexandria, VA; Mount Sinai Med Ctr, NY; et al)

J Clin Oncol 29:2121-2127, 2011

Purpose.—An American Society of Clinical Oncology (ASCO) provisional clinical opinion (PCO) offers timely clinical direction to ASCO's membership following publication or presentation of potentially practice-changing data from major studies. This PCO addresses the clinical utility of using epidermal growth factor receptor (*EGFR*) mutation testing for patients with advanced non–small-cell lung cancer (NSCLC) to predict the benefit of taking a first-line EGFR tyrosine kinase inhibitor (TKI).

Clinical Context.—Patients with *EGFR*-mutated NSCLC have a significantly higher rate of partial responses to the EGFR TKIs gefitinib and erlotinib. In the United States, approximately 15% of patients with adenocarcinoma of the lung harbor activating *EGFR* mutations. *EGFR* mutation testing is widespread at academic medical centers and in some locales in community practice. As of yet, there is no evidence of an overall survival (OS) benefit from selecting treatment based on performing this testing.

Recent Data.—One large phase III trial (the Iressa Pan-Asia Study [IPASS] trial), three smaller phase III randomized controlled trials using progression-free survival as the primary end point, and one small phase III trial with OS as the primary end point, all involving first-line EGFR TKIs and chemotherapy doublets, form the basis of this PCO.

Provisional Clinical Opinion.—On the basis of the results of five phase III randomized controlled trials, patients with NSCLC who are being considered for first-line therapy with an EGFR TKI (patients who have not previously received chemotherapy or an EGFR TKI) should have their tumor tested for *EGFR* mutations to determine whether an EGFR TKI or chemotherapy is the appropriate first-line therapy.

NOTE.—ASCO's provisional clinical opinions (PCOs) reflect expert consensus based on clinical evidence and literature available at the time they are written and are intended to assist physicians in clinical decision making and identify questions and settings for further research. Because of the rapid flow of scientific information in oncology, new evidence may have emerged since the time a PCO was submitted for publication. PCOs are not continually updated and may not reflect the most recent evidence. PCOs cannot account for individual variation among patients and cannot be considered inclusive of all proper methods of care or exclusive of other treatments. It is the responsibility of the treating physician or other health care provider, relying on independent experience and knowledge of the patient, to determine the best course of treatment for the patient. Accordingly, adherence to any PCO is voluntary, with the ultimate determination regarding its application to be made by the physician in light of each patient's individual circumstances. ASCO PCOs describe the use of procedures and therapies in clinical practice and cannot be assumed to apply to the use of these interventions in the context of clinical trials. ASCO assumes no responsibility for any injury or damage to persons or property arising out of or related to any use of ASCO's PCOs, or for any errors or omissions.

▶ The article represents a provisional clinical opinion (PCO) from the American Society of Clinical Oncology on the testing of epidermal growth factor receptor (EGFR) for patients with advanced non—small cell lung cancer (NSCLC). The authors state that PCOs are not always updated regularly and that new information may be not reflect the most recent data since their publication. The article is a review of 5 phase III randomized, controlled trials with NSCLC being considered for first-line therapy with EGFR tyrosine kinase inhibitor (TKI).

The results of the 5 studies supported their following conclusions that prolonged progression-free survival and higher response rates were seen in patients who tested positive for *EGFR*-activating mutations. There did not appear to be an overall survival benefit, though, with EGFR TKI, regardless of mutation status.

These recommendations apply mainly, but not exclusively, to patients with adenocarcinomas. The authors mention that there did not appear to be any significant difference in the types or locations of *EGFR* mutations between NSCLC of Asians and non-Asians.

T. L. Bauer II, MD

Combined use of positron emission tomography and volume doubling time in lung cancer screening with low-dose CT scanning

Ashraf H, Dirksen A, Loft A, et al (Gentofte Univ Hosp, Denmark; Univ of Copenhagen, Denmark)
Thorax 66:315-319, 2011

Background.—In lung cancer screening the ability to distinguish malignant from benign nodules is a key issue. This study evaluates the ability of positron emission tomography (PET) and volume doubling time (VDT) to discriminate between benign and malignant nodules.

Methods.—From the Danish Lung Cancer Screening Trial, participants with indeterminate nodules who were referred for a 3-month rescan were investigated. Resected nodules and indolent nodules (ie, stable for at least 2 years) were included. Between the initial scan and the 3-month rescan, participants were referred for PET. Uptake on PET was categorised as most likely benign to malignant (grades I-IV). VDT was calculated from volume measurements on repeated CT scans using semiautomated pulmonary nodule evaluation software. Receiver operating characteristic (ROC) analyses were used to determine the sensitivity and specificity of PET and VDT.

Results.—A total of 54 nodules were included. The prevalence of lung cancer was 37%. In the multivariate model both PET (OR 2.63, $p<0.01$) and VDT (OR 2.69, $p<0.01$) were associated with lung cancer. The sensitivities and specificities of both PET and VDT were 71% and 91%, respectively. Cut-off points for malignancy were PET >II and VDT <1 year, respectively. Combining PET and VDT resulted in a sensitivity of 90% and a specificity of 82%; ROC cut-off point was either PET or VDT indicating malignancy.

Conclusion.—PET and VDT predict lung cancer independently of each other. The use of both PET and VDT in combination is recommended when screening for lung cancer with low-dose CT.

▶ As CT scans become more prevalent, the management of pulmonary nodules becomes increasingly more important. There is a common urge not to miss a potential cancer, leading to unnecessary invasive biopsies or surgical resections. The authors review their results with the Danish Lung Cancer Screening Trial (DLCST). They reviewed the results of solid nodules measuring 5 to 15 mm. The patients were rescanned in 3 months. Siemens LungCARE program was used to calculate a volumetric measure and then the doubling time calculated. If the volumetric doubling time (VDT) increased more than 25%, the lesion was biopsied. The positron emission tomography (PET) scan was used for research purposes only and was not clinically available to dictate care of their patients. The VDT and PET results were placed into different categories. If both the VDT and PET were concordant, there was a 0% and 5% (positively and negatively, respectively) chance of a misdiagnosis. When they were discordant, the predictive value was 57%.

The authors recommend that when both findings are negative, a 1-year repeat CT scan be performed. All nodules that were positive on both PET and

VDT were in fact cancers and could go to resection. In the case of discordant PET and VDT studies, the nodules are recommended to be biopsied.

The authors provide a solid method to decrease unnecessary procedures in a substantial portion of their patients. In the case of smaller lesions, a longer-interval CT scan may have provided some improvement in accuracy. Physicians treating pulmonary nodules should be well versed in the literature involving PET and growth pattern analysis to minimize unnecessary procedures in CT-found pulmonary nodules.

T. L. Bauer II, MD

Genetic Abnormalities of the *EGFR* Pathway in African American Patients With Non–Small-Cell Lung Cancer

Leidner RS, Fu P, Clifford B, et al (Case Western Reserve Univ, Cleveland, OH; Yale Univ School of Medicine, New Haven, CT; Univ of Colorado Cancer Ctr, Aurora; et al)

J Clin Oncol 27:5620-5626, 2009

Purpose.—Previous studies in non–small-cell lung cancer (NSCLC) have demonstrated a wide variation in responsiveness to epidermal growth factor receptor (EGFR) –targeting agents and in genetic aberrancies of the *EGFR* pathway according to ethnic background, most notably a higher frequency of activating *EGFR* mutations among East-Asian patients. We investigated the frequency of *EGFR* pathway aberrancies among African American patients with NSCLC, for whom limited information presently exists.

Patients and Methods.—*EGFR* fluorescent in situ hybridization (FISH) was performed on archived tissues from 53 African American patients. Extracted DNA was sequenced for mutational analysis of *EGFR* exons 18 to 21 and KRAS exon 2. Results were compared by multivariate analysis to an historical control cohort of 102 white patients with NSCLC.

Results.—African Americans were significantly less likely to harbor activating mutations of *EGFR* than white patients (2% *v* 17%; $P = .022$). Only one *EGFR* mutation was identified, a novel S768N substitution. *EGFR* FISH assay was more frequently positive for African Americans than for white patients (51% *v* 32%; $P = .018$). KRAS mutational frequency did not differ between the groups (23% *v* 21%; $P = .409$).

Conclusion.—African American patients with NSCLC are significantly less likely than white counterparts to harbor activating mutations of *EGFR*, which suggests that EGFR tyrosine kinase inhibitors (TKIs) are unlikely to yield major remissions in this population. Our findings add to a growing body of evidence that points to genetic heterogeneity of the *EGFR* pathway in NSCLC among different ethnic groups and that underscores the need for consideration of these differences in the design of future trials of agents that target the *EGFR* pathway.

► The authors analyzed formalin-fixed paraffin-embedded lung cancer specimen tissue from both African-American and white cohorts for common activating mutations in epidermal growth factor receptor (EGFR). Exon 19 and L858R mutations are the most common mutations that cells are dependent on for cell growth and proliferation. These mutations have been known to occur in specific subsets of patients, most notably in women, nonsmokers, east Asians, and adenocarcinoma patients. The authors found that the African-American cohort did not have the common mutations in *EGFR* pathways. Alternatively, they found an exon 20 mutation in EGFR of the African-American cohort. This accounted for a 2% response rate in the African-American cohort compared with 17% in the white cohort. *EGFR* fluorescent in situ hybridization analysis showed increased copy number within the African-American cohort. The authors postulate that anti-*EGFR* monoclonal antibody therapy may be an effective adjunctive therapy in these patients and are planning further studies to analyze this assumption.

T. L. Bauer II, MD

Treatment-Related Mortality With Bevacizumab in Cancer Patients: A Meta-analysis

Ranpura V, Hapani S, Wu S (Stony Brook Univ Med Ctr, NY)

JAMA 305:487-494, 2011

Context.—Fatal adverse events (FAEs) have been reported in cancer patients treated with the widely used angiogenesis inhibitor bevacizumab in combination with chemotherapy. Currently, the role of bevacizumab in treatment-related mortality is not clear.

Objective.—To perform a systematic review and meta-analysis of published randomized controlled trials (RCTs) to determine the overall risk of FAEs associated with bevacizumab.

Data Sources.—PubMed, EMBASE, and Web of Science databases as well as abstracts presented at American Society of Clinical Oncology conferences from January 1966 to October 2010 were searched to identify relevant studies.

Study Selection and Data Extraction.—Eligible studies included prospective RCTs in which bevacizumab in combination with chemotherapy or biological therapy was compared with chemotherapy or biological therapy alone. Summary incidence rates, relative risks (RRs), and 95% confidence intervals (CIs) were calculated using fixed- or random-effects models.

Data Synthesis.—A total of 10 217 patients with a variety of advanced solid tumors from 16 RCTs were included in the analysis. The overall incidence of FAEs with bevacizumab was 2.5% (95% CI, 1.7%-3.9%). Compared with chemotherapy alone, the addition of bevacizumab was associated with an increased risk of FAEs, with an RR of 1.46 (95% CI, 1.09-1.94; $P=.01$; incidence, 2.5% vs 1.7%). This association varied significantly with chemotherapeutic agents ($P=.045$) but not with tumor types ($P=.13$) or bevacizumab doses (P = .16). Bevacizumab was associated with an increased risk of FAEs in patients receiving taxanes or platinum agents (RR, 3.49; 95% CI, 1.82-6.66; incidence, 3.3% vs 1.0%) but was not associated with increased risk of FAEs when used in conjunction with other agents (RR, 0.85; 95% CI, 0.25-2.88; incidence, 0.8% vs 0.9%). The most common causes of FAEs were hemorrhage (23.5%), neutropenia (12.2%), and gastrointestinal tract perforation (7.1%).

Conclusion.—In a meta-analysis of RCTs, bevacizumab in combination with chemotherapy or biological therapy, compared with chemotherapy alone, was associated with increased treatment-related mortality.

► The recent decision by the Food and Drug Administration (FDA) to remove approval for bevacizumab in breast cancer because, in its judgment, the benefits were outweighed by the risks has focused attention on the toxicity of bevacizumab and on the question of whether progression-free survival improvement provided clear evidence of clinical benefit. This article addresses the first of these concerns, the toxicity associated with the addition of bevacizumab to chemotherapy. The meta-analysis was based on 16 randomized clinical trials published or presented at American Society of Clinical Oncology (ASCO) meetings between January 2000 and October 30, 2010, and randomizing between chemotherapy and chemotherapy plus bevacizumab. The authors claim to have included all randomized clinical trials meeting these criteria. The 2 critical conclusions drawn by the authors were that the addition of bevacizumab to chemotherapy significantly increased the risk of a fatal adverse event (2.5% versus 1.7%; relative risk [RR], 1.46; $P = .01$) and that the association between bevacizumab and fatal adverse events was especially true for those receiving taxanes or platinum agents (3.3% versus 1.0%; RR, 3.49).

The results of this study, however, need to be regarded with major caution. First, the study has a glaring omission from the included randomized clinical trials. The number one plenary session article at ASCO in June 2010 was the report of the Gynecologic Oncology Group 218, a prospective randomized clinical trial of 1873 patients assigned to paclitaxel/carboplatin/placebo followed by placebo maintenance, paclitaxel/carboplatin/bevacizumab followed by placebo maintenance, or paclitaxel/carboplatin/bevacizumab followed by bevacizumab maintenance. This study showed no difference in adverse effects except for a higher frequency of hypertension among those receiving bevacizumab. All these patients received the 2 alleged high-risk drugs (a taxane and a platinum). This clearly could have affected the conclusions of the meta-analysis. Second, regarding the FDA decision in breast cancer, the meta-analysis shows an RR of 0.69 in breast cancer studies and thus suggests a decrease in fatalities among those patients with breast cancer who received bevacizumab. At least in breast cancer, there seems to be little evidence to suggest that the toxicity of bevacizumab outweighs whatever beneficial effects one might want to attribute to the improvement in progression-free survival.

J. T. Thigpen, MD

13 Neuro-Oncology

Randomized comparison of whole brain radiotherapy, 20 Gy in four daily fractions versus 40 Gy in 20 twice-daily fractions, for brain metastases

Graham PH, Bucci J, Browne L (St George Hosp, Kogarah, Australia)

Int J Radiat Oncol Biol Phys 77:648-654, 2010

Purpose.—The present study compared the intracranial control rate and quality of life for two radiation fractionation schemes for cerebral metastases.

Methods and Materials.—A total of 113 patients with a Eastern Cooperative Oncology Group performance status <3; and stable (>2 months), absent, or concurrent presentation of extracranial disease were randomized to 40 Gy in 20 twice-daily fractions (Arm A) or 20 Gy in four daily fractions (Arm B), stratified by resection status. The European Organization for Research and Treatment of Cancer Quality of Life 30-item questionnaire was administered monthly during Year 1, bimonthly during Year 2, and then every 6 months to Year 5.

Results.—The patient age range was 28–83 years (mean 62). Of the 113 patients, 41 had undergone surgical resection, and 74 patients had extracranial disease (31 concurrent and 43 stable). The median survival time was 6.1 months in Arm A and 6.6 months in Arm B, and the overall 5-year survival rate was 3.5%. Intracranial progression occurred in 44% of Arm A and 64% of Arm B patients ($p = .03$). Salvage surgery or radiotherapy was used in 4% of Arm A patients and 21% of Arm B patients ($p = .004$). Death was attributed to central nervous system progression in 32% of patients in Arm A and 52% of patients in Arm B ($p = .03$). The toxicity was minimal, with a minor increase in short-term cutaneous reactions in Arm A. The patients' quality of life was not impaired by the more intense treatment in Arm A.

Conclusion.—Intracranial disease control was improved and the quality of life was maintained with 40 Gy in 20 twice-daily fractions. This schema should be considered for better prognosis subgroups of patients with cerebral metastases.

► The use of whole brain radiotherapy in patients with cerebral metastasis has become a standard of care. Yet the overall survival for these patients remains in the range of approximately 6 months given that the short overall survival, quality of life, and time spent receiving treatment (which often affects quality of life) are important end points to study. These authors have evaluated 2 radiation fractionation schemes, 20 Gy in 4 fractions versus 40 Gy in 20 fractions (twice a day), to assess the effects on quality of life and intracranial control rates. While their data certainly support a statistical increase in intracranial control and decrease in death attributed to central nervous system progression with the use of the 40 Gy arm, overall survival was not different (6.1 vs 6.6 months).

Going forward with these results, the obvious next question is to address centers on patients with limited extracranial disease. Perhaps a randomized trial of 40 Gy in 20 fractions (twice a day) versus more standard fractionation schemes of 30 in 10 fractions or 37.5 in 15 fractions. Yet for patients with extensive extracranial disease and intracranial metastasis, 20 Gy in 4 fractions remains a reasonable option, given the overall survival rate seen in this study.

C. A. Lawton, MD

14 Head and Neck

Endoscopic spray cryotherapy for esophageal cancer: safety and efficacy

Greenwald BD, Dumot JA, Abrams JA, et al (Univ of Maryland School of Medicine and Greenebaum Cancer Ctr, Baltimore; Cleveland Clinic, Ohio; Columbia Univ Med Ctr, NY)

Gastrointest Endosc 71:686-693, 2010

Background.—Few options exist for patients with localized esophageal cancer ineligible for conventional therapies. Endoscopic spray cryotherapy with low-pressure liquid nitrogen has demonstrated efficacy in this setting in early studies.

Objective.—To assess the safety and efficacy of cryotherapy in esophageal carcinoma.

Design.—Multicenter, retrospective cohort study.

Setting.—Ten academic and community medical centers between 2006 and 2009.

Patients.—Subjects with esophageal carcinoma in whom conventional therapy failed and those who refused or were ineligible for conventional therapy.

Interventions.—Cryotherapy with follow-up biopsies. Treatment was complete when tumor eradication was confirmed by biopsy or when treatment was halted because of tumor progression, patient preference, or comorbid condition.

Main Outcome Measurements.—Complete eradication of luminal cancer and adverse events.

Results.—Seventy-nine subjects (median age 76 years, 81% male, 94% with adenocarcinoma) were treated. Tumor stage included T1-60, T2-16, and T3/4-3. Mean tumor length was 4.0 cm (range 1-15 cm). Previous treatment including endoscopic resection, photodynamic therapy, esophagectomy, chemotherapy, and radiation therapy failed in 53 subjects (67%). Forty-nine completed treatment. Complete response of intraluminal disease was seen in 31 of 49 subjects (61.2%), including 18 of 24 (75%) with mucosal cancer. Mean (standard deviation) length of follow-up after treatment was 10.6 (8.4) months overall and 11.5 (2.8) months for T1 disease. No serious adverse events were reported. Benign stricture developed in 10 (13%), with esophageal narrowing from previous endoscopic resection, radiotherapy, or photodynamic therapy noted in 9 of 10 subjects.

Limitations.—Retrospective study design, short follow-up.

Conclusions.—Spray cryotherapy is safe and well tolerated for esophageal cancer. Short-term results suggest that it is effective in those who could not receive conventional treatment, especially for those with mucosal cancer.

▶ The management of esophageal cancer requires a multimodality approach. Short of surgical resection, there are a few methods of palliation, including stenting, endoscopic mucosal resection, radio-frequency ablation, cryotherapy, and photodynamic therapy when radiation therapy is insufficient. The ablative techniques offer the potential for cure if the cancer is sufficiently localized.

The authors of this study looked retrospectively at 79 patients from 10 different institutions. All were patients with esophageal cancer in whom other therapy had failed or was refused and who were ineligible for surgery or any other therapy. They all received low-pressure liquid nitrogen therapy every 4 to 6 weeks until complete local tumor eradication was observed by appearance and lack of residual disease on endoscopic biopsy. The median number of treatments was 3 (range, 1-25).

Of the 79 patients who received treatment, no serious adverse events, including perforation and hemorrhage, were reported. Ten percent reported benign stricture, all of whom had previous tumor therapy. Only 49 of the 79 patients were available for efficacy analysis; the remaining 30 were still undergoing cryotherapy treatments. Of those 49 patients, 61.2% demonstrated a complete response at mean follow-up of 10.6 months.

The authors have shown that endoscopic spray cryotherapy is safe and effective. The authors address the limitations of their study in that it is retrospective and limited in the number of subjects and length of follow-up, but this is the largest reported series on the topic. Further studies with longer follow-up periods will be required before this therapy becomes a mainstay of treatment.

D. D'Angelo-Donovan, DO
T. L. Bauer II, MD

Human Papillomavirus and Survival of Patients with Oropharyngeal Cancer

Ang KK, Harris J, Wheeler R, et al (Univ of Texas M.D. Anderson Cancer Ctr, Houston; Radiation Therapy Oncology Group Statistical Ctr, Philadelphia, PA; Huntsman Cancer Inst, Salt Lake City, UT; et al)
N Engl J Med 363:24-35, 2010

Background.—Oropharyngeal squamous-cell carcinomas caused by human papillomavirus (HPV) are associated with favorable survival, but the independent prognostic significance of tumor HPV status remains unknown.

Methods.—We performed a retrospective analysis of the association between tumor HPV status and survival among patients with stage III or IV oropharyngeal squamous-cell carcinoma who were enrolled in a randomized trial comparing accelerated-fractionation radiotherapy (with acceleration by means of concomitant boost radiotherapy) with standard-fractionation radiotherapy, each combined with cisplatin therapy, in patients with squamous-cell carcinoma of the head and neck. Proportional-hazards models were used to compare the risk of death among patients with HPV-positive cancer and those with HPV-negative cancer.

Results.—The median follow-up period was 4.8 years. The 3-year rate of overall survival was similar in the group receiving accelerated-fractionation radiotherapy and the group receiving standard-fractionation radiotherapy (70.3% vs. 64.3%; P=0.18; hazard ratio for death with accelerated-fractionation radiotherapy, 0.90; 95% confidence interval [CI], 0.72 to 1.13), as were the rates of high-grade acute and late toxic events. A total of 63.8% of patients with oropharyngeal cancer (206 of 323) had HPV-positive tumors; these patients had better 3-year rates of overall survival (82.4%, vs. 57.1% among patients with HPV-negative tumors; P<0.001 by the log-rank test) and, after adjustment for age, race, tumor and nodal stage, tobacco exposure, and treatment assignment, had a 58% reduction in the risk of death (hazard ratio, 0.42; 95% CI, 0.27 to 0.66). The risk of death significantly increased with each additional pack-year of tobacco smoking. Using recursive-partitioning analysis, we classified our patients as having a low, intermediate, or high risk of death on the basis of four factors: HPV status, pack-years of tobacco smoking, tumor stage, and nodal stage.

Conclusions.—Tumor HPV status is a strong and independent prognostic factor for survival among patients with oropharyngeal cancer. (ClinicalTrials.gov number, NCT00047008.)

▶ The propensity of human papillomaviruses (HPVs) to stimulate development of squamous cell carcinoma has been well understood in the context of cervical cancer. Unfortunately, there are a growing number of HPV-positive patients who have developed squamous cell carcinoma of the head and neck region, especially the oropharynx. One plus of these HPV-associated oropharyngeal cancers is that the prognosis in terms of survival is better than non-HPV–associated oropharyngeal squamous cell carcinomas. Yet until these data, the exact relationship of HPV versus other risk factors such as smoking, tumor, and nodal stage was not well understood.

One of the many benefits of data sets of large cooperative groups is the ability to do meta-analyses such as was performed here. The data and therefore the results are strengthened by the fact that single-institution biases are lessened dramatically and thus the results carry more statistical power.

These authors are to be commended for this work, which clearly demonstrates tumor HPV status as a strong independent prognostic factor for improved survival in patients with oropharyngeal squamous cell carcinoma. The next question will be, can these patients be treated differently, perhaps less intensively and still see excellent survival outcomes?

C. A. Lawton, MD

15 Late Effects of Therapy

Long-term risk for subsequent leukemia after treatment for childhood cancer: a report from the Childhood Cancer Survivor Study

Nottage K, Lanctot J, Li Z, et al (St Jude Children's Res Hosp, Memphis, TN; et al)

Blood 117:6315-6318, 2011

Previous investigations of cancer survivors report that the cumulative incidence of subsequent leukemia plateaus between 10 and 15 years after primary therapy. Risk beyond 15 years has not been comprehensively assessed, primarily because of lack of long-term follow-up. Among 5-year survivors from the Childhood Cancer Survivor Study cohort, 13 pathologically confirmed cases of subsequent leukemia occurred ≥ 15 years after primary malignancy, with a mean latency of 21.6 years (range, 15-32 years). Seven were acute myeloid leukemia (2 acute promyelocytic leukemia with t(15;17), 2 with confirmed preceding myelodysplastic syndrome), 4 acute lymphoblastic leukemia (2 pre-B lineage, 1 T cell, 1 unknown), and 2 other. Two acute myeloid leukemia cases had the 7q− deletion. The standardized incidence ratio was 3.5 (95% confidence interval, 1.9-6.0). Median survival from diagnosis of subsequent leukemia was 2 years. This is the first description of a statistically significant increased risk of subsequent leukemia ≥ 15 years from primary diagnosis of childhood cancer.

▶ The risk of secondary malignancies in survivors of childhood cancers has been extensively studied through individual institutional studies as well as more recently large, national registry—oriented investigations. Most results have emphasized the increased risk of secondary leukemias during the first 5 years following therapy, with solid tumors then becoming more predominant. Such conclusions have also been drawn from the studies of outcome in survivors of the atomic bombs being dropped on Hiroshima and Nagasaki. By studying survivors beyond 15 years after their therapy for cancer, the report by Nottage et al provides the important observation that leukemias still develop at a standardized incidence ratio of 3.5 and a 6-fold risk of developing leukemia compared with that in the general population (Fig 1A in original article). Most of these leukemias were of the myeloid lineage. Survival after the development of the secondary leukemia showed a median of only 2 years. Although the overall number of leukemias identified was small and the treatments received by the patients for the leukemia were not ascertained, the observation provides important information to help direct follow-up of such patients. We can hope that more modern treatments will reduce the long-term risk of such leukemias and other secondary malignancies in cancer survivors.

R. J. Arceci, MD, PhD

16 Miscellaneous

What Constitutes Reasonable Evidence of Efficacy and Effectiveness to Guide Oncology Treatment Decisions?

Sargent D (Mayo Clinic, Rochester, MN)

Oncologist 15:19-23, 2010

The need to practice evidence-based medicine is the current prevailing paradigm within the medical community. Evidence to guide practice can and should come from a variety of sources, including clinical trials, observational studies, and meta-analyses of both or either. This paper discusses the relative strengths and weaknesses of data that arise from these various sources. The different types of evidence required to demonstrate "efficacy" versus "effectiveness," a critical and often overlooked distinction, are discussed. In the genomic age, in which targeted therapies with or without specific biomarkers are emerging in cancer care, new approaches are necessary to generate the evidence required for decision making.

▶ Practicing evidence-based medicine is a goal of most physicians. Even the Accreditation Council for Graduate Medical Education, which governs residency education, requires program directors of all specialties to teach evidence-based medicine. In addition, the insurance companies and the Federal government want evidence of efficacy to agree to pay for medical care. Yet what level of evidence is required to show efficacy and is that the same as effectiveness?

This article is a review of this topic and is an excellent overview of the type of evidence available to evaluate efficacy and effectiveness. It is important for clinicians to understand the levels of evidence I to III and the meaning of each. The reality is that for many treatment decisions we make as oncologists, we do not have randomized trials (ie, level I evidence). The other reality is that even when we do have level I data, the effectiveness of a particular treatment may still not be known because patients in the randomized clinical trials providing the level I data often are not representative of the general population of patients who might receive a therapy. This is why there is a great need for oncologic registries such as the old Patterns of Care and now Quality Research in Radiation Oncology data. These registries (data sources) help us to understand how a given oncologic treatment impacts cancer in the real world. It is this type of data that the payers are looking for as we try to cost-justify oncologic care.

C. A. Lawton, MD

Article Index

Chapter 1: Supportive Care

Chapter 2: Breast Cancer

Chapter 3: Gynecology

Chapter 4: Genitourinary

Chapter 5: Hematologic Malignancies

Chapter 6: Lymphoproliferative Disorders and Lymphoma

Chapter 7: Thoracic Cancer

Chapter 8: Gastrointestinal

Chapter 9: Cancer Biology

Chapter 10: Sarcoma

Chapter 11: Melanoma

Chapter 12: Cancer Therapies

Chapter 13: Neuro-Oncology

Chapter 14: Head and Neck

Chapter 15: Late Effects of Therapy

Chapter 16: Miscellaneous

Author Index

Z

Printed and bound by CPI Group (UK) Ltd, Croydon, CR0 4YY
08/05/2025
01864677-0001